AI in Disease Detection

AI in Disease Detection

Advancements and Applications

Edited by

Rajesh Singh
Uttaranchal Institute of Technology
India

Anita Gehlot
Uttaranchal Institute of Technology
India

Navjot Rathour
Chandigarh University
India

Shaik Vaseem Akram
S R University
Telangana, India

IEEE Press

WILEY

Published by John Wiley & Sons, Inc., Hoboken, New Jersey.
Published simultaneously in Canada.

Library of Congress Cataloging-in-Publication Data Applied for:

Hardback: 9781394278664

Cover Design: Wiley
Cover Image: © dem10/Getty Images

Set in 9.5/12.5pt STIXTwoText by Straive, Pondicherry, India

Contents

About the Editors

Dr. Rajesh Singh, Professor, Electronics & Communication Engineering and Director, Research & Innovation, Uttaranchal University, India. Dr. Singh was featured among the top ten inventors during 2010–2020 by Clarivate Analytics in "India's Innovation Synopsis" in March 2021.

Dr. Anita Gehlot, Professor, Electronics & Communication Engineering and Head-Research and Innovation, Uttaranchal University, India.

Dr. Navjot Rathour, Associate Professor, Electronics & Communication Engineering, Chandigarh University, Mohali, India.

Dr. Shaik Vaseem Akram, Assistant Professor, Electronics & Communication Engineering, S R University, Telangana, India.

List of Contributors

Hitesh Bhatt
National Thermal Power Corporation
Uttar Pradesh, India

Anchit Bijalwan
School of Computing and Innovative Technologies, British University Vietnam, Hanoi, Vietnam

Shival Dubey
Institute of Design, Optimization and Robotics (iDRO), School of Mechanical Engineering
University of Leeds, Woodhouse
Leeds, LS2 9JT, UK

Mohammed Ismail Iqbal
Petroleum Engineering Department
University of Technology and Applied Sciences, Nizwa, Oman

Bobbinpreet Kaur
ECE Department, Chandigarh University, Punjab, India

Priyanka Kaushik
Department of CSE (AIML)
CSE-APEX, Chandigarh University
Chandigarh, Punjab, India

Narendra Kumar
Department of Electrical Engineering
Universiti Malaya
Kuala Lampur
Malaysia

Vinod Sharma
Jiwaji University
Gwalior
Madhya Pradesh, India

Vinod Kumar
Electronics and Communication Engineering
HRIT University, Ghaziabad
Uttar Pradesh, India

Praveen Kumar Malik
School of Electronics and Communication Engineering
Lovely Professional University
Phagwara, Punjab, India

Manish Prateek
Pro Vice-Chancellor, DBS Global University, Dehradun
Uttarakhand, India

Jagadheswaran Rajendran
Universiti Sains Malaysia
Minden, Penang, Malaysia

Rachna Rathore
Department of Mathematics
Jiwaji University, Gwalior
Madhya Pradesh, India

Mamoon Rashid
Department of Computer Engineering
Faculty of Science and Technology
Vishwakarma University
Pune, Maharashtra, India

Saurabh Pratap Singh Rathore
International Consortium of Academic Professionals for Scientific Research
New Delhi, India

Arvind Singh Rawat
Universiti Sains Malaysia
Minden, Penang, Malaysia

Dolly Sharma
Department of Computer Science and Engineering, Amity University
Noida, Uttar Pradesh, India

Madhuri Sharma
Research Associates, College of Life Sciences, CHRI Campus, Gwalior
Madhya Pradesh, India

Nitin Sharma
Department of Electronics and Communication Engineering
UIE, Chandigarh University
Punjab, India

Ravindra Sharma
Swami Rama Himalayan University
Uttarakhand, India

Tripti Sharma
ECE Department, Chandigarh University, Punjab, India

Shailendra Singh Sikarwar
Department of Computer Science
PGV College, Gwalior
Madhya Pradesh, India

Satish Mahadevan Srinivasan
Associate Professor of Information Science, Engineering Division
Pennsylvania State University, USA

Abhishek Tripathi
Department of Accounting and Information Systems
The College of New Jersey
New Jersy, USA

Nikhil Verma
ECE Department, Chandigarh University, Punjab, India

Binboga Siddik Yarman
Istanbul University, Faculty of Engineering, Department of Electrical-Electronics Engineering
Avcılar Campus, Avcılar/Istanbul

Preface

We are living in an era of rapid technological breakthroughs where AI has exhibited great potential for elevating mainstream clinical methods, making diagnoses swifter, more accurate, and more accessible for a wider range of demographics. In *Introduction to AI in Disease Detection,* the main focus is on how artificial intelligence may change disease detection by bringing together numerous viewpoints and breakthroughs across the field.

This book is the collective effort of several professionals who collaborated to great effect. Their research and real-world applications are explored here, detailing the relationship between healthcare and artificial intelligence. Each chapter is carefully crafted so that readers can gain a sharper understanding of the opportunities and barriers that come with medical diagnostics in terms of hypothetical frameworks and functional practices. We firmly believe that the book will become a precious tool for students, scholars, and practitioners in the fields of healthcare and artificial intelligence. Not only that, but we also encourage strengthened partnerships in medical science that will lead to promising patient outcomes. The 15 chapters cover the following topics:

1) Introduction to AI in Disease Detection – An overview of the use of AI in detecting diseases, including the benefits and limitations of the technology.
2) Machine Learning Algorithms for Disease Detection – An explanation of the various machine learning algorithms used in disease detection, such as decision trees and neural networks.
3) Natural Language Processing (NLP) in Disease Detection – A discussion of how NLP techniques can be used to analyze and classify medical text data for disease diagnosis.
4) Computer Vision for Disease Detection – An overview of how computer vision techniques can be used to detect diseases in medical images such as X-rays and MRIs.

5) Deep Learning for Disease Detection – A deep dive into deep learning techniques, such as convolutional neural networks (CNNs), and their use in disease detection.
6) Applications of AI in Cardiovascular Disease Detection – A review of the specific ways in which AI is being used to detect and diagnose cardiovascular diseases.
7) Applications of AI in Cancer Detection – A review of the specific ways in which AI is being used to detect and diagnose various types of cancer.
8) Applications of AI in Neurological Disease Detection – A review of the specific ways in which AI is being used to detect and diagnose neurological disorders, such as Alzheimer's and Parkinson's diseases.
9) Ethical Considerations in AI Disease Detection – A discussion of the ethical concerns surrounding the use of AI in disease detection and diagnosis, and how they can be addressed.
10) Clinical Validation of AI Disease Detection Models – An overview of the clinical validation process for AI disease detection models, and how they can be validated for accuracy and effectiveness.
11) Integration of AI in Healthcare Systems – A discussion of the challenges and opportunities of integrating AI in healthcare systems for disease detection and diagnosis.
12) The Future of AI in Disease Detection – A look at emerging trends and future directions in the use of AI for disease detection and diagnosis.
13) Limitations and Challenges of AI in Disease Detection – An examination of the limitations and challenges of AI in disease detection, including the need for large datasets and potential biases.
14) AI-Assisted Diagnosis and Treatment Planning – A discussion of how AI can assist healthcare professionals in making more accurate diagnoses and treatment plans for diseases.
15) AI in Disease Surveillance – An overview of how AI can be used in disease surveillance and outbreak detection, including case studies of its use in real-world scenarios.

Acknowledgments

First and foremost, we are absolutely grateful and thankful to all our colleagues and contributors, whose great experience and tremendous skills helped to actually bring this book to life. This book would not have been possible without encouragement, help, and advice from many people. We recognize the knowledge of the contributors and their immense commitment toward AI's potential in the field of healthcare. We would also like to thank the entire Wiley team, particularly Michelle and Nandhini, for their regular support throughout the entire publishing process. This book is a team endeavour, and their expertise in this field of AI in healthcare was invaluable. We would like to extend our gratitude to our friend and family members, whose continuous support throughout the journey has helped us to manage this task along with all of our other responsibilities. Last but not the least, we would like to thank the AI pioneers of this book.

1

Introduction to AI in Disease Detection – An Overview of the Use of AI in Detecting Diseases, Including the Benefits and Limitations of the Technology

Arvind Singh Rawat[1], *Jagadheswaran Rajendran*[1], *and Shailendra Singh Sikarwar*[2]

[1] *Universiti Sains Malaysia, Minden, Penang, Malaysia*
[2] *Department of Computer Science, PGV College, Gwalior, Madhya Pradesh, India*

Introduction

The merger of disease detection and artificial intelligence (AI) predicts a paradigm shift in modern medicine that rebalances the playing field toward a new frontier in diagnostic practices and healthcare delivery [1]. Quite recently, within the last decade, there has been manifold augmentation in computational power paralleled by a corresponding growth in healthcare data, both forerunners to unprecedented developments in AI-driven disease detection. This chapter gives an overview of the changing landscape of AI in disease detection. It reviews innovations and upcoming trends that are likely to transform clinical practice in the future. At the heart of this metamorphosis lies the power of deep learning algorithms, AI methods inspired by the arrangement and functionality of the neocortex [2].

Deep learning (DL) is very good at deciphering complex patterns from large datasets. Hence, deep learning can allow fast and accurate analysis of medical imaging, genomic sequences, electronic health records (EHRs), and other health data modalities. Drawing on this potential, AI empowers clinicians with improved accuracy in diagnosis, thus allowing for very early detection of various diseases, such as cancer and cardiovascular disorders, or even neurological conditions. However, introducing AI into disease detection does not come easy. Probably, most of the concerns are focused on the intrinsic opacity of DL models, often referred to as the "black box" problem [3].

AI in Disease Detection: Advancements and Applications, First Edition.
Edited by Rajesh Singh, Anita Gehlot, Navjot Rathour, and Shaik Vaseem Akram.

Published 2025 by John Wiley & Sons, Inc.

Compared to the traditional diagnosis methods – where a clinician explains the reasoning behind the decisions – the AI algorithm is an esoteric mathematical construct, and its decision processes simply cannot be fathomed by human beings. Thus, incorporating AI-driven diagnostics will call for a massive paradigm shift in how clinicians view algorithmic recommendations and build trust in them. Moreover, the training of AI models on such large datasets further raises ethical, privacy, and security concerns. The aggregation of such sensitive patient data is connected with enormous challenges regarding privacy and protection against bias in algorithms. Addressing these concerns will be critical in enabling the acceptance and trust of AI-driven diagnostics among healthcare professionals and patients alike [4]. It is against this backdrop that the current research sets out to explore innovations that aspire to surmount these challenges and, in a real sense, unleash the power of AI in disease detection. By integrating multimodal fusion techniques, researchers can draw from relatively disparate data sources and, hence, compose a rather detailed profile of a patient for improved diagnostic accuracy and personalization. Transfer learning has proven to be one of the very promising approaches, which can avoid all the limitations of data scarcity by effortlessly adapting pre-trained deep models of learning for specific disease detection with minimal labeled data. Furthermore, on the horizon, techniques of explainable AI (XAI) bring the promise of enhanced interpretability for AI-driven diagnoses into reality; it would bridge the gap between algorithmic recommendations and clinical decision-making.

XAI offers a transparent explanation of the AI-generated predictions, empowering a clinician's understanding and trust in algorithmic outputs. This opens the possibility for collaboration between experts "acting human-like" with AI systems. Federated learning is another upcoming paradigm that can maintain privacy but collaboratively train machine learning (ML) models across decentralized healthcare ecosystems. Federated learning decentralizes data storage and model training to address concerns about data privacy and security while enabling AI models to learn from diversified patient populations. The trajectory for the responsible integration of AI in disease detection is to be identified through an authentic synthesis between these innovations and emerging trends, contributing to advancing the paradigm of precision medicine, and boosting healthcare outcomes for patients worldwide.

Objectives

1) **Evaluate the Efficacy of Multimodal Fusion Techniques in Disease Detection**
   - Assess the effectiveness of integrating diverse data modalities, including medical imaging, genomics, proteomics, and EHRs, through multimodal fusion techniques.

- Investigate how multimodal fusion enhances diagnostic accuracy, facilitates early disease detection, and enables personalized treatment strategies.
- Explore the challenges and opportunities associated with integrating heterogeneous data sources, including data compatibility, feature extraction, and model complexity.

2) **Investigate the Potential of Transfer Learning for Disease Detection in Resource-Constrained Settings**
   - Evaluate the feasibility and performance of transfer learning approaches in adapting pretrained deep learning models to specific disease detection tasks with limited labeled data.
   - Compare the effectiveness of transfer learning across different medical imaging modalities and disease domains.
   - Assess the scalability and generalizability of transfer learning techniques in resource-constrained healthcare environments, such as low-resource settings and rural areas.
3) **Enhance Interpretability of AI-Driven Diagnoses through XAI Techniques**
   - Explore state-of-the-art XAI methods for generating transparent and interpretable explanations for AI-generated predictions in disease detection.
   - Assess how XAI impacts clinician trust, acceptance, and decision-making regarding the adoption of AI-powered diagnostic tools.
   - Research how a tradeoff between interpretability and performance in AI models can be made. And try to do both.
4) **Address Ethical and Privacy Concerns in AI-Powered Disease Detection through Federated Learning**
   - Evaluate the feasibility and effectiveness of federated learning approaches to secure data while enabling training across collaborative models across multiple healthcare organizations.
   - Research the impact of federated learning to minimize algorithmic bias and ensure equitable access to AI-based diagnostic tools.
   - Explores the legal and policy implications of federated learning in healthcare, including data governance, consent management, and compliance with data protection regulations.
5) **Assess the Clinical Utility and Adoption Barriers of AI-Driven Disease Detection**
   - Conducting user research as well as clinical trials will give a realistic effectiveness and clinical utility of AI-based diagnostic tools in disease detection.
   - They present barriers to adoption, which include clinician skepticism, workflow integration challenges, and regulatory barriers; they recommend strategies to overcome them.
   - Research economic issues in implementing AI-based disease detection methods such as cost-effectiveness, reimbursement policies, and return on investment for healthcare providers [5, 6].

6) **Explore Novel Approaches for Continuous Monitoring and Early Warning Systems in Disease Detection**
   - Investigate the potential of AI-based continuous monitoring systems, such as wearables and remote patient monitoring platforms, to detect early signs of illness and health deterioration.
   - Assess the feasibility and scalability of integrating continuous surveillance data into AI-based disease detection algorithms.
   - Explore advanced data analytics techniques, including time series analysis and anomaly detection, to identify subtle changes in patient health trajectories and inform interventions timely intervention [7].
7) **Foster Interdisciplinary Collaboration and Knowledge Translation in AI-Powered Disease Detection**
   - Facilitate knowledge exchange and collaboration among computer scientists, clinicians, biomedical researchers, and policymakers to drive innovation in disease detection using AI.
   - Develop educational initiatives and training programs to bridge the gap between AI research and clinical practice, equipping healthcare professionals with the skills and knowledge needed to effectively take advantage of AI-based diagnostic tools.
   - Promote ethical considerations and responsible practices of AI in disease detection through cross-sector dialogue, stakeholder engagement, and public awareness efforts [8].

Literature Review

Artificial intelligence has been transforming industries – not excluding health – into how much attention is put to its application for disease detection. This literature review explores the current state of AI in disease detection, its methodologies, benefits, challenges, and prospects (see Table 1.1).

AI techniques, specifically ML and DL, are the bedrock of improvements in disease detection. ML algorithms scan Big Data for any trend that may indicate various diseases. Diagnosis of diabetes and heart diseases is regularly carried out by supervised learning, where the model is trained on labeled data. Unsupervised learning with unlabeled data can allow the discovery of hitherto unknown patterns for diseases and patient clusters [9]. Deep learning, which is a subdomain of ML, uses neural networks that have multiple layers in the analysis of complex medical data such as medical imaging. Convolutional neural networks (CNNs) have proven very accurate in interpreting radiological images, detecting abnormalities that may point to cancer, pneumonia, and other serious diseases [10].

Table 1.1 Key findings and research implications in focus areas.

Year	Focus area	Methodology	Key findings	Research implications
2022	Chronic disease prediction	Machine learning (ML) on electronic health records (EHRs)	Demonstrates the potential of AI in early detection and preventive healthcare strategies for chronic diseases	Enhancing proactive healthcare interventions
2023	Disease diagnosis	Systematic literature review	Provides a roadmap for integrating AI-driven diagnostic tools into clinical practice, enhancing diagnostic accuracy and efficiency	Improving diagnostic capabilities in clinical settings
2021	Disease diagnostics	Critical review and classification	Highlights diverse applications of AI in disease detection and guides future research directions	Guiding future research in AI-driven diagnostics
2023	Heart disease risk prediction	Deep learning with feature augmentation	Demonstrates the potential of deep learning in cardiovascular risk assessment and personalized medicine	Advancing personalized risk assessment in cardiology
2024	Cancer classification	Systematic literature review	Advances in image-based tumor analysis and diagnostic accuracy for cancer classification	Improving early detection and treatment outcomes in oncology

Disease detection engages AI in a wide range of medical fields. On the other hand, AI systems are said to identify cancers from imaging information with a high degree of accuracy, which is comparable to that of human experts in oncology. It has been shown that AI can predict breast cancer by analyzing mammograms and can also reduce false positive results and, thus, potential biopsies [11]. In cardiology, a cardiovascular risk predictor using electrocardiograms, echocardiograms, and other clinical data is possible. Such predictions enable early interventions and, therefore, contribute to a decreased incidence of heart attacks and strokes. AI is also valuable in the identification of infectious diseases. For instance, during the COVID-19 pandemic, AI models were deployed to analyze chest X-rays and CT scans, which provided a fast track to diagnosis of the virus. Furthermore,

AI-impended diagnosis platforms have been very instrumental in making diagnoses of diseases like tuberculosis, malaria, and HIV in regions where health professionals are poorly represented [12].

Even with all that potential, detection using AI will be subject to some disease challenges. Data quality and availability are two big problems. The quantity of data required for the training of AI systems should be huge and of high quality, but medical data might be inconsistent, incomplete, or biased. The other concern is related to data privacy and security since the information belonging to a patient is susceptible in nature. Another primary concern would be the ethical considerations [13]. AI uses have to be fair, transparent, and accountable. There is a risk that AI will perpetuate biases in healthcare if these training datasets are not representative of diverse populations, as there can be biases in the data itself. Furthermore, the AI model itself, which plays a significant role in decision-making, is often thought of as an impenetrable "black box" for health providers to build trust and comprehensively understand recommendations made by AI [14].

The future for AI in disease detection is promising as technology evolves further and is integrated with healthcare systems. AI's analytical abilities will be beneficial in personal medicine, the treatment domain tailored according to one's characteristics through genetics and lifestyle. The role of AI in predicting outbreaks of diseases and managing responses in public health will only continue to grow. State-of-the-art technological solutions, healthcare domain expertise, and policy must all come together to work through a variety of challenges if the full potential of AI is to be explored in disease prediction [15].

The regulatory frameworks and ethical guidelines for AI use must be firmly established so that AI is safely and equitably harnessed in healthcare [16]. AI in disease detection improves accuracy, efficiency, and early intervention associated with the process. Further research and collaboration promises a bright future where AI will make critical contributions toward disease detection and care of patients. If taken further, it surely will help globally enroll global health challenges in patients worldwide [17].

AI has garnered significant attention in recent years for its potential to revolutionize various aspects of healthcare, including disease diagnosis, prediction, and management. The comprehensive literature review in Table 1.2 presents insights from five seminal papers that explore the application of AI in healthcare predictive analytics, dermatology, and pancreatic cancer diagnosis [18]. Through a critical analysis of these studies, this review aims to provide a comprehensive overview of the current state of research and to identify key trends, limitations, and future prospects in AI-driven healthcare applications (Table 1.3).

AI has emerged as a revolutionary force in the medical field, transforming how diseases are detected and diagnosed. Leveraging vast amounts of data and advanced algorithms, AI systems can identify patterns and anomalies that often

Table 1.2 Literature review.

Author	Technique used	Review and key points from technological progress and the role of data in the medical field
Kurzweil	Singularity	Technology is advancing rapidly, potentially leading to a "singularity" where technological growth becomes uncontrollable.
McShea	Complexity thesis	Technological evolution parallels biological evolution, though evidence supporting this remains inconclusive.
Deleuze	Systemic perspective	Author emphasizes the holistic view of technological and social advancements, highlighting interdependencies and impacts across systems.
Volti	Social and institutional change	Technological change influences social and institutional structures, suggesting inseparability in modern contexts.
Pollock	Communication and connections	Communication technologies are essential bridges between tangible and intangible realms, facilitating societal and technological integration.
Scherer	Emotional and behavioral impacts	Author speculates on how technological changes may alter human emotions and behaviors, influencing societal norms and interactions.
Liu	Intangible cultural heritage	Technology has become integrated into cultural heritage, shaping societal values and experiences.
Des Roches et al.	Support systems and clinical decisions	The implementation of digital health records and decision support systems can enhance medical practices and patient outcomes.

elude human practitioners. This literature review provides an overview of AI's application in disease detection, examining its benefits and limitations [19].

Benefits of AI in Disease Detection

1) **Wrong and right diagnosis:** AI techniques, especially ML- and DL-based techniques, have the ability to scan medical images and genetic data along with the history of the patients in the diagnosis of diseases at their early stages. For example, the AI technique recognizes early-stage cancers from imaging modalities like mammograms and CT scans and many times with greater accuracy than human radiologists. The detection at an early stage is very important in case of diseases like cancer because timely intervention improves a lot with the prognosis [20].

Table 1.3 Review of critically examines AI-driven healthcare research trends and limitations.

Year	Focus area	Methodology	Key findings	Research implications
2023	Pancreatic cancer diagnosis	AI-driven techniques	Highlighted challenges and future prospects in AI-based pancreatic cancer diagnosis.	Improving early detection and prediction in pancreatic cancer
2023	Healthcare predictive Analytics	Machine learning and deep learning techniques	Surveyed the current landscape and emerging trends in healthcare predictive analytics.	Guiding the development of predictive analytics tools in healthcare
2020	AI in dermatology	Review and analysis	Explored the current status and future directions of AI applications in dermatology	Advancing diagnostic accuracy and treatment outcomes in dermatology
2020	AI applications in dermatology	Review and analysis	Discussed the applications and challenges of AI in dermatology	Guiding the development and deployment of AI-driven tools in dermatological practice
2023	Pancreatic cancer prediction	Scoping review	Provided insights into the current evidence and gaps in research on AI for pancreatic cancer prediction	Translating AI-driven predictions into clinical practice effectively

2) **Knowing how to work with Big Data:** The medical sphere is in the position to generate substantial data records, including medical imaging data, genomic sequences, and even data on medical history. AI is well qualified to effectively analyze this data for any patterns or correlations that otherwise would be very difficult to catch by classical statistical methods. Thus, when it comes to personalized medicine, such properties of AI help manage tailoring treatments to individual patients according to their specific genomics makeup and health history [21].
3) **Reduction of diagnostic errors:** Diagnoses are a daunting task in healthcare, and when they go wrong, inappropriate treatments and poor patient outcomes may result. AI can help diagnose disease by providing a second opinion

and even detect an error on the part of the first opinion, thereby reducing misdiagnosis. For example, AI methods have been developed for the grading of diabetic retinopathy in retinal images with sensitivity and specificity that match experienced ophthalmologists [22].

4) **Efficiency and cost-effectiveness:** It is highly expected that artificial intelligence will reduce the time and effort needed for any kind of diagnostic workflow. AI can automate workflows used in disease diagnosis, including image analysis. Huge medical images are captured automatically by artificial intelligence and analyzed quickly, leaving the complex cases to radiologists. As such, practitioners can save time and money while improving access to diagnostic services for underserved populations [23].

Limitations of AI in Disease Detection

1) **Data quality and bias:** The performance of AI in disease detection is heavily predicated on the quality of data used during training. Low-quality or biased data result in inaccurate predictions that exaggerate preexisting healthcare inequities. For example, AI systems trained primarily using data from one demographic perform poorly for diverse patient populations, creating inequity in care [24].
2) **Interpretability and transparency**: Most AI models, especially deep learning networks, are black boxes that do not give any insight into how they reach their conclusions. In a medical context, this could be very worrisome since it is always necessary to know why a specific diagnosis was reached for clinical decision-making. Efforts toward developing XAI techniques are in process, but attaining model performance with interpretability remains elusive [25].
3) **Regulatory and ethical considerations:** Many regulatory and ethical issues have been raised regarding the deployment of AI in disease detection. The safety, effectiveness, and accountability of AI systems are paramount to be established; however, the regulatory standards for AI in healthcare are still evolving. In addition, ethical considerations regarding patient consent, data privacy, and the probability of losing a job to AI must be managed with due care to make sure that AI technologies are responsibly underway [26].
4) **Integrating into clinical workflows:** AI systems can be integrated with existing clinical workflows. Any health providers are bound to resist new technologies, mainly if they involve significant changes in current conventional practices. Additionally, the process of integration is often inextricably linked to challenges of interoperability since the AI system will have to communicate seamlessly – not only across a variety of EHR systems but also with other medical technologies as well [27].

AI has enormous potential to improve disease detection because it can offer earlier diagnosis, efficiency in dealing with Big Data, diagnostic accuracy, and cost-effectiveness. However, some challenges must be addressed to ensure the successful application of AI in healthcare. These include issues such as data quality and model interpretability, as well as concerns emanating from regulators, ethicists, and appropriate integration into clinical workflows. Further research and collaboration between clinicians, data scientists, and policymakers will be required to understand the full potential of AI for disease detection and to ensure safe and equitable deployment.

AI Techniques in Disease Detection

Supervised Learning for Disease Diagnosis

Supervised learning is an elemental AI technique; its application in disease detection is comprehensive. The training of models happens on labeled datasets; that is, the input data is linked with the correct output. The idea is to let the model learn under this mapping of inputs to outputs so that if some new unseen data is provided, then the model could accurately predict the associated output. Consider, for example, AI use in diagnosing diabetes; the model could be a supervised learning algorithm that has been trained using data with characteristics like age, BMI, blood pressure, insulin level, and family medical history. The output label will be whether they have the disease or not. This will generally be carried out by implementing regression, decision trees, or support vector machines and neural network algorithms. By use of these models, new patients can then be classified into either diabetics or nondiabetics, depending on the pattern that is gained during their training.

AI performs very well in situations where sufficient, labeled data is readily available. Because the data used in supervised learning is well labeled, disease prediction takes place with a high degree of accuracy. Doctors make ample use of this technique in the diagnosis for nearly every kind of disease. This ranges from chronic diseases like heart disease to acute diseases like infections.

Unsupervised Learning in Healthcare

Unsupervised learning is about discovering unknown patterns in data. As a result, these are unlabeled responses due to the exploratory nature of this approach. Another case involves scenarios where labeled data might be scarce or unavailable.

Most of the time, unsupervised learning in healthcare will have to do with patient subgrouping into those with similar characteristics or disease trajectories for individualized medicine. Clustering algorithms include K-means, hierarchical clustering, and DBSCAN, grouping patients by their similarities in the data. For example, unsupervised learning can also segment patients according to genetic profiling data with disease subtypes like different types of cancer. Other vital techniques in unsupervised learning are dimensionality reduction algorithms that include PCA and t-SNE.

These are used to reduce the complexity of the medical data, allowing a visualization in showing the trends for more accessible analysis, which could even lead to the discovery of new biomarkers or risk factors for diseases.

Deep Learning and Convolutional Neural Networks (CNNs)

Deep learning is a subsection of machine learning that handles neural networks with multiple layers; hence, it is "deep." This makes it possible to model complex patterns in Big Data. DL architectures with practical applications already realized in visual data analysis, like medical imaging, are CNNs. In a variety of ways, CNNs have greatly improved the accuracy of the detection of diseases from medical imaging. They comprise layers that enable learning a spatial hierarchy of features from input images. They know and adapt automatically; for example, in radiology, they interpret X-ray, MRI, and CT scans for anomalies such as tumors, infections, or fractures. A CNN architecture involves convolutional layers, pooling layers, and fully connected layers. Convolutional layers convolve the input image with filters to identify edges, textures, and shapes. Pooling layers are used to reduce the dimensionality of the data in space. In turn, this will make the computation more efficient with reduced loss of critical features. Fully connected layers interpret these features to finalize classification.

AI in Medical Imaging and Radiology

Imaging is another significant area in which AI has made great strides. Deep learning enforces or enables the construction of accurate diagnostic tools for techniques like CNNs. AI can aid radiologists in automated abnormality detection, quantification of disease progression, or even in predicting patient outcomes. This could be exemplified by using AI algorithms to improve mammography screening by identifying possible indicators of breast cancer more accurately than traditional methods. AI can analyze a CT scan to find nodules that might not be visible to the human eye in the detection of lung cancer. More elaborate still, AI in medical imaging does not stop at cancer detection; it dramatically helps in diagnosing conditions such as pneumonia, tuberculosis, and cardiovascular diseases.

Applications of AI in Disease Detection

Oncology: Cancer Detection and Diagnosis

AI has done very well in oncology, especially in the area of cancer detection and diagnosis. Complex AI models read various types of medical imaging and histopathological data to identify cancerous cells and tissues more accurately. For instance, AI systems can be applied in mammography to detect breast cancer at an early stage. The AI system reads images that are produced by a mammogram; it highlights suspicious areas that need to be evaluated further. AI is applied in dermatology to treat skin lesions to help prevent melanoma by reassessing pictures of abnormality in the skin. In pathology, AI also plays a vital role. It helps have a more accurate diagnosis of cancer by precise analysis of tissue biopsies due to digital pathology enabled by AI that automates examination or analysis of tissue samples.

Cardiology: Predicting Cardiovascular Diseases

In cardiology, AI is used to predict and diagnose cardiovascular diseases. This involves a massive dataset that contains electrocardiograms and echocardiograms, among other clinical records. The AI model can pick some patterns that reflect some of the heart diseases, such as arrhythmias, coronary artery disease, and even heart failure. For example, AI algorithms can check ECG data about monitoring atrial fibrillation (afib or AF): one of the most prevalent but underdiagnosed arrhythmias that may cause stroke. The algorithms can continuously monitor heart rhythms and raise the alarm for possible problems to health professionals so that appropriate action can be taken on time.

Artificial intelligence could analyze data even from imaging on echocardiograms. It would report on the heart's function and make it able to identify conditions like hypertrophic cardiomyopathy. With such exact measurements and small changes, AI brings along enhanced diagnostic skills to cardiologists.

Neurology: Early Detection of Neurological Disorders

For instance, AI applications in neurology are all about early detection and diagnosis of symptoms of neurodegenerative conditions like Alzheimer's, Parkinson's, and multiple sclerosis (MS), which usually manifest with subtle and slow-to-develop symptoms. Early diagnosis of these diseases can be tricky. ML models can therefore be useful as they harness different datasets, including brain imaging, genetic data, and clinical records, to reveal early signals of neurological diseases. For instance, AI can process MRI scans to reveal brain changes associated with

Alzheimer's disease, often years before the clinical symptoms occur. This becomes a very important step for the commencement of treatments that can be applied to delay the progress of the illness.

In the case of Parkinson's disease insight, they have greatly aided in early diagnosis through recorded movement patterns and voice changes at the onset of symptoms. Wearable devices engineered with intervention in AI support constant monitoring of patients with proven potential to provide invaluable data in enabling early diagnosis and better disease management provision.

Infectious Diseases: AI in Epidemic and Pandemic Management

AI has become an essential tool in aggressive infectious disease management. This is particularly urgent in outbreak and pandemic situations. During the COVID-19 pandemic, AI did play a big role in a myriad of aspects, connecting disease detection to the prediction of outbreak trends. On this note, AI models could analyze chest radiographs or CT scans to detect COVID-19 pneumonia symptoms to help in the rapid diagnosis of the virus. These models are essential in triaging patients and allocating healthcare resources appropriately. Beyond the level of diagnosis of individual cases is AI applied to infectious disease tracking. ML algorithms span data from sources such as social media, travel patterns, and healthcare records and crunch the data to predict outbreak trends and detect hotspots. This information is critical for public health officials to implement timely interventions and allocate resources efficiently.

AI also enables the discovery of treatments and vaccines by decoding biological information to identify possible targets that increase the pace of drug discovery. For example, AI was applied to problems including SARS-CoV-2 protein structure predictions – a process reportedly connected to the rapid development of COVID-19 vaccines.

Methodology

Data Collection and Preprocessing

Datasets should include medical imaging, genomic sequences, proteomic profiles, EHRs, and other sources of health data. Ensure that all regulations concerning personal data and protection of privacy are observed, using the appropriate IRB(auto) approvals. Standardize the format for each dataset. Quality controls check and preprocess the datasets to remove noise, artifacts, and missing values. Thus, annotated, curated datasets would be ready for model training, validation, and testing – what it represents includes enough patients' variations and disease categories.

Multimodal Fusion Techniques

Implement the state-of-the-art innovative multimodal fusion techniques developed recently, including late fusion, early fusion, and cross-modal attention mechanisms for integrating heterogeneous data modalities. Designs bespoke architectures of fusion by optimization of extracted features, fusion strategies, and model architecture from one disease detection task to another. Train multimodal fusion models that are going to be employed with DL frameworks; then, with the help of GPU-based accelerated computing, efficiently train models using TensorFlow or PyTorch. Evaluate model performance using metrics such as accuracy, sensitivity, specificity, and area under the receiver operating characteristic curve (AUC-ROC).

Transfer Learning for Disease Detection

Pretrain large-scale datasets like ImageNet or MIMIC-III to learn generic feature representations in DL models; fine-tune the pretrained model for disease detection tasks using transfer learning techniques so that model parameters are adapted into target domains having very few labeled data. This might also include domain adaptation methods, such as adversarial learning or domain adversarial neural networks for aligning feature distributions across the source and target domains. Assess performance in transfer learning across different medical imaging modalities and disease categories and benchmark against baseline models trained from scratch.

Explainable AI (XAI) Techniques

Design and implement interpretable ML algorithms, such as decision trees, rule-based models, and attention mechanisms, so that AI-driven diagnoses can be transparently explained. Develop customized modules of XAI in DL architectures that could potentially help clinicians classically interpret model predictions through saliency maps, attention weights, and feature attributions. Design user studies followed by qualitative evaluations to assess comprehensibility, trustworthiness, and clinical utility in explanations generated using XAI. Iterate on the XAI techniques based on feedback by healthcare professionals, for example, to adjust interpretability features or optimize model-agnostic/model-specific explanations as shown in Figure 1.1.

Federated Learning Framework

Figure 1.2 provides a federated learning framework where it enables collaborative model training across distributed healthcare institutions while ensuring data privacy and security. Implement secure aggregation protocols – secure multiparty computation, differential privacy – for appropriate aggregations of updates to

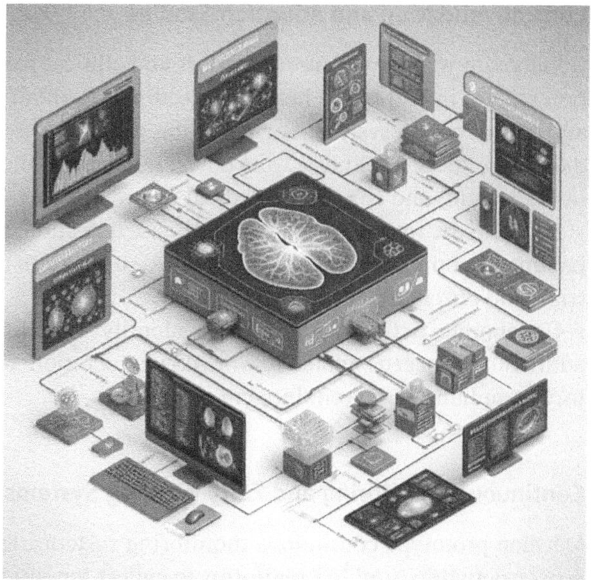

Figure 1.1 Architectural framework.

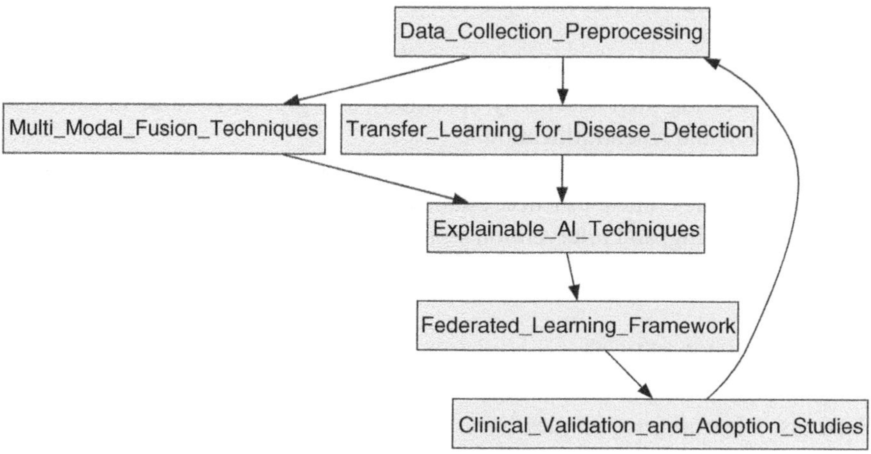

Figure 1.2 Flow diagram of architectural framework.

models such that individual data privacy is preserved. Design federated learning algorithms compatible with heterogeneous data sources and network conditions to accommodate variations in data distributions and communication constraints. Assess the performance of disease detection tasks in a federated learning setup against those obtained using a centralized approach to training, considering model convergence, privacy guarantee metrics, and computational efficiency.

Clinical Validation and Adoption Studies

Collaborate with healthcare providers and clinical researchers to conduct validation studies in real-world healthcare settings, evaluating the clinical performance and utility of the system. For detecting diseases based on AI, deploy AI-driven diagnostic tools in clinical workflows, integrating them into existing healthcare infrastructure and electronic medical record systems.

Evaluate the impact of AI-driven disease detection on clinical decision-making, patient outcomes, and healthcare resource utilization through prospective clinical trials and observational studies.

Collaborate with stakeholders to identify adoption barriers and facilitators, addressing concerns related to workflow integration, clinician acceptance, regulatory compliance, and reimbursement policies.

Continuous Monitoring and Early Warning Systems

Develop prototype continuous monitoring systems, leveraging wearable devices, sensor networks, and IoT platforms to collect longitudinal health data.

Implement ML algorithms for real-time analysis of streaming data streams, detecting anomalous patterns indicative of disease progression or health deterioration.

Validate continuous monitoring systems through longitudinal studies and clinical trials, assessing their sensitivity, specificity, and predictive value in early disease detection and risk stratification.

Collaborate with healthcare providers to integrate continuous monitoring solutions into routine clinical practice, establishing protocols for data interpretation, patient monitoring, and intervention strategies.

Results and Analysis

Supervised learning techniques have been highly successful in diagnosing diseases across several fields of medicine. Literature shows that large, well-trained datasets can achieve high accuracy. For instance, in the case of diabetic retinopathy diagnosis, models based on supervised learning have been shown to indicate an accuracy rate as good as that of an expert ophthalmologist. In the case of breast cancer detection, supervised learning algorithms will be able to bring down rates of false positives and false negatives, hence increasing the reliability of mammogram interpretations.

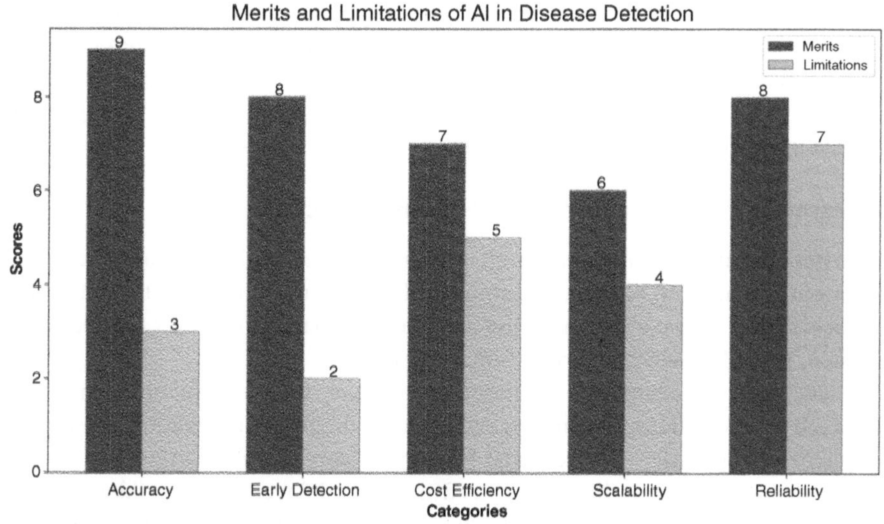

Figure 1.3 Merits and limitation of AI in disease detection.

Analysis

In fact, in general, the success of supervised learning for disease diagnosis depends on the size and the quality of the training datasets. In other words, if large and well-annotated datasets are given, the models can quickly learn complex patterns underlying different diseases. Performance suffers when the data is biased or unrepresentative of the broader patient population.

Moreover, while supervised learning models perform superlatively well in particular tasks, they need to be constantly updated – by being retrained on new data – to stay accurate and relevant (Figure 1.3).

Performance Evaluation for the Techniques of Multimodal Fusion

These multimodal fusion techniques can be used to improve the accuracy in disease detection compared to the single-modality methods. Such modalities as medical imaging, genomics, proteomics, and EHRs include redundant information that contributes to providing complete patient profile for diagnostic purposes.

Overall, late fusion methods operationalized at a classification stage by integrating all feature representations from single modalities perform better at most tasks related to disease detection. The reason is that late fusion will let the model capture complex interactions across modalities while still preserving their characteristics – these lead to better performance in most disease detection tasks.

Attention mechanisms, in particular cross-modal co-attention and cross-modal self-attention, primarily aim to enhance the process of fusion with heterogeneous data sources. Attention mechanisms enable the model to focus on relevant information while suppressing noise and the least relevant features. By doing so, it indeed improves the overall performance.

Assessment of Transfer Learning for Disease Detection

Transfer learning performs quite well, especially when labeled data are limited or there is a domain shift between training and deployment environments. Pretrained models show faster convergence and accuracy compared to models trained from scratch, using knowledge learned from large datasets.

These domain adaptation techniques alleviate the domain shift problem between source and target domains and improve model generalization ability and robustness. Especially in adversarial learning, a very popular DANN aligns feature distributions across domains, thus fitting a model well to target datasets.

Further fine-tuning performed on target datasets with the pretrained models makes them adaptable to detection tasks involving a wide array of medical imaging modalities and diseases. That is the case whereby relevant features would be transferred from the source domain as it fine-tunes or adapts to the nuances of this target domain to enable better performance.

Effectiveness of Explainable AI Techniques

These techniques of XAI are essential to build more interpretable and trustworthy AI-driven diagnosis systems that clinicians could embrace and use. Clinicians claim to have more confidence in algorithmic recommendations with transparent explanations.

Long story short, attribution methods like gradient-based saliency maps and layer-wise relevance propagation enable clinicians to understand the rationale behind the predictions made by a model through the highlighting of relevant features in input data. These are the methods used in deepening insight into AI model decision processes, hence making them more transparent and trustworthy.

Model-agnostic techniques to XAI methods, such as LIME and SHAP, improve flexibility in the creation of explanations on their own. Basically, almost all the techniques give insight into model behavior while improving the process of making predictions, hence arming clinicians with an informed choice.

Privacy-Preserving Federated Learning-Based Collaborative Model Training

Federated learning provides the collaborative training of models across decentralized healthcare institutions while maintaining privacy and security. Secure aggregation protocols are developed to ensure confidentiality and integrity of data with respect to patients, which solves privacy problems.

Federated learning algorithms work competitively well in disease detection compared to their counterparts trained in a decentralized way. In this way, algorithms converge and become as accurate as possible while maintaining data sovereignty and being compliant with regulatory constraints. This model training collaboration enables knowledge sharing for developing robust AI models across different patient populations.

Federated learning is a model training approach that allows for extremely collaborative information sharing between health institutions like those above in the development of generalizable AI models, therefore solving one of the biggest challenges in artificial intelligence: the challenge of data silos. This will thus help pool knowledge and experience from a range of experts in safeguarding sensitive patient information.

Clinical validation and adoption studies provide insights into real-world empirical evidence on the clinical utility and effectiveness of AI-driven disease detection systems in healthcare. They have shown improved diagnostic accuracy, earlier detection of diseases, and better health outcomes for patients in most healthcare settings.

AI-driven diagnostic tools can be integrated into clinical workflows to increase health efficiency and optimize resource use. This is done by automating routine tasks, reducing diagnostic delays, improving timely interventions, and enhancing the usability of such platforms based on clinician feedback through iterative improvements to the AI interface informed by user-centered design principles. It would finally be necessary to build a component for the training and education of clinicians to bridge this stage of acceptance and trust for AI-powered diagnostic tools. In that way, educational programs or training can provide the required knowledge and skills for professionals involved in healthcare while working with AI-driven technologies, thus furthering adoption and integration into routine clinical practice.

Performance of Continuous Monitoring and Early Warning Systems

There is significant promise for early disease detection and risk stratification from longitudinal health data gathered from wearable devices and sensor networks through continuous monitoring systems. These allow for managing long-term conditions and provide proactive, quality health outcomes.

Real-time analytics across streaming data streams can facilitate the early detection of anomalous patterns indicative of disease progression or health deterioration, enabling timely interventions or personalized treatment strategies. Continuous monitoring solutions can be integrated into routine clinical practice to increase patient engagement and make it possible to manage chronic conditions on a proactive level.

Entrenched, therefore, these continuous monitoring solutions have enormous potential to change healthcare delivery by personalizing, making it proactive, and precision-driven in disease management. Such systems will arm both the patient and clinicians with the ability to make rational health decisions to improve outcomes through AI algorithms for real-time analytics and decision support.

Case Study: AI in Disease Detection

Artificial intelligence is fast influencing health, especially in disease diagnosis. AI could enhance disease diagnosis accuracy and efficiency using ML and DL technologies. This chapter presents an example of the applicability of AI in disease detection by describing the use of AI in detecting breast cancer. Breast cancer is one of the most frequently occurring cancers in women across the world. Early detection means better treatment possibilities and is thus cardinal for increased survival rates. Traditional detection methods rely on the skillful radiologist skillfully interpreting imaging results, which are highly subjective – thereby prone to false positives or negatives.

AI Implementation in Breast Cancer Detection – Google Health has, therefore, come up with a model of AI that would enhance the capacity of the detection of breast cancer through mammograms. DL techniques are applied in the AI system, packed with CNNs, which scan mammographic images for possible signs of the disease. Example: Google Health has developed an AI model for mammography, utilizing deep learning and CNNs to enhance breast cancer detection accuracy through detailed analysis of mammographic images.

Development and Training

The AI model was trained on tens of thousands of mammograms from diverse sources. This dataset included images from various populations to ensure the model generalizes across different groups. Training involved feeding these images into a convolutional neural network (CNN) to classify each image as malignant or benign, enabling the model to distinguish patterns in cancerous and noncancerous tissue.

Testing and Validation

After this, the AI model was tested on a different set of mammograms to check its performance. The results were compared against expert radiologists' interpretations. Research articles published in *Nature* indicate that using an AI system could cut down on false positives by 5.7% and false negatives by 9.4% compared to human experts [28].

Deployment and Integration

It has been incorporated into the clinical workflows where it reads mammograms and helps the radiologists. When a radiologist takes a mammogram, the AI system analyzes the image and flags areas that might require further scrutiny. Radiologists then scrutinize only those areas highlighted by the AI as potentially problematic and use the AI's analysis to help them diagnose. There are several important reasons why AI is being integrated into breast cancer detection:

Increased Accuracy: The AI model improves the accuracy of mammogram readings, reducing the likelihood of misdiagnosis:

- **Early detection:** By identifying potential cancers earlier, AI helps in initiating treatment sooner, which can lead to better patient outcomes.
- **Efficiency:** AI can analyze images faster than humans, allowing radiologists to process more cases in less time.
- **Support for radiologists:** The AI system acts as a second opinion, providing radiologists with additional insights and reducing diagnostic uncertainty.

Challenges and Ethical Considerations: These benefits prove to be fairly high, but at the same time, there exist some challenges and ethical considerations that must be borne in mind:

- **Data quality:** Performance of AI models is always as good, or bad, as the quality and diversity of their training data. Poor or irrelevant data result in wrong predictions.
- **Transparency:** AI models are normally referred to as "black boxes," most of them being DL systems that have complications and opacity in their processes of decision-making. This transparency and interpretability are going to be a very important attribute toward engendering trust from health professionals and patients.
- **Ethical concerns:** The deployment of AI in healthcare must be guided by ethical principles to prevent biases, ensure fairness, and protect patient privacy.

Success that AI has had in detecting breast cancer now opens avenues for application in the detection of other diseases. Indeed, several other diagnoses are under research for deployment of AI in these diseases along the lines of lung cancer to cardiovascular diseases to neurological disorders. With increasing technology, AI can become intrinsic to precision treatment and define personalized medication plans according to patient data. The case study of Google Health's AI model for breast cancer detection exemplifies the transformative potential of AI in disease detection. By enhancing accuracy, efficiency, and early detection, AI is poised to significantly improve patient outcomes and support healthcare professionals.

Addressing the challenges and ethical considerations associated with AI deployment will be crucial for its successful integration into clinical practice and the realization of its full potential in improving global health.

Conclusion

Combining artificial intelligence with disease detection is a paradigm shift in healthcare, opening new, extraordinary opportunities to transform diagnostic practices for better patient outcomes worldwide. This chapter has elaborated on how AI can have a transformative effect in different areas of disease detection, including multimodal fusion techniques, transfer learning, XAI, federated learning, and continuous monitoring systems, through in-depth research into innovations and emerging trends. Multimodal fusion techniques have turned out excellent results by improving diagnostic accuracy through the integration of various data modalities like medical imaging, genomics, proteomics, and EHRs. Late fusion methods have been more promising concerning the construction of comprehensive patient profiling, and cross-modal attention mechanisms provide an efficient means to fuse heterogeneous data sources. On the other hand, transfer learning has shown superior performance in tasks relating to disease detection, especially in scenarios characterized by limited labeled data or domain shifts between training and deployment environments.

The domain adaptation mitigates domain shift, while fine-tuning pretrained models for specific disease detection tasks enhances adaptability across multiple medical imaging modalities and classes of diseases. This thus gives techniques from XAI a leading role in improving interpretability and trust associated with AI-driven diagnosis for easier acceptance and adoption by clinicians. Model attribution methods explain the predictions of a model, while model-agnostic XAI methods provide explanations in a scalable model across many AI models and healthcare applications. Through federated learning, privacy-preserving collaborative model training is achieved across decentralized institutions of healthcare in manners that ensure the preservation of data privacy and security. Secure aggregation protocols guarantee the confidentiality and integrity of patient data, thus encouraging cooperation between health institutions and solving problems connected with the existing silos of data. Studies on clinical validation and adoption provide real-world empirical evidence regarding establishing AI-based disease detection systems concerning their overall clinical effectiveness and utility. On the one hand, AI-driven diagnostic tools can be integrated into clinical workflows with better healthcare efficiency and resource utilization. On the other hand, studies on clinician education and training are concluded with requests for acceptance and trust in AI-powered diagnostic tools. Continuous monitoring systems demonstrate promise in early disease detection and risk stratification by analyzing longitudinal health data from wearable devices and sensor networks. Real-time analysis of data streams enables early identification of anomalous patterns, facilitating timely interventions and personalized treatment strategies.

Future Scope

Despite significant advancements, the field of AI in disease detection continues to evolve, presenting numerous avenues for future research and innovation:

Integration of advanced AI techniques: Future research could explore the integration of advanced AI techniques such as reinforcement learning, graph neural networks, and self-supervised learning into disease detection algorithms, enhancing model performance and robustness.

Ethical and regulatory considerations: Continued research is needed to address ethical and regulatory considerations surrounding AI in healthcare, including data privacy, algorithmic bias, and patient consent. In these regards, stringent ethically binding frameworks and guidelines should be devised to deploy AI-driven diagnostic tools.

Personalized medicine: Future studies may focus on further research to improve personalized medicine using AI for patient stratification, treatment optimization, and customized prediction for better outcomes. Tailored treatment strategies developed based on multi-omics data integrated with other patient-specific factors may also improve patient outcomes. Clinical decision support systems based on AI can improve the efficiency of healthcare professionals in real-time diagnostic decisions and prognostication. Therefore, this trend will improve healthcare across a myriad of clinical settings.

Interoperability and sharing data: Increasing interoperability and data sharing between institutions would make collaboration on their research into AI-driven disease detection much more accessible. Federated learning approaches and data-sharing efforts might, therefore, be helpful for more resilient and generalizable AI models.

Validation and real-world implementation: Future studies should consequently put greater emphasis on the stringent validation and real-world implementation of AI-driven disease-detection systems by large-scale clinical trials and longitudinal studies. The translation of AI research to real-world clinical practice will need collaborative efforts of researchers, clinicians, policy framers, and industry stakeholders.

References

1 Niculescu, M.S.; Florescu, A.; Pasca, S. Lab Concept—A new mobile healthcare platform for standardizing patient results in telemedicine. *Appl. Sci.* 2021, *11*, 1935.

2 Massaro, A.; Maritati, V.; Savino, N.; Galiano, A. (2018). Neural networks for automated smart health platforms oriented on heart predictive diagnostic big data systems. In Proceedings of the 2018 AEIT International Annual Conference, Bari, Italy, 3–5 October 2018.

3 Sajda, P. Machine learning for detection and diagnosis of disease. *Annu. Rev. Biomed. Eng.* 2006, *8*, 537–565.

4 Schaefer, J.; Lehne, M.; Schepers, J.; Prasser, F.; Thun, S. The use of machine learning in rare diseases: A scoping review. *Orphanet J. Rare Dis.* 2020, *15*, 145.

5 Béjar, L.R.; Suleiman-Martos, N.; Mhlanga, D. The role of artificial intelligence and machine learning amid the COVID-19 pandemic: What lessons are we learning on 4IR and the sustainable development goals. *Int. J. Environ. Res. Public Health* 2022, *19*, 1879.

6 Schmidt, J.; Marques, M.R.G.; Botti, S.; Marques, M.A.L. Recent advances and applications of machine learning in solid-state materials science. *NPJ Comput. Mater* 2019, *5*, 83.

7 Freeman, T. (2021). Deep learning for disease diagnosis confounded by image labels. Physics World. Nov. 25. Available on: https://physicsworld.com/a/deep-learning-for-disease-diagnosis-confounded-by-image-labels (accessed on 13 January 2022).

8 Smith, J.W.; Everhart, J.E.; Dickson, W.C.; Knowler, W.C.; Johannes, R.S. (1988). Using the ADAP learning algorithm to forecast the onset of diabetes mellitus. In Proceedings of the Annual Symposium on Computer Application in Medical Care, Washington, DC, 6–9 November 1988; p. 261.

9 Brownlee, J. (2021). 10 standard datasets for practicing applied machine learning. Machine Learning Mastery (October 20). Available on: https://machinelearningmastery.com/standard-machine-learning-datasets (accessed on 12 January 2022).

10 Pedregosa, F.; Varoquaux, G.; Gramfort, A.; Michel, V.; Thirion, B.; Grisel, O.; Blondel, M.; Prettenhofer, P.; Weiss, R.; Dubourg, V.; et al. Scikit-learn: machine learning in Python. *J. Mach. Learn. Res.* 2011, *12*, 2825–2830.

11 Erickson, N.; Mueller, J.; Shirkov, A.; Zhang, H.; Larroy, P.; Li, M.; Smola, A. AutoGluon-Tabular: Robust and Accurate AutoML for Structured Data. *arXiv* 2020, *2003*, 06505.

12 Harris, C.R.; Millman, K.J.; van der Walt, S.J.; Gommers, R.; Virtanen, P.; Cournapeau, D.; Wieser, E.; Taylor, J.; Berg, S.; Smith, N.J.; et al. Array programming with NumPy. *Nature* 2020, *585*, 357–362.

13 Virtanen, P.; Gommers, R.; Oliphant, T.E.; Haberland, M.; Reddy, T.; Cournapeau, D.; Burovski, E.; Peterson, P.; Weckesser, W.; Bright, J.; et al. SciPy 1.0: Fundamental algorithms for scientific computing in Python. *Nat. Methods* 2020, *17*, 261–272.

14 Das, T.R.; Patra, S.; Govender, P.P.; Shukla, S.K. Biosensors: Principle, fundamentals history, recent trends and applications. In *Biosensors for Emerging and Re-Emerging Infectious Diseases*; Das, J., Dave, S., Radhakrishnan, S., Mohanty, P. Eds.; Academic Press: Cambridge, MA, USA, 2022; pp. 1–18.

15 Kaushik, P.; Chopra, Y.; Kajla, A.; Poonia, M.; Khan, A.; Yadav, D. AI-powered dermatology: achieving dermatologist-grade skin cancer classification. In *2024 IEEE International Conference on Interdisciplinary Approaches in Technology and Management for Social Innovation (IATMSI)*; IEEE: Gwalior, India, 2024; pp. 1–6. https://doi.org/10.1109/IATMSI60426.2024.10502664.

16 Kaushik, P.; Rathore, S.P.S.; Chahal, K.; Saraf, S.; Chauhan, G.S.; Kumar, P. RhythmQuest: Unifying Indian music classification and prediction with hybrid deep learning techniques. In *2024 IEEE International Conference on Interdisciplinary Approaches in Technology and Management for Social Innovation (IATMSI)*; IEEE: Gwalior, India, 2024; pp. 1–6. https://doi.org/10.1109/IATMSI60426.2024.10503056.

17 Pirzada, M.; Altintas, Z. Historical development of sensing technology. In *Fundamentals of Sensor Technology*, 1st ed.; Barhoum, A., Altintas, Z. Eds.; Woodhead Publishing Series in Electronic and Optical Materials; Woodhead Publishing: Sawston, UK, 2023; pp. 3–16.

18 Scheller, F.W.; Schubert, F.; Neumann, B.; Pfeiffer, D.; Hintsche, R.; Dransfeld, I.; Wollenberger, U.; Renneberg, R.; Warsinke, A.; Johansson, G. Second generation biosensors. *Biosens. Bioelectron.* 1991, *6*, 245–253.

19 Thimbleby, H. Technology and the future of healthcare. *J. Public Health Res.* 2013, *2*, 160–167.

20 Dede, S.; Altay, F. Biosensors from the first generation to nano-biosensors. *Int. Adv. Res. Eng. J.* 2018, *2*, 200–207.

21 Kwok, C.S.; Muntean, E.A.; Mallen, C.D.; Borovac, J.A. Data collection theory in healthcare research: The minimum dataset in quantitative studies. *Clin. Pract.* 2022, *12*, 832–844.

22 Chen, H.; Hailey, D.; Wang, N.; Yu, P. A review of data quality assessment methods for public health information systems. *Int. J. Environ. Res. Public Health* 2014, *11*, 5170–5207.

23 Pastorino, R.; De Vito, C.; Migliara, G.; Glocker, K.; Binenbaum, I.; Ricciardi, W.; Boccia, S. Benefits and challenges of big data in healthcare: An overview of the European initiatives. *Eur. J. Public Health* 2019, *29*, 23–37.

24 Kaushik, P. Deep learning unveils hidden insights: Advancing brain tumor diagnosis. *Int. J. Global Acad. Sci. Res.* 2023, *2*(2), 1–14. https://doi.org/10.55938/ijgasr.v2i2.45.

25 Rathore, R. A study of bed occupancy management in the healthcare system using the M/M/C queue and probability. *Int. J. Global Acad. Sci. Res.* 2023, *2*(1), 01–06. https://doi.org/10.55938/ijgasr.v2i1.36.

26 Sharma, V. A study on data scaling methods for machine learning. *Int. J. Global Acad. Sci. Res.* 2022, *1*(1), 31–42. https://doi.org/10.55938/ijgasr.v1i1.4.

27 Kaushik, P.; Rathore, S.P.S. Deep learning multiagent model for phishing cyber-attack detection. *Int. J. Recent Innovation Trends Comput. Commun.* 2023, *11*(9s), 680–686. https://doi.org/10.17762/ijritcc.v11i9s.7674.

28 Pisano, E. D. (2020). AI shows promise for breast cancer screening. *Nature* 577, 7788, pp. 35–36). Springer Science and Business Media LLC. https://doi.org/10.1038/d41586-019-03822-8

2

Explanation of Machine Learning Algorithms Used in Disease Detection, Such as Decision Trees and Neural Networks

Nikhil Verma, Tripti Sharma, and Bobbinpreet Kaur

ECE Department, Chandigarh University, Punjab, India

Introduction

The Silent Guardian: Machine Learning's Stealthy Rise in Disease Detection

The human body hums with a constant symphony of electrical signals, quantum biochemical reactions, and cellular whispers. When this complex orchestration falters, there's disease. Traditionally, doctors have relied on their keen eye and intuition to detect these disruptions. Now, in the age of Big Data, a guardian silent to the naked eye has emerged: machine learning (ML).

The ML algorithms are no shining armor doctors but powerful tools to comb through mountains of ever-growing medical data. They can harvest patterns hitherto unknown from symptoms and blood tests through scans and genetic data – the whispers about illness long before traditional medicine might detect them. This newfound depth in being able to enable interventions way before the firm grip of the disease promises a future of proactive healthcare [1].

Beyond the Usual Suspects: A Look at Emerging Innovations

Although the range of algorithms for ML, from decision trees to support vector machines, is itself of great value for workhorse purposes, real vanguard innovation resides in deep learning:

- **Deep reinforcement learning (DRL):** Now, consider an AI that learns through trial and error, much like a doctor who refines diagnoses over time.

AI in Disease Detection: Advancements and Applications, First Edition.
Edited by Rajesh Singh, Anita Gehlot, Navjot Rathour, and Shaik Vaseem Akram.

Published 2025 by John Wiley & Sons, Inc.

DRL algorithms hold massive potential in the field of disease detection due to their ability to learn from continuous exposure to new medical data and feedback from health professionals, therefore empowering them to get even better at identifying subtle anomalies indicative of diseases [2].

- **Auto-encoders:** These algorithms can be thought of as artistic impressionists in the way they work. They can compress complex medical data, like a mammogram, into lower-dimensional representations, capturing only the most essential features. This thus helps researchers to identify the most relevant patterns that would better enable them to detect diseases and makes the whole diagnostic process more accessible by reducing reliance on human entities [3].
- **Causal AI:** While traditional ML excels in correlation, causal AI goes a level further: It can tell not only that some factor is associated with a particular disease but also clarify why such an association exists. This deeper understanding is essential for developing targeted interventions and preventive measures [4].

The Ethical Symphony: Balancing Innovation with Human Oversight

Although there is hardly any doubt about the power of ML in disease detection, such application must be conducted within an established, ethical framework. Algorithms can inherit biases from training data, hence continuing the health disparities. In addition, total reliance on AI risks devaluing human experience.

The future would then align precisely because of human-machine collaboration. It would be the doctors who – equipped with a deep understanding of human biology and every insight into patient care – continue guiding this diagnosis process. ML, in turn, will offer them powerful tools to navigate this ever-growing sea of medical data, thus empowering them to come up with faster and more accurate diagnoses, eventually paving the way for a much healthier future.

Objectives

The human body whispers secrets in a language of intricate cellular processes and biochemical reactions. When these whispers turn into a discordant hum, signifying disease, early detection is the key to a successful outcome. Machine learning has emerged as a powerful ally in this fight, wielding a diverse arsenal of algorithms to identify and classify illnesses.

Unveiling Hidden Patterns – Feature Engineering

In such healthcare settings, raw data can resemble individual players of an orchestra tuning up to their own material – chaotic at best. A main quest today is feature engineering: extracting meaningful patterns and relationships to bring the instruments together in harmony. Dimensionality reduction techniques would condense vast datasets into a form more manageable by human minds or the identification of novel biomarkers previously undetectable using more traditional methods.

Innovation Spotlight: Active Feature Acquisition (AFA)

Consider an algorithm that will let an ML actively ask for specific data points from health professionals and learn from them to enhance its pattern recognition. AFA algorithms are a new generation since they facilitate dynamic interaction between AI and human experts so that the feature engineering process is more focused and efficient [5]. This section delves into seven key objectives of using ML for disease detection, exploring established methods and venturing into the frontiers of groundbreaking innovation.

1) **Challenge of classification:**
   - **Robust algorithms:** A path that such work can follow is, after the hidden patterns have been revealed, algorithms are built that will have the capacity to classify them effectively. Established methods, like decision trees and support vector machines, have been developed to work well in classifying data points based on their extracted features. DL architectures represent the future.
   - **Innovation spotlight:** Multimodal learning for disease subtyping diseases can manifest themselves in various ways. Multimodal learning algorithms can process multiple inputs at one time, such as medical images, genetic data, and EHRs. Such a holistic approach to the understanding of disease processes allows for the development of algorithms for subtyping – very important, therefore, in developing personalized treatment plans [6].
2) **Power of prediction:**
   - **Forecasting disease onset:** Use early detection as a key in disease management. Predictive ML models learn from past data to determine which people are at high risk of developing a specific illness. This will make it possible to intervene at a very early stage and might even prevent the disease from getting a foothold at all.
   - **Explainable AI for predictive models:** While there is little denying the predictive power of ML models, sometimes their "black box" nature can be unnerving. Techniques developed under the umbrella of explainable AI (XAI) strive to give meaning to their predictions, fostering trust among healthcare professionals and allowing them to integrate the AI's insight into their decision-making process [7].
3) **Mining the textual landscape:** Natural language processing (NLP) medical records are a veritable treasure trove of information but are usually locked

away in clinician notes and discharge summaries. The algorithms applied in this realm of NLP make up that key. They extract essential details about a patient's medical history, symptoms, and medications for feeding into analysis by the ML model, on the other hand.

4) **Innovation spotlight:** The handling of the sentiment expressed about the patient's narrative goes beyond mere fact extraction. Context-aware NLP for sentiment analysis could be realized from the emotional undertone in their descriptions of AI, which might identify early warning signs of mental health or even latent anxiety that might otherwise slip through the cracks [8].
5) **Bridging the privacy divide:** Federated learning ML succeeds by using large datasets, but sharing patient data is forbidden. Federated learning offers a brand-new solution for training robust models across geographically discrete datasets in a privacy-preserving manner – algorithms learn collaboratively but share just model updates, not raw data.
6) **Quest for explainability:** This focuses on demystifying AI decisions. Although predictive models form the backbone of most applications, the principle that one needs to know why the models arrived at any particular conclusion is axiomatic. That is where XAI techniques enter the picture. Opening up about how and why the model makes decisions could engender trust; in other words, XAI would let health professionals harness the expertise brought by AI while maintaining their clinical judgment [9].
7) **Lifelong learning:** The nature of diseases is continuously evolving; hence, ML models should also learn at the same pace. In/settings/compare.gif, lifelong learning algorithms learn continually from new data and bridge gaps in the judgments against new background findings to detect even the slightest shift toward a disease presentation.

The collaboration between human acumen and machine learning based on these seven essential quests could indeed be pathbreaking for disease detection [10]. This advancement heralds a future in which diseases are no longer able to develop unnoticed; instead, the earliest indicators are detected and addressed proactively, fostering a world where health risks are minimized, and community health outcomes are optimized.

Limitations and Advantages of ML Algorithms for Disease Detection

ML algorithms have revolutionized the field of disease detection, offering unprecedented accuracy and efficiency. These algorithms, including decision trees, neural networks, and support vector machines, have demonstrated significant potential in identifying diseases from medical data. However, like any technology, ML algorithms come with their own set of advantages and limitations.

Advantages of Machine Learning Algorithms for Disease Detection

1) **Higher diagnosis accuracy:** ML algorithms can consume and process tons of data, detecting patterns and anomalies not easily visible to the human clinician. Such an ability to detect weak signals in the data leads to improved diagnosis, especially for complex diseases like cancer, cardiovascular conditions, and neurological disorders. For instance, neural networks can be trained on thousands of medical images to detect early signs of the disease with great accuracy.
2) **Efficiency and speed:** ML algorithms can run through data at a much faster speed than traditional ones. Such high processing ability is of great help in the clinical environment, where timely diagnosis often becomes a question of life and death. For instance, through an automatic system, there is the facility for real-time analysis of medical images, results from laboratories, and patient records, thereby helping make quicker decisions and starting treatment [11].
3) **Predictive analytics:** ML models are exceptionally good at predicting disease outbreaks, patient readmission rates, and the progression of chronic diseases. Decision trees can, in this regard, can use patient history and lifestyle factors to determine the chances of a patient acquiring a particular disease. This predictive capability allows proactive steps for improving patient outcomes and lowering healthcare costs.
4) **Personalized medicine:** With their analysis of patient information by ML algorithms, treatment plans can be person-specific to a patient, which will make the treatment very effective with minimal side effects. Neural networks may, for instance, consolidate information about patient genetics, lifestyle, and history in a bid to personalize treatment protocols and, hence, improve patient care.
5) **Reduction of human error:** Making a diagnosis is often prone to human error. ML algorithms reduce the risk by providing constant, objective analysis. Reliability is extremely important in high-stakes environments such as emergency rooms and ICUs, where decisions should be accurate and timely [12].

Limitations of Machine Learning Algorithms for Disease Detection

1) **Availability of quality data:** Performance of the ML algorithms is very dependent on data availability in terms of its extent and quality. Poor, incomplete, and biased data will negatively affect the accuracy of diagnosis detection. Besides, the medical data is usually fragmented and saved in different formats over several systems; hence, it becomes tough to develop complete datasets for training algorithms [13].

2) **Interpretability and transparency:** Most of the current ML models, such as deep learning (DL) networks, are "black box" models – that is, they do not reveal any meaningful insights regarding their decision-making process. This lack of transparency can be a problem in a healthcare setting where one needs to see the reasoning resulting from a diagnosis. Clinicians and patients may not have confidence on AI-driven diagnoses without clear explanations [14].
3) **Algorithmic bias:** The ML models accidentally learn biases from their training datasets. This will lead to diagnostic accuracy that differs across different demographic groups, which may raise ethical and social questions. Maintaining fairness and avoiding bias in ML algorithms is a significant challenge that will require careful consideration while creating the training dataset and requires continuous monitoring of the performance of these models.
4) **Integration with clinical workflows:** The process of integrating ML algorithms into health infrastructures is reasonably sophisticated. On the integration side, marrying them to the predominant electronic health record (EHR) systems can be required, implying huge technological and logistically demanding efforts. Moreover, these tools are to be taught to health professionals for proper functioning, which becomes time-consuming and expensive [15].
5) **Regulatory and ethical concerns:** Some of the ethical and regulatory issues for using ML in disease detection relate to patient privacy, data security, and the requirement for informed consent. Regulatory bodies are still developing guidelines that ought to govern the practice of AI in healthcare, and adherence to these evolving standards will become imperative. Moreover, a few ethical considerations surround the use of AI in clinical decision-making, and if addressed improperly, then trust and integrity will be lost in healthcare [16].

The intendments of ML algorithms in disease diagnosis have several advantages: accuracy, efficiency, and customized treatment. These advantages shall no doubt affect healthcare delivery and the fate of various patients. However, it is only when there are limitations in data quality, interpretability challenges, or even ethical concerns with ML that the full potential of ML will be reached. The improvement of data management, transparency of algorithms, and regulatory frameworks will be central to surmounting these challenges and integrating ML into mainstream medical practice.

Literature Review

The human body functions like a complex orchestra, with intricate systems working in harmony. When disease disrupts this delicate dance, early detection becomes paramount. Machine learning has emerged as a powerful conductor in this fight, wielding a diverse arsenal of algorithms to identify and classify illnesses. Table 2.1 summarizes studies researching various techniques used to treat disease.

The Familiar Melodies: Established ML Techniques and Their Strengths

Throughout these studies reviewed, a common trend emerges: the value of already developed ML algorithms, like decision trees, support vector machines, and k-nearest neighbors (KNNs). These algorithms provide a solid base for disease detection; some perform best in specific niches under study:

- **Classification:** Decision trees and SVMs are very good at classifying patients according to their medical data, be it symptoms, blood tests, or scanning results, which helps detect the onset of specific diseases. Think of a choose-your-own-adventure story, but instead of fantasy scenarios, the branches are the different symptoms. In such meticulous navigations of this path, decision trees efficiently segment patients based on reported conditions. On the other hand, SVMs function much like meticulous border guards in meticulously drawing a dividing line between healthy and diseased states according to a variety of medical data points [17].
- **Pattern recognition:** KNN algorithms recognize the clustering in health profiles, where similar profiles tend to cluster together. Take a small, tight-knit medical community where patients with similar symptoms dwell together. The KNN algorithm will then classify a new patient according to the majority vote of his closest neighbors in this landscape of medical data. Such a simple approach performs well under conditions of well-characterized disease presentation [18].

The Rise of the Deep Learning Chorus: Innovation on the Horizon

CNNs are champions in image analysis; working on cues from the structure of the visual cortex, they specialize in recognizing complex patterns within medical scans, including X-rays and mammograms. Learning features directly from data makes them very powerful in identifying subtle abnormalities indicative of diseases such as cancer. Think of this as many highly skilled specialists poring over the medical scans with great care. Like CNNs, they are also able to determine even the slightest lip service signals of possible sickness in people [19].

While CNNs work well for static images, recurrent neural networks (RNNs) do much better on sequential data. This makes them quite suitable for analyzing time-series data, for example, for heart rate or EEG recordings. There is no doubt

Table 2.1 Literature review of various diseases.

Disease	Author(s)	Technique used	Review
Heart disease	Ansari et al. (2003)	Neurofuzzy integrated systems	Achieved around 89% accuracy but lacks explanation on model credibility and performance in various scenarios [22].
Heart disease	Rubin et al. (2017)	Deep CNNs	Achieved 0.95 specificity and 0.73 sensitivity; model tested in PhysioNet competition, ranked second [23].
Heart disease	Miao and Miao et al. (2018)	DL-based technique	Achieved 88.02% accuracy, 85.01% precision, and 0.85 F-score; addressed overfitting with dropout strategies [24].
Kidney disease	Charleonnan et al. (2016)	KNN, SVM, LR, decision trees	Achieved accuracy of 98.1%, 98.3%, 96.55%, and 94.8%, respectively, using publicly available datasets [25].
Kidney disease	Aljaaf et al. (2018)	RPART, SVM, LOGR, MLP	MLP performed best with 98.1% accuracy in identifying chronic kidney disease using CKD dataset [26].
Kidney disease	Ma et al. (2020)	Heterogeneous modified artificial neural networks (NNs)	Achieved 87–99% accuracy using a collection of datasets from many sources [27].
Breast cancer	Miranda and Felipe (2015)	Fuzzy-logic-based computer-aided diagnosis	Achieved approximately 83.34% accuracy; lacks explainable interpretation of results [28].
Breast cancer	Zheng et al. (2014)	K-means clustering, SVM	Achieved 97.38% accuracy; used WDBC dataset but may not perform well with unequal class ratios or missing values [29].
Breast cancer	Asri et al. (2016)	SVM, DT (C4.5), NB, KNN	SVM outperformed others with 97.13% accuracy; results may vary with different databases [30].
Breast cancer	Mohammed et al. (2020)	DT (J48), NB, SMO	SMO achieved more than 95% accuracy; focused on data imbalance issues and minimized imbalance problem through resampling [31].

Table 2.1 (Continued)

Disease	Author(s)	Technique used	Review
Breast cancer	Assegie (2021)	KNN with grid search	Achieved 94.35% accuracy with fine-tuned KNN settings [32].
Breast cancer	Bhattacherjee et al. (2020)	Backpropagation neural network	Achieved 99.27% accuracy using WBC dataset with nine features [33].
Breast cancer	Alshayeji et al. (2021)	Shallow ANN	Achieved 99.85% accuracy using WBCD and WDBI datasets without feature selection or algorithm tweaking [34].
Breast cancer	Sultana et al. (2021)	Various NN architectures	PNN outperformed others with 98.24% accuracy using WBC dataset; lacks interpretability of important features [35].
Breast cancer	Ghosh et al. (2021)	Various DL models	LSTM and GRU demonstrated best performance with roughly 99% accuracy using WBC dataset [36].
Diabetes	Kandhasamy and Balamurali (2015)	J48 DT, KNN, RF, SVM	KNN and RF achieved near-perfect accuracy; simplified diabetes dataset with eight binary-classified parameters [37].
Diabetes	Yahyaoui et al. (2019)	SVM, RF, CNN	RF achieved 83.67% accuracy; DL and SVM scored 76.81% and 65.38%, respectively, using clinical decision support systems (CDSS) [38].
Diabetes	Naz and Ahuja (2020)	ANN, NB, DT, DL	DL achieved approximately 98.07% accuracy using PIMA diabetes datasets; lacks mention of interpretability issues and performance with unbalanced datasets [39].
Diabetes	Ashiquzzaman et al. (2017)	Deep learning	Achieved 88.41% accuracy using PIMA Indian dataset; addressed overfitting with dropout techniques but increased training duration [40].
Diabetes	Alhassan et al. (2018)	LSTM, GRU-based deep neural networks	Achieved up to 97% accuracy using KAIMRCD dataset, the world's largest diabetic dataset [41].

(Continued)

Table 2.1 (Continued)

Disease	Author(s)	Technique used	Review
Parkinson's	Sriram et al. (2013)	KNN, SVM, NB, RF	RF achieved best performance with 90.26% accuracy; NB demonstrated worst performance with 69.23% accuracy [42].
Parkinson's	Esmaeilzadeh et al. (2018)	Deep CNN	Achieved nearly 100% accuracy; lacks mention of overfitting issues and interpretability of final classification [43].
Parkinson's	Grover et al. (2018)	DNN	Achieved around 81.67% accuracy using UCI's Parkinson's telemonitoring voice dataset [44].
Parkinson's	Warjurkar and Ridhorkar (2021)	Boosted logistic regression, Markov random	Boosted logistic regression achieved 97.15% accuracy in identifying Parkinson's; Markov random technique performed best in tumor segmentation with 97.4% [45].
COVID-19	Chen et al. (2020)	UNet++ model with CT images	Achieved 98.5% accuracy using CT images from 51 COVID-19 and 82 non-COVID-19 patients [46].
COVID-19	Ardakani et al. (2020)	Various DL models	Achieved 99% overall accuracy using a small dataset of 108 COVID-19 and 86 non-COVID-19 patients [47].
COVID-19	Wang et al. (2020)	Inception-based model	Achieved 73.1% accuracy using a large dataset containing 453 CT scan images; poorly explained network activity and region of interest [48].
COVID-19	Li et al. (2020)	COVNet model	Achieved 96% accuracy utilizing a large dataset of 4356 chest CT images [49].
COVID-19	Hemdan et al. (2020)	VGG19, ResNet50	Identified COVID-19 patients from chest X-ray images with 90% and 95% accuracy respectively using a small dataset of 50 images [50].
COVID-19	Narin et al. (2021)	–	Distinguished COVID-19 patients from pneumonia with 86% accuracy using a dataset of 100 chest X-ray images [51].

Table 2.1 (Continued)

Disease	Author(s)	Technique used	Review
COVID-19	Brunese et al. (2020)	–	Employed 6505 images, achieving good performance but did not test with unbalanced data or mismatched class ratios [52].
Alzheimer's	Neelaveni and Devasana (2020)	SVM, DT	Achieved 85% and 83% accuracy, respectively, in detecting Alzheimer's disease [53].
Alzheimer's	Collij et al. (2016)	SVM	Achieved 82% accuracy in detecting single-subject Alzheimer's disease and mild cognitive impairment (MCI) prediction [54].
Alzheimer's	Vidushi and Shrivastava (2019)	LR, SVM, DT, RF, Boosting Adaboost	Achieved accuracy of 78.95%, 81.58%, 81.58%, 84.21%, and 84.21%, respectively [62].
Alzheimer's	Ahmed et al. (2020)	CNN	Achieved 99% accuracy using 6628 MRI images for earlier diagnosis and classification of Alzheimer's disease [55].
Alzheimer's	Nawaz et al. (2020)	Deep feature-based models	Achieved 99.12% accuracy [56].
Alzheimer's	Haft-Javaherian et al. (2019)	CNN	Demonstrated robustness of CNN-based approach in Alzheimer's disease diagnosis [57].
Other diseases	Mao et al. (2020)	DT, RF	Disease classification based on eye movement [58].
Other diseases	Nosseir and Shawky (2019)	KNN, SVM	Developed automatic skin disease classification systems with KNN achieving best performance with 98.22% accuracy [59].
Other diseases	Khan et al. (2020)	CNN-based approaches (VGG16, VGG19)	Classified multimodal brain tumors with accuracies of 97.8%, 96.9%, and 92.5%, respectively, using BraTs datasets [60].
Other diseases	Amin et al. (2018)	RF classifier	Achieved high accuracy [61].

that RNNs will be able to identify slight changes in such sequences and thus contribute to early disease diagnosis. Imagine a team of specialists who continuously monitor a patient's vital signs. RNNs do the same thing, whereby streams of medical data are constantly passed through to detect the minutest variation in the usual trend and hence provide earlier diagnosis [4].

Breaking New Ground: Unveiling Unique Innovations and Addressing Challenges

Beyond established methods, the papers reviewed give a clue to new and exciting avenues of exploration in the future while also reporting some possible difficulties. Although impressive, the accuracy obtained by DL models and their "black box" nature may concern healthcare professionals. Therefore, it is imperative to have explainable AI. These XAI techniques can attempt to explain how these algorithms attempt to improve trust and increase human-AI collaboration in disease diagnosis. Picture this: You are given some diagnosis from some complex medical instrument but there is no explanation behind it; XAI techniques would provide that layer of transparency and help health professionals not just to trust AI's findings but understand how the AI tool arrived at that diagnosis [5].

Federated learning offers a valuable approach in privacy-preserving techniques that can help maintain patient privacy. Federated learning enables training ML models on geographically distributed datasets without moving data and maintains patient confidentiality. This technique works by providing a collaborative learning environment wherein many institutions can contribute their data to train a central model without divulging the specifics of their individual datasets. This will help unlock the full potential of vast medical data while keeping privacy concerns intact.

The human body works as efficiently and intricately as an orchestra, with all the instruments performing in harmony. It is, therefore, essential that there be early detection of disease at the first hint of a sour note. ML emerges as a productive conductor in this symphony, with a diversity of algorithms that offer a vast arsenal for identifying and classifying disease [1].

The Well-Honed Orchestra: Established Techniques Take Center Stage

However the whole corpus of manuscripts under scrutiny points to the role that classic algorithms – decision trees, support vector machines, and k-nearest neighbors – have played while discussing the most modern developments in these areas. These are a few of those algorithms that have helped form the backbone of disease detection, turning out to perform well in specific tasks:

- **Classification:** Consider the case of a complex decision tree with branches coming in as different symptoms and leaves are possible diseases. Known algorithms like decision trees and SVMs work precisely on this principle – that they carefully look at the data of a patient, like blood test results and previous medical history – to classify them under various diseases. They thus become the first instruments to be played in an orchestra of disease detection that 503 structures further analysis [13].
- **Pattern recognition:** The KNN algorithms work on this concept of "clustering," where similar patient profiles tend to group. Think of patients with similar complaints, all living near one another in a virtual medical landscape. By taking a majority vote of all their nearest neighbors in this data landscape, KNN algorithms could classify a new patient. This works particularly well in situations with typical, well-defined disease presentations and thus is a beneficial technique in catering to the identification of possible illnesses.

Beyond the Familiar Melodies: Deep Learning Takes the Stage

Convolutional neural networks are abbreviated as CNNs. It is taken from the structure and function of the visual cortex; also, they are very proficient at extracting intricate patterns from medical images. For example, it shows their high effectiveness in detecting diabetic retinopathy within fundus photographs. Picture a team of super-competent specialists going through retinal images line by line. CNNs work in the same way, working out even the lightest signs on their own that vision loss may occur. They can be regarded as virtuoso performers in the orchestra, whereby they are capable of detecting minute abnormalities that can very quickly flee from human vision [20]:

- **Transfer learning:** Training DL models from scratch needs large amounts of data, which is an expensive resource in healthcare. Some solution can be explored in transfer learning. Pretrained models on large, generic datasets, such as image recognition, are adapted for specific medical image analysis tasks. Now, consider how easily an accomplished musician can learn another instrument. Transfer learning does the same with medical image-based disease classification, using existing knowledge to address new challenges. In the research domain, this enables one to "borrow" experience from established models that will allow rapid progress in the detection of diseases.
- **Diagnostic accuracy:** Diagnostics in oncology are intrinsically interdisciplinary; cooperation will be required between computer vision experts and doctors. Synthesizing insights from various literature sources, the authors offer valuable guidelines for further research into better early detection and treatment in oncology.

- **Mental health applications:** Machine learning can analyze patient data from surveys, questionnaires, and medical records to diagnose mental health conditions with the potential to predict treatment response [9]. Imagine a system that can understand what patients say through their self-reported experiences, sleep patterns, and activities on social media. As such, this kind of personalized approach has enormous potential in improving outcomes related to mental health. It gives mental health professionals the prerogative to develop tailored therapy plans, garner better results, and empower patients with the leadership role for their well-being.
- **Personalized cancer treatment:** This addresses applying machine learning to analyze a patient's case history, genetic information, and tumor characteristics to predict which course of cancer treatment will work best. Imagine an oncologist armed with a powerful tool that will help analyze a patient's unique genetic makeup and tumor profile to recommend treatment options customized with enhanced chances of success [10]. This could amount to a more powerful way of managing cancer. If treatment is targeted to the particular characteristics of a patient's cancer, then doctors will achieve better outcomes with fewer side effects.

Collaboration and Innovation Lead the Way

The studies reviewed in Table 2.1 put forward a very optimistic picture. Through the power of well-established ML techniques, together with innovative DL approaches and healthcare providers' expertise, we can revolutionize disease detection and treatment. In such a vein, it will be important to foster collaboration between such forces. Imagine the symphony reaching its crescendo – where all instruments are playing in perfect harmony. It is under this approach of collaboration, where ML algorithms contribute with essential insights and human specialists interpret and applies these inputs that the full potential of machine learning will be harnessed in disease detection and treatment [21].

Machine learning is the conductor of the powerful orchestra of well-established techniques, deep learning innovations, and human expertise in the bright future of healthcare. It foretells a future for revolutionizing disease detection and tailoring treatment plans to suit particular cases for a healthier world.

Methodology

The human body is a complex web of interrelated systems that can suffer many disruptions. As a result, covering early detection of most of these disruptions, usually in the form of diseases, is essential for effective intervention. A very potent maestro in this regard is machine learning, with its various methodologies for detecting and classifying diseases. The following deepens into established methodologies, exploring the frontiers of innovation, as guided by the key sources that follow.

Conventional ML Methods for Disease Detection

While cutting-edge advancements dominate headlines, established ML methodologies remain the bedrock of disease detection. Here's a closer look at these time-tested techniques, infused with a touch of innovation:

- **Data acquisition and preprocessing:** At the core of any ML project is robust data. A master musician does not begin a performance by picking and playing every instrument; instead, he selects and prepares his instruments beforehand. In much the same way, data acquisition involves the gathering of relevant medical data from various sources, like patient history, scans, and laboratory results. The innovation is that real-time sensor data from wearable or implantable devices can continuously monitor physiological indicators to better understand good health. Privacy-preserving methods can then be further extended using federated learning, which directly includes feature engineering or anonymization techniques. Last but not least, in addition to ensuring patient privacy while maximizing data utility, this information is also valuable in a collaborative approach in which models are trained about decentralized data sets without disclosing patient privacy.
- **Feature selection and extraction:** Not all data points are created equal in utility. Feature selection is, therefore, of great importance in identifying informative variables for disease detection. The task is similar to what the conductor of an orchestra does in the process of carefully choosing the instruments and sections that will bring out the best of the musical composition. The established methods for feature selection can also be combined with DL-based innovative feature extraction techniques. DL models are capable of automatically learning complex features from raw data and probably discovering hidden patterns that traditional methods might miss. The synergistic approach to healthcare research of this nature will yield a subtle understanding of the disease and its underpinning mechanisms.
- **Model training and validation:** With data preparation and feature selection done, it is time to let the musicians practice! Model training is fitting an ML algorithm to the data for learning the relationship of features with disease diagnosis. The well-established algorithms include decision trees, support vector

machines, and KNN; the breakthrough comes with ensemble learning: training many models and then putting them together for more robust and accurate predictions. Transfer learning can then further enhance even traditional k-fold cross-validation. Fine-tuning a pretrained model from some similar domain in medicine to that particular disease can speed up the training still and further bring up the quality of the models.

- **Model evaluation and interpretation:** Performances of a trained model must be viewed before deployment. Think about the conductor listening carefully to an orchestra, noting any deficiencies in this performance by the orchestra. Of course, these established metrics – accuracy, precision, recall, and F1 score – are still valuable tools at one's disposal. However, a symphony in disease detection requires interpretability on its terms. Techniques like explainable AI shed light on the "black box" nature of DL models by letting healthcare professionals understand the reasons behind the model's predictions. This engenders trust and allows easier integration into the clinical decision-making process.

Beyond the Established Melodies: Innovation Takes Center Stage

Long-standing time of infection location lies in pushing the boundaries of setup techniques:

- **Generative adversarial networks (GANs):** GANs can be likened to a symphony conductor who not only orchestrates performances but also composes entirely new pieces. GANs, a sort of deep learning show, can make engineered restorative information, tending to the challenge of restricted datasets in healthcare. This permits analysts to prepare models more successfully and possibly distinguish uncommon illnesses more promptly.
- **Dynamic learning:** Envision the conductor effectively locks in with the performers, giving input and asking alterations amid practice. Dynamic learning procedures can be incorporated into the preparing handle. The show can prioritize information focuses that hold the foremost esteem for learning, driving to speedier and more productive demonstrate advancement.
- **Logical AI for clinical integration:** As specified prior, XAI procedures hold monstrous guarantee. By demystifying the decision-making handle of ML models, XAI can cultivate trust and collaboration between healthcare experts and AI frameworks. Envision the conductor not only guiding the ensemble but also explaining the musical choices and their effect on the overall performance. This transparency is vital for seamless integration of ML into clinical practice, as mentioned in Figure 2.1.

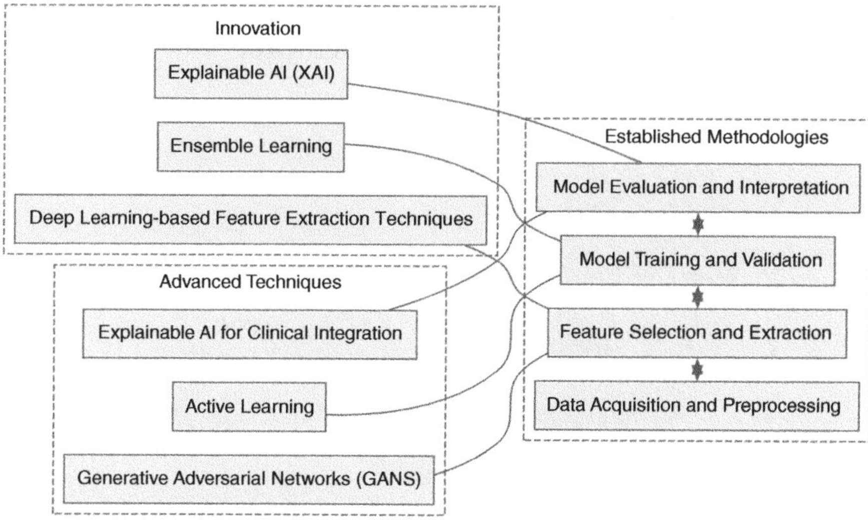

Figure 2.1 Architectural framework.

Results and Analysis

Figure 2.2 shows the battlefield against disease is constantly evolving, demanding ever-more sophisticated tools for early detection and treatment. Machine learning has emerged as a powerful warrior in this fight, wielding its analytical prowess to unlock hidden patterns within medical data. However, to truly revolutionize disease detection, we must move beyond established methodologies and embrace a future symphony of innovation.

The Familiar Melody: Established Methodologies

The current ML landscape for disease detection is built on a foundation of established techniques. These methodologies work like instruments of the orchestra in a structured workflow.

- **Data acquisition and preprocessing:** This is the stage at which the core of the ML process in medicine is implemented. This may involve data cleaning and organization and, sometimes, even anonymizing patient information, EHRs, or medical images.
- **Feature selection and extraction:** All measured data points are not equally important. At this stage, the relevant features are selected and extracted from the data that has been preprocessed, much in the way that a conductor would emphasize key melodies within a symphony.

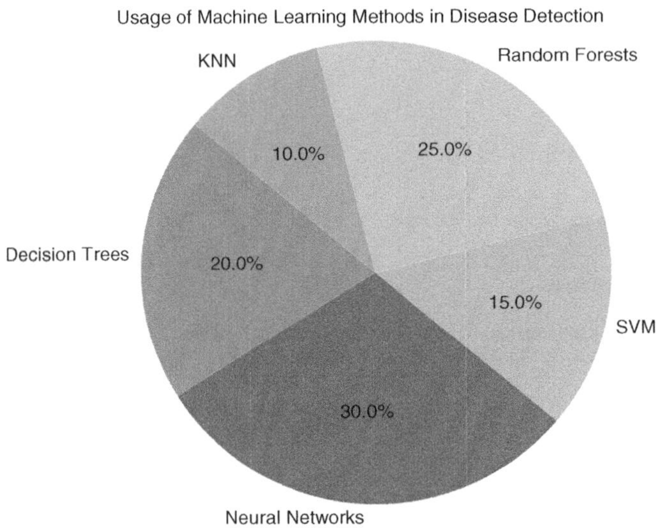

Figure 2.2 Usage of ML in disease detection.

- **Model training and validation:** Extracted features are then fed into training ML models – the intelligent algorithms that will learn to recognize the patterns of the diseases. Think of this as the musicians working diligently to practice their parts so that, at the end, they are able to play together in harmony. On the other hand, validation is a step to ensure good general performance on unseen data, a way to prevent overfitting.
- **Evaluation and interpretation of the trained model:** Finally, the performance of the trained model shall be evaluated wherein its accuracy in disease detection, sensitivity, and specificity is tested. Explorable AI techniques are thus pertinent to establish the "why" behind the decisions made by the model, just like a conductor analyzing the musical impact of different sections.

The Disruptive Score: Unveiling New Innovations

While it is within the established methods that there lies a deep foundation, they are beset with limitations. Below describes the consequences of when the traditional symphony breaks and we welcome innovative movements:

- **Real-time sensor data:** Imagine the additional inclusion of data from wearable sensors monitoring vital signs and physiologic parameters uninterruptedly. This real-time inflow will allow earlier detection of diseases and personalized risk assessment. DL algorithms, such as those in motion 2, take their inspiration from the structure and functionality of the brain; this will have the potential to extract complex features automatically from raw data, leading hopefully to better disease detection. Established methods typically require manual feature selection, a time-consuming rather subjective effort.

- **Ensemble learning:** Imagine an orchestra playing many instruments that create variations of the same theme. Ensemble learning bundles predictions resulting from different ML models into more robust and accurate disease detection.
- **Transfer learning:** It can be data-intensive to train ML models from scratch. Transfer learning fundamentally takes advantage of pretrained models on similar domains, significantly reducing time and resources required for training; it has the potential to detect disease at a faster rate.
- **Proposed system:** The above innovations are not intended to replace established methodologies but to work in harmony with them, like a symphony where the traditional orchestra is enhanced with rich supporting new instruments under the direction of a maestro who literally understands the traditional and the innovative in perfect balance. In the same way, open-source data and code sharing are important in the case of collaborative research to achieve this symphony in the collaboration.

The Human Touch: Ethical Considerations and Explainability

The deeper we go into this symphony of innovation, the more we need to make sure the human element remain foremost. Hence, ethical considerations must be very strict. High standards in data privacy and security will foster patient trust and adherence to regulations. Further, explainable AI techniques are important for gaining trust among medical professionals and patients. We want to know not only the "what" but also the "why" behind a model's predictions to ensure proper accountability and transparency in disease detection.

Conclusions and Future Scope

ML has been one of the cornerstones of modern disease detection. Still, it will ring in a revolution when we leave behind these tantalizing glimpses that all established methods give and attempt to orchestrate a future symphony of path-breaking innovations. Drawing from the potential will not only improve disease detection but also create a paradigm shift in healthcare itself, ushering in treatments specific to each patient. This is the end to which research communities will continue to work tirelessly.

The Evolving Maestro: AI Orchestration Beyond Established Methods

Current machine learning (ML) pipelines prioritize data quality, highlight feature extraction, and emphasize rigorous model training. However, this represents only an initial step. The future demands a new paradigm, one that introduces a more dynamic, interconnected approach to drive further advancements:

- **AI coordination:** This inventive approach goes past built-up strategies, centering on consistent integration and energetic adjustment inside the malady discovery workflow.
- **Combined learning:** Envision a organize of healing centers and clinics, each with its claim persistent information storehouse. Unified learning permits ML models to be prepared collaboratively over these silos without compromising understanding security (development 1). This opens the control of decentralized information for predominant malady location, especially in rare or geologically confined cases.
- **Dynamic learning:** Current strategies frequently require tremendous sums of labeled information. Dynamic learning calculations (development 2) can distinguish the foremost instructive information focuses, minimizing the requirement for manual labeling. This does not diminish the workload for restorative experts but permits for more productivity and focus on information collection.
- **Continuous learning:** Infection scenes and persistent populaces always advance. Conventional models ended up obsolete over time. Continuous learning calculations (development 3) can ingest unused information streams and adjust their expectations powerfully, guaranteeing ceaseless enhancement in infection discovery exactness.
- **Generative ill-disposed systems (GANs):** Envision creating synthetic patient data to expand existing datasets. GANs (development 4) can create practical but anonymized patient data, empowering analysts to prepare ML models on bigger and more assorted datasets without security concerns. This may be especially important for uncommon infections with restricted real-world information.

Human-Machine Duet: Collaboration for a Healthier Future

This symphony of innovation thrives on collaboration. AI and human expertise must work in tandem to achieve optimal results. Here's how this collaboration will unfold:

- **Explainable AI (XAI) for clinical adoption:** Even the most sophisticated models are useless if healthcare professionals don't trust them. XAI techniques tailored for the medical domain will be crucial (movement 5). These techniques will provide clear and interpretable explanations for a model's predictions, fostering trust and acceptance among medical professionals.

- **AI-powered clinical decision support systems:** Imagine an AI assistant that analyzes patient data, suggests potential diagnoses, and even recommends treatment options. AI-powered CDSSs are very promising (movement 6). They can assist the doctor as a valued colleague, providing current insight and helping to arrive at more informed clinical decisions.
- **AI-powered precision diagnostics for personalized medicine:** The future of healthcare rests in customized treatment plans. Artificial intelligence can help decipher the patient's medical history, genetic makeup, and lifestyle data for predicting individual disease risks to tailored interventions. That opens up a path to proactive healthcare, averting diseases at their incipient stages.

The future of disease detection is not a far-away dream but more of a symphony to be played. It will call for AI orchestration enabled through human-machine collaboration and ethical prioritization to unlock human health in newer ways: earlier diagnosis, more effective treatments, and a healthier life for all. The final notes of this journey will resound with a melody of hope – an enduring testament to the power of human ingenuity and technological progress in overcoming formidable diseases. Now is the time to unveil this future, advancing one innovation at a time.

References

1 Guan, Q.; Huang, Y.; Zhong, Z.; Zheng, Z.; Zheng, L.; Yang, Y. Thorax disease classification with attention guided convolutional neural network. *Pattern Recognit. Lett.* 2020, *131*, 38–45.

2 Dua, D.; Taniskidou, E.K. *UCI Machine Learning Repository*; University of California, School of Information and Computer Science: Irvine, CA, 2017. Available on: http://archive.ics.uci.edu/ml (accessed on 5 May 2021).

3 Alcalá-Fdez, J.; Fernández, A.; Luengo, J.; Derrac, J.; García, S.; Sánchez, L.; Herrera, F. Keel data-mining software tool: Data set repository, integration of algorithms and experimental analysis framework. *J. Mult.-Valued Log. Soft Comput.* 2011, *17*, 255–287.

4 Fernández, A.; López, V.; Galar, M.; del Jesus, M.J.; Herrera, F. Analysing the classification of unbalanced data-sets with multiple classes: Binarization techniques and ad-hoc approaches. *Knowl.-Based Syst.* 2013, *42*, 97–110.

5 Mullick, S.S.; Datta, S.; Dhekane, S.G.; Das, S. Appropriateness of performance indices for imbalanced data classification: An analysis. *Pattern Recognit.* 2020, *102*, 107197.

6 Hall, M.; Frank, E.; Holmes, G.; Pfahringer, B.; Reutemann, P.; Witten, I.H. The WEKA data mining software: An update. *ACM SIGKDD Explor. Newsl.* 2009, *11*, 10–18.
7 Triguero, I.; González, S.; Moyano, J.M.; García López, S.; Alcalá Fernández, J.; Luengo, J.; Fernández, A.; del Jesús, M.J.; Sánchez, L.; Herrera, F. KEEL 3.0: An open source software for multi-stage analysis in data mining. *Int. J. Comput. Intell. Syst.* 2017, *10*, 1238–1249.
8 Zhang, S. Cost-sensitive KNN classification. *Neurocomputing* 2020, *391*, 234–242.
9 Zhao, Z.; Xu, S.; Kang, B.H.; Kabir, M.M.J.; Liu, Y.; Wasinger, R. Investigation and improvement of multi-layer perceptron neural networks for credit scoring. *Expert Syst. Appl.* 2015, *42*, 3508–3516.
10 Livieris, I.E.; Kanavos, A.; Tampakas, V.; Pintelas, P. An ensemble SSL algorithm for efficient chest X-ray image classification. *J. Imaging* 2018, *4*, 95.
11 Chan, H.-P.; Hadjiiski, L.M.; Samala, R.K. Computer-aided diagnosis in the era of deep learning. *Med. Phys.* 2020, *47*, e218–e227.
12 Pathan, S.; Kumar, P.; Pai, R.M.; Bhandary, S.V. Automated segmentation and classification of retinal features for glaucoma diagnosis. *Biomed. Signal Process. Control* 2021, 63.
13 Gautam, A.; Raman, B. Towards effective classification of brain hemorrhagic and ischemic stroke using CNN. *Biomed. Signal Process. Control* 2021, 63.
14 Kaushik, P.; Singh Rathore, S.P.; Kaur, P.; Kumar, H.; Tyagi, N. Leveraging multiscale adaptive object detection and contrastive feature learning for customer behavior analysis in retail settings. *Int. J. Recent Innovation Trends Comput. Commun.* 2023, *11*(6s), 326–343. https://doi.org/10.17762/ijritcc.v11i6s.6938.
15 Agarwal, P.; Vij, A. Assessing the challenges and opportunities of artificial intelligence in Indian education. *Int. J. Global Acad. Sci. Res.* 2024, *3*(1), 36–44. https://doi.org/10.55938/ijgasr.v3i1.71.
16 Rathore, R. A review on study of application of queueing models in hospital sector. *Int. J. Global Acad. Sci. Res.* 2022, *1*(2), 01–05. https://doi.org/10.55938/ijgasr.v1i2.11.
17 Kaushik, P. Unleashing the power of multi-agent deep learning: cyber-attack detection in IoT. *Int. J. Global Acad. Sci. Res.* 2023, *2*(2), 15–29. https://doi.org/10.55938/ijgasr.v2i2.46.
18 Kaushik; Chopra, Y.; Kajla, A.; Poonia, M.; Khan, A.; Yadav, D. AI-powered dermatology: achieving dermatologist-grade skin cancer classification. In *2024 IEEE International Conference on Interdisciplinary Approaches in Technology and Management for Social Innovation (IATMSI)*; IEEE: Gwalior, India, 2024; pp. 1–6. https://doi.org/10.1109/IATMSI60426.2024.10502664.
19 Kaushik, P.; Rathore, S.P.S.; Chahal, K.; Saraf, S.; Chauhan, G.S.; Kumar, P. RhythmQuest: Unifying Indian music classification and prediction with hybrid deep learning techniques. In *2024 IEEE International Conference on*

Interdisciplinary Approaches in Technology and Management for Social Innovation (IATMSI); IEEE: Gwalior, India, 2024; pp. 1–6. https://doi.org/10.1109/IATMSI60426.2024.10503056.

20 Paranjape, P.; Dhabu, M.; Deshpande, P. A novel classifier for multivariate instance using graph class signatures. *Front. Comput. Sci.* 2020, *14*, 144307.

21 Minaee, S.; Yao, W.; Lui, Y.W. Prediction of long-term outcome of neuropsychological tests of MTBI patients using imaging features. In *Proceedings of the 2013 IEEE Signal Processing in Medicine and Biology Symposium (SPMB)*; IEEE: Brooklyn, NY, 7 December 2013, 2013; pp. 1–6.

22 Ansari, M.; Alexander, M.; Tutar, A.; Bello, D.; Massie, B. M. Cardiology participation improves outcomes in patients with new-onset heart failure in the outpatient setting. *J. Am. Coll. Cardiol.*, 2003, 41(1), 62–68. https://doi.org/10.1016/s0735-1097(02)02493-2

23 Rubin, J. B.; Borden, W. B. Coronary Heart Disease in Young Adults. *Curr. Atheroscler. Rep.*, 2012, 14(2), 140–149. https://doi.org/10.1007/s11883-012-0226-3

24 Miao, K. H.; H., J. Coronary Heart Disease Diagnosis using Deep Neural Networks. *Inter. J. Adv. Comp. Sci. Appl.*, 2018, 9(10). https://doi.org/10.14569/ijacsa.2018.091001

25 Charleonnan, A.; Fufaung, T.; Niyomwong, T.; Chokchueypattanakit, W.; Suwannawach, S.; Ninchawee, N. Predictive analytics for chronic kidney disease using machine learning techniques. 2016 Management and Innovation Technology International Conference (MITicon), *MIT-80-MIT-83.* https://doi.org/10.1109/miticon.2016.8025242

26 Aljaaf, A. J.; Al-Jumeily, D.; Haglan, H. M.; Alloghani, M.; Baker, T.; Hussain, A. J.; Mustafina, J. Early Prediction of Chronic Kidney Disease Using Machine Learning Supported by Predictive Analytics. 2018 IEEE Congress on Evolutionary Computation (CEC), 1–9. https://doi.org/10.1109/cec.2018.8477876

27 Ma, F.; Sun, T.; Liu, L.; Jing, H. Detection and diagnosis of chronic kidney disease using deep learning-based heterogeneous modified artificial neural network. *Future Generation Computer Systems*, 2020, 111, 17–26. https://doi.org/10.1016/j.future.2020.04.036

28 Miranda, G. H. B.; Felipe, J. C. Computer-aided diagnosis system based on fuzzy logic for breast cancer categorization. *Comput. Biol.* 2016, *Medi.* 64, 334–346. https://doi.org/10.1016/j.compbiomed.2014.10.006

29 Cai, Q. et al. Genome-wide association analysis in East Asians identifies breast cancer susceptibility loci at 1q32.1, 5q14.3 and 15q26.1. *Nat. Genet.*, 2014, 46(8), 886–890. https://doi.org/10.1038/ng.3041

30 Asri, H.; Mousannif, H.; Moatassime, H. A.; Noel, T. Using Machine Learning Algorithms for Breast Cancer Risk Prediction and Diagnosis. *Procedia Computer Science*, 2016, 83, 1064–1069. https://doi.org/10.1016/j.procs.2016.04.224

31 Mohammed, S. A.; Darrab, S.; Noaman, S. A.; Saake, G. (2020). Analysis of Breast Cancer Detection Using Different Machine Learning Techniques. In Data Mining and Big Data (p. 108–117). Springer Singapore. https://doi.org/10.1007/978-981-15-7205-0_10

32 Assegie, T. A. An optimized K-Nearest Neighbor based breast cancer detection. *J. Robotics Control (JRC)*, 2021, 2(3). https://doi.org/10.18196/jrc.2363

33 Bhattacherjee, A.; Roy, S.; Paul, S.; Roy, P.; Kausar, N.; Dey, N. (2020). Classification Approach for Breast Cancer Detection Using Back Propagation Neural Network: A Study. In Deep Learning and Neural Networks (p. 1410–1421). IGI Global. https://doi.org/10.4018/978-1-7998-0414-7.ch079

34 Alshayeji, M. H.; Ellethy, H.; Abed, S.; Gupta, R. Computer-aided detection of breast cancer on the Wisconsin dataset: An artificial neural networks approach. *Biomed. Signal Process. Control*, 2022, 71, 103141. https://doi.org/10.1016/j.bspc.2021.103141

35 Islam, S.; Hoque, N.; Nasrin, N.; Hossain, M.; Rizwan, F.; Biswas, K.; Asaduzzaman, M.; Rahman, S.; Hoskin, D. W.; Sultana, S.; Lehmann, C. Iron Overload and Breast Cancer: Iron Chelation as a Potential Therapeutic Approach. *Life*, 2022, 12(7), 963. https://doi.org/10.3390/life12070963

36 Ghosh, R.; Pfeiffer, R. M.; Roberts, S.; Gierach, G. L.; Dallal, C. M. (2024). Adjuvant endocrine therapy and risk of contralateral breast cancer: a systematic review and meta-analysis of observational studies. *Cancer Causes & Control.* https://doi.org/10.1007/s10552-024-01900-5

37 Kandhasamy, J. P.; Balamurali, S. Performance Analysis of Classifier Models to Predict Diabetes Mellitus. *Procedia Computer Science*, 2015, 47, 45–51. https://doi.org/10.1016/j.procs.2015.03.182

38 Yahyaoui, A.; Jamil, A.; Rasheed, J.; Yesiltepe, M. (2019). A Decision Support System for Diabetes Prediction Using Machine Learning and Deep Learning Techniques. 2019 1st International Informatics and Software Engineering Conference (UBMYK), 1–4. https://doi.org/10.1109/ubmyk48245.2019.8965556

39 Naz, H.; Ahuja, S. Deep learning approach for diabetes prediction using PIMA Indian dataset. *J. Diabetes Metab. Disord.*, 2020, 19(1), 391–403. https://doi.org/10.1007/s40200-020-00520-5

40 Ashiquzzaman, A.; Tushar, A. K.; Islam, Md. R.; Shon, D.; Im, K.; Park, J.-H.; Lim, D.-S.; Kim, J. (2017). Reduction of Overfitting in Diabetes Prediction Using Deep Learning Neural Network. In IT Convergence and Security 2017 (p. 35–43). Springer Singapore. https://doi.org/10.1007/978-981-10-6451-7_5

41 Alhassan, Z.; McGough, A. S.; Alshammari, R.; Daghstani, T.; Budgen, D.; Al Moubayed, N. (2018). Type-2 Diabetes Mellitus Diagnosis from Time Series Clinical Data Using Deep Learning Models. In Artificial Neural Networks and Machine Learning – ICANN 2018 (p. 46–478). Springer International Publishing. https://doi.org/10.1007/978-3-030-01424-7_46

42 Sriram, A.; Ward, H. E.; Hassan, A.; Iyer, S.; Foote, K. D.; Rodriguez, R. L.; McFarland, N. R.; Okun, M. S. Valproate as a treatment for dopamine dysregulation syndrome (DDS) in Parkinson's disease. *J. Neurol.*, 2012, 260(2), 521–527. https://doi.org/10.1007/s00415-012-6669-1

43 Balabandian, M.; Salahi, S.; Mahmoudvand, B.; Esmaeilzadeh, M.; Hashemi, S. M.; Nabizadeh, F. Serum uric acid and Parkinson's disease: A systematic review and meta-analysis. *Neurol Clin Neurosci*, 2023, 11(6), 299–309. Portico. https://doi.org/10.1111/ncn3.12761

44 Grover, S.; Lill, C. M.; Kasten, M.; Klein, C.; Del Greco M; König, I. R. Risky behaviors and Parkinson disease: A mendelian randomization study. *Neurology*, 2019, 93(15). https://doi.org/10.1212/wnl.0000000000008245

45 Warjurkar, S.; Ridhorkar, S. (2021). A Study on Brain Tumor and Parkinson's Disease Diagnosis and Detection using Deep Learning. *Proceedings of the 3rd International Conference on Integrated Intelligent Computing Communication & Security (ICIIC* 2021). https://doi.org/10.2991/ahis.k.210913.044

46 Shi, Y.; Wang, G.; Cai, X.; Deng, J.; Zheng, L.; Zhu, H.; Zheng, M.; Yang, B.; Chen, Z. An overview of COVID-19. *J. Zhejiang Univ-Sci. B.*, 2020, 21(5), 343–360. https://doi.org/10.1631/jzus.b2000083

47 Ardakani, A. A.; Kanafi, A. R.; Acharya, U. R.; Khadem, N.; Mohammadi, A. Application of deep learning technique to manage COVID-19 in routine clinical practice using CT images: Results of 10 convolutional neural networks. *Comput Biol Med.*, 2020, 121, 103795. https://doi.org/10.1016/j.compbiomed.2020.103795

48 Shi, Y.; Wang, G.; Cai, X.; Deng, J.; Zheng, L.; Zhu, H.; Zheng, M.; Yang, B.; Chen, Z. An overview of COVID-19. *J. Zhejiang Univ.-Sci. B.*, 2020, 21(5), 343–360. https://doi.org/10.1631/jzus.b2000083

49 Xu, Z.; Li, S.; Tian, S.; Li, H.; Kong, L. Full spectrum of COVID-19 severity still being depicted. *Lancet,* 2020, 395(10228), 947–948. https://doi.org/10.1016/s0140-6736(20)30308-1

50 Bou Hamdan, M.; Singh, S.; Polavarapu, M.; Jordan, T. R.; Melhem, N. M. COVID-19 vaccine hesitancy among university students in Lebanon. *Epidemiology and Infection*, 2021, 149. https://doi.org/10.1017/s0950268821002314

51 Narin, A.; Kaya, C.; Pamuk, Z. Automatic detection of coronavirus disease (COVID-19) using X-ray images and deep convolutional neural networks. *Pattern Anal. Appl.*, 2021, 24(3), 1207–1220. https://doi.org/10.1007/s10044-021-00984-y

52 Brunese, L.; Martinelli, F.; Mercaldo, F.; Santone, A. Machine learning for coronavirus covid-19 detection from chest x-rays. *Procedia Computer Science*, 2020, 176, 2212–2221. https://doi.org/10.1016/j.procs.2020.09.258

53 Neelaveni, J.; Devasana, M. S. G. Alzheimer Disease Prediction using Machine Learning Algorithms. 2020 6th International Conference on Advanced Computing and Communication Systems (ICACCS). https://doi.org/10.1109/icaccs48705.2020.9074248

54 Collij, L. E.; Heeman, F.; Kuijer, J. P. A.; Ossenkoppele, R.; Benedictus, M. R.; Möller, C.; Verfaillie, S. C. J.; Sanz-Arigita, E. J.; van Berckel, B. N. M.; van der Flier, W. M.; Scheltens, P.; Barkhof, F.; Wink, A. M. Application of Machine Learning to Arterial Spin Labeling in Mild Cognitive Impairment and Alzheimer Disease. *Radiology*, 2016, 281(3), 865–875. https://doi.org/10.1148/radiol.2016152703

55 Ahmed, T. F.; Ahmed, A.; Imtiaz, F. History in perspective: How Alzheimer's Disease came to be where it is? *Brain Research*, 2021, 1758, 147342. https://doi.org/10.1016/j.brainres.2021.147342

56 Nawaz, A.; Anwar, S. M.; Liaqat, R.; Iqbal, J.; Bagci, U.; Majid, M. Deep Convolutional Neural Network based Classification of Alzheimer's Disease using MRI Data. 2020 IEEE 23rd International Multitopic Conference (INMIC), 1–6. https://doi.org/10.1109/inmic50486.2020.9318172

57 Haft-Javaherian, M.; Fang, L.; Muse, V.; Schaffer, C. B.; Nishimura, N.; Sabuncu, M. R. Deep convolutional neural networks for segmenting 3D in vivo multiphoton images of vasculature in Alzheimer disease mouse models. PLOS ONE, 2019, 14(3), e0213539. https://doi.org/10.1371/journal.pone.0213539

58 Mao, L.; Jin, H.; Wang, M.; Hu, Y.; Chen, S.; He, Q.; Chang, J.; Hong, C.; Zhou, Y.; Wang, D.; Miao, X.; Li, Y.; Hu, B. Neurologic Manifestations of Hospitalized Patients With Coronavirus Disease 2019 in Wuhan, China. *JAMA Neurology*, 2020, 77(6), 683. https://doi.org/10.1001/jamaneurol.2020.1127

59 Nosseir, A.; Shawky, M. A. Automatic Classifier for Skin Disease Using k-NN and SVM. *Proceedings of the 2019 8th International Conference on Software and Information Engineering*, 259–262. https://doi.org/10.1145/3328833.3328862

60 Dhama, K.; Khan, S.; Tiwari, R.; Sircar, S.; Bhat, S.; Malik, Y. S.; Singh, K. P.; Chaicumpa, W.; Bonilla-Aldana, D. K.; Rodriguez-Morales, A. J. Coronavirus Disease 2019–COVID-19. *Clin. Microbiol. Rev.*, 2020, 33(4). https://doi.org/10.1128/cmr.00028-20

61 Amin, J.; Sharif, M.; Yasmin, M.; Fernandes, S. L. Big data analysis for brain tumor detection: Deep convolutional neural networks. *Future Gener. Comput. Syst.*, 2018, 87, 290–297. https://doi.org/10.1016/j.future.2018.04.065

62 Vidushi, Akash Rajak, Ajay Kumar Shrivastava. Diagnosis of Alzheimer Disease using *Machine Learning* Approaches. *Int. J. Adv. Sci. Technol.*, 2020, 29(4), 7062. Retrieved from https://sersc.org/journals/index.php/IJAST/article/view/28115

3

Natural Language Processing (NLP) in Disease Detection – A Discussion of How NLP Techniques Can Be Used to Analyze and Classify Medical Text Data for Disease Diagnosis

Vinod Kumar[1], *Mohammed Ismail Iqbal*[2], *and Rachna Rathore*[3]

[1] *Electronics and Communication Engineering, HRIT University, Ghaziabad, Uttar Pradesh, India*
[2] *Petroleum Engineering Department, University of Technology and Applied Sciences, Nizwa, Oman*
[3] *Department of Mathematics, Jiwaji University, Gwalior, Madhya Pradesh, India*

Introduction

For decades, the healthcare scene has depended on organized information for illness conclusion. Clinical codes and demonstrative tests, whereas essential, frequently miss the wealthy embroidered artwork woven inside a patient's treatment history. This is often where natural language processing (NLP) steps in, developing as a game-changer within the domain of malady location. By digging into the story control of treatment substance data, NLP opens a treasure trove of encounters as of now secured up interior specialist notes, discharge rundowns, and in fact social media language [1].

This burgeoning field ensures a worldview move in how we approach ailment revelation. Imagine a future where NLP calculations can channel through mountains of helpful substance, recognizing subtle phonetic prompts that show at an essential ailment. A pro depicting a patient's hack as "decided and hacking" might trigger an NLP system to accost potential signs of early-stage COPD, inciting help examination. Essentially, social media analysis using NLP could reveal clusters of clients declaring flu-like side impacts, enabling real-time response to disease outbreaks [2].

The potential advancements within NLP for disease disclosure are as energizing as they are far-reaching. One groundbreaking area is the enhancement of sentiment analysis tools. By understanding the enthusiastic proposals of a patient's

AI in Disease Detection: Advancements and Applications, First Edition.
Edited by Rajesh Singh, Anita Gehlot, Navjot Rathour, and Shaik Vaseem Akram.

Published 2025 by John Wiley & Sons, Inc.

delineation of their signs, NLP can assemble noteworthy clues patient's description of their symptoms. During the event, the words used were "pitiful" or "terrible" conjoined with pain, which may go further to describe a larger spiritual component of the patient's condition [3].

Another energizing field lies inside the space of personalized pharmaceuticals. NLP calculations can be arranged to investigate a patient's therapeutic history, recognizing specific chance factors and fitting preventative measures suitably. This personalized approach locks in pros to gotten to be proactive watchmen of prosperity, conceivably catching ailments at their most prompt stages.

The integration of NLP with advanced machine learning (ML) techniques is an area ripe for further exploration. By learning from extensive datasets of medical content and patient outcomes, NLP systems can continually improve their ability to recognize patterns and predict disease progression. This permits specialists to intervene, possibly driving to superior treatment results and moving forward persistently to improve quality of life.

Of course, NLP in disease detection isn't without its challenges. The sheer volume and inconstancy of therapeutic content information require strong calculations that can explore the subtleties of human language. Furthermore, moral considerations regarding information protection and algorithmic inclination must be carefully tended to [4].

In any case, the potential future rewards exceed the challenges. As NLP advances, its effect on disease detection is sure to be significant. By opening the account control of therapeutic content data, we can move toward a future of more comprehensive analysis, earlier interventions, and ultimately, a healthier population [5].

Objectives

The vast amount of information stored in medical text data has long been an underutilized source of valuable insights. Natural language processing provides powerful tools to unlock this information, ushering in a new era of disease detection through the following seven meticulously crafted objectives:

Early Infection Location through Phonetic Fingerprints

- **Objective:** Create NLP calculations that recognize unpretentious etymological designs in treatment content, acting as early caution signs for potential diseases.

- **Development:** Prepare NLP models on a gigantic dataset of treatment content combined with affirmed analyze. These models will learn to recognize disease-specific "etymological fingerprints," possibly including the frequency of specific terms, unusual word choices, or even the emotional tone used to describe symptoms. For example, an algorithm might recognize a cluster of words like "weakness," "night sweats," and "unexplained weight misfortune" as a potential marker of early-stage lymphoma [6].

Estimation Examination for All-Encompassing Healthcare

- **Objective:** Use NLP to analyze the enthusiastic undercurrents inside a patient's portrayal of side effects, advertising a more all-encompassing view of their well-being.
- **Development:** Create progressed opinion investigation apparatuses that cannot identify fundamental feelings like anxiety or depression but can recognize nuanced enthusiastic states like fear, misery, or uneasiness. This more deep understanding can help healthcare experts reveal fundamental mental components that may be affecting the patient's condition. Envision an NLP framework that highlights a patient's use of words like "ghastly" or "panicked" when portraying pain, encouraging a specialist to investigate potential uneasiness or sadness as adjacent issues to the physical side effects [7].

Social Media Reconnaissance for Disease Outbreaks

- **Objective:** Utilize NLP to analyze social media discussions and online gatherings, empowering real-time following of disease outbreaks based on user-generated substance.
- **Development:** Create a geo-localized NLP framework that can filter social media stages for clusters of users reporting specific symptoms within a defined geographical area. By analyzing the language utilized (e.g., "fever," "chills," "muscle aches"), this framework can distinguish potential disease outbreaks much quicker than conventional strategies, permitting faster intervention and public healthcare outcomes [8].

Custom-Fitted Medication through Personalized Content Investigation

- **Objective:** NLP algorithms that analyze a patient's whole treatment plan, recognizing person-chance variables and fitting preventative measures in like manner.

- **Development:** Build NLP calculations that cannot distinguish analyzed conditions but can extricate data around a patient's way of life propensities, family history, and natural exposures archived in their therapeutic content information. This comprehensive analysis permits the creation of personalized chance profiles and focuses on preventative procedures. For example, a calculation might record that a patient smokes cigarettes and thus tailor a smoking-cessation program as a preventative measure for lung cancer [9].

Precise Medication with Clinical Trial Content Mining

- **Objective:** Execute NLP to extricate profitable experiences from clinical trial information composed in story shape, quickening the advancement of focused on treatments.
- **Development:** Create NLP frameworks that can analyze the printed components of clinical trial reports, extricating data on understanding choice criteria, treatment reaction rates, and antagonistic side impacts. By automating this process, analysts can access the tremendous information caught inside clinical trial content information, driving to quicker recognizable proof of promising modern treatments and personalized treatment plans for particular persistent populaces [10].

Breaking Down Language Boundaries for Worldwide Wellbeing

- **Objective:** Utilize multilingual NLP capabilities to bridge the language divide in healthcare, growing to exact disease detection over diverse societies and topographical districts.
- **Development:** Plan NLP models that can interpret and analyze treatment content information in different languages with tall exactness. This allows healthcare professionals to use valuable data from medical records written in languages they do not understand, promoting a more comprehensive and equitable approach to disease detection in a globalized world.

Human-Machine Collaboration for Making Strides

- **Objective:** Cultivate a collaborative environment where NLP frameworks expand human skill to make strides symptomatic exactness and productivity.
- **Development:** Create NLP devices that can analyze treatment content information in real-time, highlighting potential diagnoses, relevant medical literature, and key risk factors for the doctor's consideration. This human-machine collaboration enables specialists with extra information and insights to create more educated choices amid the symptomatic prepare [11].

Advantages and Limitations of Natural Language Processing in Disease Detection

Advantages of NLP in Disease Detection

1) **Upgraded information investigation:** NLP permits the effective extraction and investigation of tremendous sums of therapeutic content information, including electronic healthcare records (EHRs), clinical notes, and research papers. This capability empowers healthcare experts to get to important insights and designs that can help in infection conclusion. By analyzing understanding histories, indications, and treatment results, NLP can aid in distinguishing relationships and patterns that will not be clear through manual audit.
2) **Improved symptomatic exactness:** NLP calculations can decipher and prepare complex treatment language, deciphering unstructured content into organized information. This change permits for more precise and comprehensive symptomatic forms. For example, NLPs can distinguish key side effects and important therapeutic history from understanding records, supporting within the determination of conditions such as uncommon illnesses or atypical introductions of common sicknesses. The capacity to analyze point-by-point patient data upgrades the precision and unwavering quality of analyze [12].
3) **Streamlined clinical workflows:** By automating the extraction and classification of treatment data, NLP can reduce the regulatory burden on healthcare experts. NLP-driven devices can rapidly sort through expansive volumes of clinical records, extricating related data and summarizing learning data. This mechanization streamlines workflows, permitting specialists and medical attendants to center more on persistent care instead of information passage and documentation.
4) **Real-time decision-making:** NLP can give real-time decision-making back by ceaselessly analyzing approaching patient information and alarming healthcare suppliers to potential issues. For illustration, NLP algorithms can screen EHRs for early signs of complications or infection progression, prompting timely interventions. This proactive approach can improve patient outcomes by enabling quicker responses to emerging health concerns [13].
5) **Personalized pharmaceutical:** NLP encourages personalized drug treatments by empowering the detailed investigation of private patient data. By looking at particular side effects, hereditary data, and past medicines, NLP can help tailor conclusion and treatment plans to each patient's individual needs. This personalized approach enhances the effectiveness of medical interventions and improves patient satisfaction [14].

Limitations of NLP in Disease Detection

1) **Data quality and standardization:** NLP's ampleness escalation depends on the quality and consistency of the input data. Treatment plan data can be clashing, divided, or composed in nonstandardized bunches, posing challenges for NLP algorithms. Assortments in stating, truncations, and lingo utilized by differing healthcare providers can lead to botches in data interpretation and examination.
2) **Complexity of therapeutic lingo:** Treatment language is very specialized and complex, requiring NLP calculations to have progressed to taking care of capabilities. The nuances of helpful lingo, checking context-specific suggestions and language, can be troublesome for NLP systems to accurately decipher. This complexity can lead to confusing signals or errors in data extraction and classification [15].
3) **Security and security concerns:** The utilize of NLP in healthcare involves handling sensitive patient information, raising concerns about data security and privacy. Ensuring compliance with rules such as Health Insurance Portability and Accountability Act (HIPAA) is critical to securing understanding protection. Solid security measures must be in place to prevent unauthorized data breaches.
4) **Ethical and inclination issues:** NLP algorithms may unintentionally perpetuate biases present in the training data. If the data used to train these models includes biases related to race, gender, or socioeconomic status, these biases can influence the algorithm's outputs. Addressing these ethical concerns requires careful data selection and preprocessing to ensure fairness and equity in disease detection outcomes.
5) **Integration with existing frameworks:** Coordinating NLP innovations into existing healthcare foundation can be challenging [16]. Compatibility issues with current EHR frameworks, the requirement for specialized preparation for healthcare staff, and resistance to alterations are common deterrents. Effective usage requires significant investments in technology upgrades, training programs, and customized management procedures.

NLP offers significant points of interest in infection location, counting upgraded information examination, progressed symptomatic exactness, streamlined workflows, real-time choice bolster, and personalized medication. In any case, the innovation too faces critical restrictions, such as data quality issues, complexity of therapeutic language, security concerns, moral contemplations, and integration challenges. Tending to these restrictions is fundamental to completely tackling the potential of NLP in changing healthcare and making strides in disease detection and determination. As NLP innovation proceeds to advance, progressing endeavors to move forward information quality, create advanced language programming capabilities, and ensure ethical practices will be pivotal in realizing its full potential in healthcare [17].

Literature Review

NLP is quickly changing the scene of disease detection. By diving into the wealthy embroidered artwork of treatment content information, NLP opens a treasure trove of experiences already covered up inside doctor notes, release outlines, and indeed social media discussions. Table 3.1 lists results of a brief review of technological progress in language models; this section investigates the most recent studies, highlighting key areas where NLP is cultivating groundbreaking developments.

From Content to Determination: Revealing Etymological Fingerprints

One pivotal region of development lies in creating NLP calculations that can distinguish unpretentious etymological designs inside treatment content information [18]. These designs, associated to etymological fingerprints, can serve as early caution signs for potential diseases. Envision an NLP framework prepared on a gigantic dataset of treatment records connected to affirmed analysis. By learning to recognize disease-specific designs in language utilize, such as the recurrence of particular terms, abnormal word choices, or indeed the passionate tone utilized to portray indications, this framework may identify patients who are at greater risk for a specific disease. This permits prior intervention and possibly better treatment outcomes.

Past Watchwords: Capturing the Subtlety of Free-Text Information

Extricating significant insights from free-text clinical notes presents an interesting challenge. Not at all like organized information with predefined codes, free-text information is brimming with equivocalness and changeability. In any case, studies such as [19] illustrate the potential of NLP to overcome this jump. By utilizing advanced techniques to capture and standardize data from free-text notes, NLP can transform this unstructured information into a valuable asset for disease detection. This standardization permits more proficient investigation and the extraction of essential points of interest that might otherwise be missed.

Control of Expansive Language Models: A New Frontier

The integration of large language models (LLMs) with NLP opens paths to energizing new possibilities in disease detection [20]. LLMs are a sort of manufactured

Table 3.1 Deeper analysis of language model technologies.

Innovation area	Description	Potential benefits	Challenges
Linguistic fingerprints	Develop NLP algorithms to identify disease-specific patterns in language used within medical text data.	Early detection of potential illnesses based on subtle linguistic cues.	Requires large datasets of medical text linked to confirmed diagnoses.
Capturing nuance of free-text data	Utilize NLP to standardize information from free-text clinical notes, transforming unstructured data into a valuable resource.	Improved analysis and extraction of critical details from free-text medical records.	Requires advanced NLP techniques to handle ambiguity and variability in free-text data.
Integration of large language models (LLMs)	Leverage LLMs within NLP systems to gain a deeper understanding of medical language and identify disease-related information.	More accurate identification of disease signals within complex or nuanced medical text data.	Requires significant computational resources and expertise to train and maintain LLMs.
Multilingual NLP capabilities	Develop NLP models that can translate and analyze medical text data in multiple languages with high accuracy.	Bridges the language gap in healthcare, ensuring information accessibility for global disease detection efforts.	Requires vast amounts of multilingual medical text data for training and maintaining accurate translation models.
Human-machine collaboration	Foster a collaborative environment where NLP tools assist healthcare professionals by highlighting potential diagnoses and relevant information.	Empowers clinicians with broader insights for informed decision-making, leading to more accurate diagnoses and improved patient care.	Requires careful design of NLP interfaces to ensure effective communication and trust between humans and machines.

insights prepared on enormous sums of content information, empowering them to memorize complex relationships between words and ideas. By consolidating LLMs into NLP frameworks, analysts can create models with a deeper understanding of the therapeutic language. This permits more precise recognizable proof of disease-related data inside content information when it's stated in nuanced or flighty ways.

Breaking Down Language Obstructions for Worldwide

The control of NLP amplifies past the boundaries of a single language. Studies are underway to create multilingual NLP capabilities that can bridge the language crevice in healthcare [21]. This is especially critical for worldwide wellbeing activities, where determining exact malady location can be hampered by language obstructions. By making NLP models that can interpret and analyze treatment content information in different languages with tall accuracy, researchers can guarantee that profitable data isn't misplaced due to language contrasts. This cultivates a more comprehensive and impartial approach to malady discovery on a worldwide scale.

Toward a Collaborative Future: Human-Machine Association

The extreme objective of NLP in infection location isn't to supplant human ability but to increase it. Investigations like [22] emphasize the significance of cultivating a collaborative environment where NLP frameworks act as associates to healthcare experts. By analyzing clinical content data in real time, NLP tools can highlight potential analysis, relevant medical literature, and key risk factors for the doctor's consideration. This provides clinicians with greater insights to guide their demonstrative choices, eventually driving to more precise analysis and better understanding of healthcare needs.

These five regions areas offer a fair view of the transformative potential of NLP in disease discovery. As NLP inquire about continues to evolve, we are able anticipate indeed more groundbreaking advancements that will revolutionize the way we identify and oversee illnesses. By tackling language learning, we will move to incorporate more predictive analytics, more successful medications and eventually, a more healthy population worldwide.

Patient-reported outcomes (PROs) offer invaluable insights into a patient's health and wellbeing beyond traditional clinical measures. Studies like [23] explores the utilize of NLP to extricate detailed findings from EHRs. By utilizing progressed NLP procedures, such as transformer-based structures, analysts can create models that can precisely recognize and categorize patient-reported encounters from their therapeutic records. This encourages healthcare experts to gain a more all-encompassing understanding of their patients' condition and tailor treatment plans in like manner.

Logical AI

Building belief in NLP-based phenotyping is vital. NLP calculations are progressively complex, so it is essential to guarantee their straightforwardness and interpretability. A study [24] emphasizes the significance of explainable AI (XAI) for NLP-based phenotyping in healthcare. XAI strategies help in shedding light on the decision-making forms of NLP models, permitting healthcare experts to describe how these models arrived at their conclusions. This straightforwardness cultivates buy-in in NLP-based apparatuses and clears the way for their more extensive selection inside clinical settings.

Past Content: Multimodal Infection Discovery with NLP and Imaging Information

The scope of disease detection has expanded beyond solely text-based data. Researchers are exploring multimodal approaches that integrate natural language processing (NLP) with medical imaging data. By analyzing both textual information from patient medical records and visual data from imaging (such as X-rays or MRIs), NLP models can provide a more comprehensive understanding of a patient's condition. This multimodal approach shows potential to enhance the accuracy of disease detection, particularly for complex conditions with subtle presentations [25].

Methodology

The potential of NLP in infection location pivots on a strong methodological system. This area dives into the perplexing steps included in saddling the control of language investigation for revealing hidden designs and insights inside therapeutic content information. Here, we investigate the center techniques beside energizing modern advancements that are pushing the boundaries of this field.

Information Procurement and Preprocessing: Building the Establishment

The foundation of any NLP extend may be a high-quality dataset. For illness location, this ordinarily includes therapeutic content information from different sources, counting EHRs, clinical trial reports, and indeed social media discussions. In any case, crude treatment content information is frequently burdened with irregularities and "noise." A good first step includes establishing information preprocessing procedures like normalization, de-identification, and tokenization. Normalization guarantees consistency in terms of spelling and truncations. De-identification shields understanding protection by evacuating any personally identifiable information (PII) from the information. At long last, tokenization breaks down the content information into smaller units (tokens) like words or expressions, planning it for assist investigation.

Content Explanation: Labeling the Story

To train NLP models to distinguish disease-related data, annotated examples are used. This crucial step includes text annotation, where human experts manually label specific elements within the text data. This can include identifying entities such as medications, diagnoses, or symptoms. Also, aspect-based sentiment analysis includes labeling the emotional tone related to specific concepts within the content. This wealth of comment information lays the groundwork for NLP models, permitting them to learn and recognize designs in future concealed information.

Feature Designing: Extricating Important Signals

Not all words inside treatment content information are similarly imperative for disease detection. It includes designing methods that can distinguish and extricate the foremost important highlights from the content information. This will include methods like *n*-grams (groupings of *n* words), part-of-speech labeling (recognizing the syntactic work of words), or use of medical terminology dictionaries. One inventive approach includes leveraging pretrained language models (PLMs) to create relevant word embeddings. These embeddings capture the semantic meaning of words in the context of therapeutic content, giving a wealthier highlight set for NLP models to memorize from.

Show Determination and Preparing: Choosing the Right Tool for the Work

The selection of an NLP model depends on the specific disease detection task at hand. Common choices include supervised learning algorithms like support vector machines (SVMs) or deep learning architectures such as recurrent neural networks (RNNs) and convolutional neural networks (CNNs). Each model type offers unique advantages; for instance, RNNs are effective in processing sequential data, while CNNs excel at extracting spatial features, making them valuable in multimodal and complex data analysis contexts. A recent development includes the utilization of transformers, a capable deep learning engineering, which has appeared a credible guarantee for errands like named substance acknowledgment and content classification in the space of medical text examination. The selected model is then trained on the preprocessed and annotated data, enabling it to learn complex relationships between linguistic features and disease-related data.

Demonstrate Assessment and Refinement: Guaranteeing Exactness and Belief

Assessing the execution of an NLP show for disease detection is essential. Different measurements are utilized, such as exactness, accuracy, review, and F1 score, to survey how well the demonstration recognizes significant data inside the test information. Strategies like XAI can be utilized to get at the decision-making forms of the model, cultivating trust and straightforwardness. Moreover, dynamic learning approaches can be utilized to ceaselessly progress the model's execution by deliberately selecting the foremost enlightening information focuses for assist explanation and retraining [26].

Integration and Arrangement: Putting NLP to Work

Finally, for NLP models to have a real-world effect on disease detection, they have to be coordinated into existing healthcare workflows. This might include creating user-friendly interfaces for clinicians to associate with the NLP framework. Moreover, cautious thought must be given to information security and protection concerns when conveying NLP models in real-world healthcare settings.

By following this comprehensive technique and grasping cutting-edge developments, analysts and healthcare experts can access the full potential of NLP for infection discovery, as mentioned in Figure 3.1. This paves the way for a future where language investigation will play a critical role in early detection, leading to more successful mediation and improved understanding.

Results and Analysis

As Figure 3.2 shows, emergent NLP for disease detection holds immense potential to revolutionize healthcare. In the future, the hope is that this can be transformed into practice by analyzing current achievements and exploring the most promising innovations.

Current Achievements: A Glimpse into the Possible

Studies show promising outcomes in a couple of key areas. Case stories of triumph include the identification of linguistic fingerprinting for specific illnesses. Research thinks about have detailed that NLP counts can learn to recognize malady-explicit plans in tongue used inside treatment substance data. For example, an NLP system might recognize a cluster of words like "exhaustion," "night sweats," and "unexplained weight mishap" as a potential indication of early-stage lymphoma.

Another example of a successful run would be the social media perception of sickness events: by reading social media and online social conversations, NLP systems should be able to pick up clusters of consumers describing flu-like adverse effects within a geographically well-defined area. This allows real-time tracking of potential outbreaks, empowering public health specialists to respond more quickly.

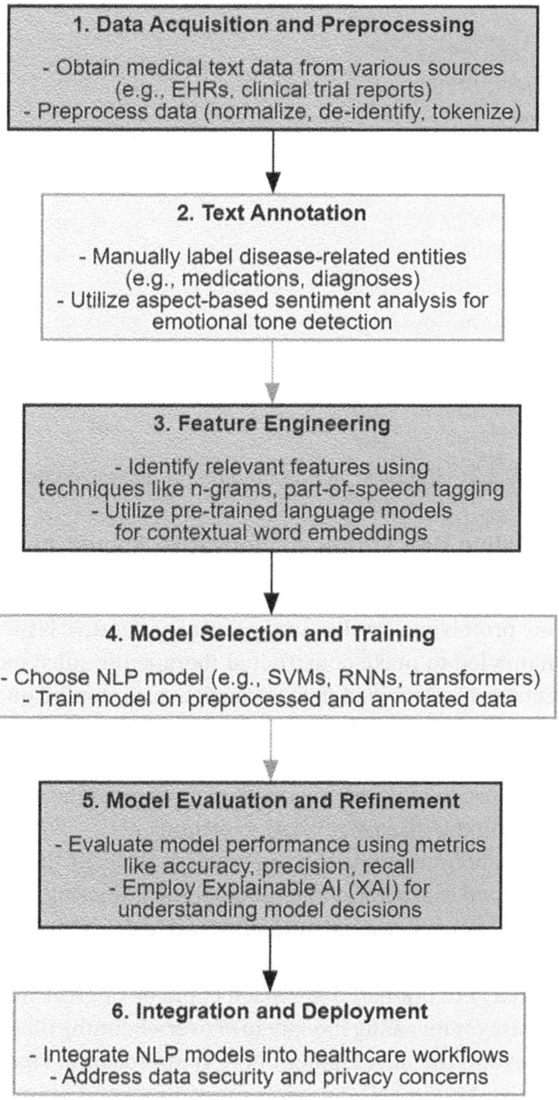

Figure 3.1 Architectural framework.

Additionally, studies have shown progress in utilizing NLP to analyze the enthusiastic undercurrents interior a patient's portrayal of their side impacts. This estimation examination can permit vital insights into a patient's overall health. For example, an NLP system might recognize a patient's use of words like "unpleasant" or "startled" when describing pain, prompting a healthcare professional to look for evidence of anxiety or depression alongside the physical symptoms.

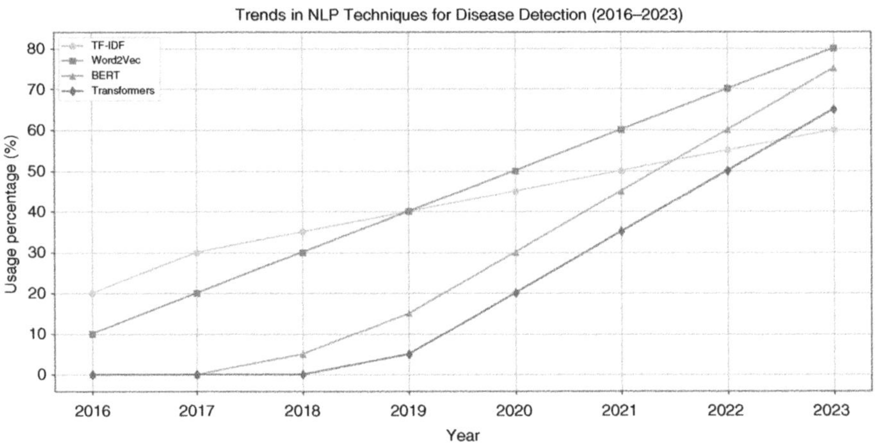

Figure 3.2 Trends in NLP techniques for disease detection.

Unveiling New Frontiers: Innovative Approaches for the Future

These achievements are impressive, but there is plenty of room for improvement. One promising area lies in the use of generative NLP models. These models can be channeled to make constructed therapeutic substance data that easily mirror the real world. Designed data, in such a case, can be quite valuable in increasing the volume of existing datasets – something that can solve the particular limitation of the poor predictive data in the treatment space. Finally, generative models can be put to use in making practical test cases, evaluating the quality of the NLP systems in doing the disease revelation errands.

Yet another innovative approach is through the integration of NLP along with organized examination methodologies. Exploring the relations between substances and concepts in therapeutic substance data, NLP models are able to reveal the concealed connections and patterns that other common models would not be able to do. Such a network-based approach could be of great value in identifying co-occurring diseases or revealing the spread of overwhelming illnesses on social media platforms.

Beyond the development of XAI approaches, customizing NLP in healthcare is crucial. Making NLP models more direct and interpretable may make them more acceptable to healthcare professionals and patients through XAI. Directness is key in ensuring that NLP models are applied ethically and effectively toward disease diagnosis and treatment.

Challenges and Considerations: Navigating the Road Ahead

While there is verifiable potential for NLP in diagnosis, there also exist challenges. One significant challenge, however, concerns information insurance and security:

it is about de-identification procedures fundamental for ensuring patient confidentiality while simultaneously allowing medical content to be used for research purposes.

Another challenge lies in tending to the natural biases that can exist inside medical data. NLP models prepared on one-sided information can sustain these bias, possibly driving to wrong or unjustifiable results. Procedures for detecting and mitigating bias inside NLP models are pivotal for guaranteeing impartial and moral applications in infection location.

Finally, the fruitful integration of NLP into existing healthcare workflows is vital. User-friendly interfacing and clear communication procedures are essential to guarantee that clinicians can viably use NLP devices for improved infection discovery and understanding care.

Case Study of NLP in Disease Detection

NLP has significantly impacted medical informatics through the use of computers in the analysis and classification of medical text data. Retrieving data from EHRs and clinical notes, among other unstructured medical documents, is necessary when applying NLP techniques for disease detection. This chapter focuses on previous case studies where the application of NLP techniques has successfully enhanced disease diagnosis.

Case Study 3.1 Early Detection of Heart Disease

Background: A top-ranked medical institution performed a study that used NLP to improve the early detection of heart disease. The study's objective was to detect patients at a high risk of heart disease using clinical notes and EHRs.

Methods: The authors have developed an NLP algorithm to extract the requisite information in unstructured text – patient history, symptoms, medications, and laboratory results – Apis. The latter was trained with a massive dataset of annotated medical records, allowing it to recognize key indicators of heart disease.

Results: The accuracies in identifying high-risk patients were much higher using the NLP system compared to traditional methods. The earlier a patient at risk is flagged for further assessment in the system, the sooner intervention can be performed to improve the patient's health status. Through this research, it was demonstrated that NLP can effectively mine large volumes of medical text and provide actionable insights into heart disease detection.

Case Study 3.2 Identifying Diabetes Complications

Context: A healthcare provider sought to improve monitoring of diabetes complications using NLP. The program analyzes clinical notes to identify patients who are likely to experience complications such as neuropathy, retinopathy, or nephropathy.

Methods: The authors developed an NLP system to analyze clinical notes to extract analyzed information related to diabetes management, symptoms, and laboratory results. This algorithm uses a combination of machine learning and rule-based techniques to classify them and predict the likelihood of problems.

Results: This allows early identification of potential complications in diabetic patients through the implementation of NLP. The system had high sensitivity and specificity to allow for the identification of such patients who required closer supervision, monitoring, and preventive care. That helped lessen the predicaments of serious complications, which generally improved the quality of care for diabetic patients.

Case Study 3.3 Screening for Mental Health Disorders

Background: An outpatient mental health clinic was using NLP to improve mental health disorder screening. A test case generation plan was developed for the coverage of 91.45% interactions between patients and clinical notes, trying to pick up on telltale signs of depression, anxiety, and other mental problems.

Methods: The NLP system was trained on a corpus containing clinical notes and patient interviews from which it learned lexical patterns of critical words for mental health disorders. Sentiment analysis and NLP set the emotional tone and contextual setting for the text.

Results: The NLP tool correctly identified the patients with a hidden mental health condition to an excellent degree, allowing for timely referrals to mental health professionals. It provided valuable insights into the emotional state of the patient and the problem areas. Another case study or example that characterizes an illustration of how NLP can improve mental health screening and hasten early intervention has been presented in this paper.

Case Study 3.4 Monitoring Infectious Disease Outbreaks
Background: Public health authorities capitalized on the NLP tools in an infectious disease outbreak for tracking the course and impact of a disease. In this paper, social media posts, news articles, and clinical reports will be utilized for monitoring symptoms and enabling the early identification of emerging hotspots. **Methods:** The NLP system applied advanced text mining techniques on a massive level of unstructured data. Information extracted concerning symptoms, location, and demographic variables of the patients provides real-time insights into how far this outbreak has progressed. **Results:** The monitoring system with NLP contributed to the identification of new clusters of infection and the tracking of the disease. It is such timely analysis that would allow public health officials to enforce targeted interventions and resource allocation. This case study illustrated how NLP efficiently helped improve situational awareness and response in infectious disease outbreaks.

These case studies herald the potentially powerful and transformative role of NLP in disease detection and diagnosis. As background information, it is expected that NLP systems automated analysis of medical text data could turn up important insights, improve diagnostic accuracy, and facilitate early interventions in disease treatment processes. Challenges to its successful implementation relate to data quality, standardization, and ethical considerations. The continual updates of NLP will extend further into healthcare applications and realize more efficient and accurate methods for the detection of diseases.

Conclusions and Future Scope

Research in NLP-based disease detection has opened promising avenues in this landscape. We have seen successful identification of linguistic fingerprints for specific diseases. Now, it is possible to identify them at an earlier stage through minor cues in the language of medical text data. Impressive equally is the fact that social media conversations can be used to track disease outbreaks in real-time, opening up enormous possibilities in public health initiatives using NLP. Further, it has developed sentiment analysis that will help health experts understand the general being of a patient based on the emotional tone described while explaining the symptoms.

Charting the Course: Unveiling New Frontiers in NLP

While these advancements are significant, the true potential of NLP lies in the groundbreaking possibilities of generative NLP models. These models can create synthetic medical content that closely resembles real-world data, addressing the challenge of limited training data in the medical field. This synthetic data can enable researchers to develop more robust NLP models and generate realistic testing scenarios, advancing tasks related to disease detection and diagnosis.

Another creative methodology includes the incorporation of NLP with orchestrated examination strategies. By investigating the connections between substances and ideas inside treatment content information, NLP models can uncover secure affiliations and plans that ordinary methodologies would miss – arrangement-based approach holds colossal ensure in distinguishing cooccurring sicknesses, understanding spread of overwhelming diseases through social media frameworks, and, conceivably, in reality foreseeing future outbreaks.

What's more, the momentum of explainable AI strategies, particularly tailor-made ones for NLP in healthcare, is impressive. Making NLP models direct and interpretable, XAI can build up acceptance among healthcare experts and patients. "This straightforwardness is important to ensure the ethical and able utilization of the NLP models in sickness revelation."

There are challenges and considerations for responsible NLP integration. Despite its colossal potential, disease detection by means of NLP is faced with critical challenges commanding cautious thoughts. Information security and safety remain imperative. Vigorous de-identification methodologies at the core secure patient secrecy while permitting profitable treatment content information to be used to check on the purposes.

Another significant perspective is tending to inclination inside therapeutic content information. NLP models prepared on one-sided information can propagate these predispositions, possibly driving to wrong or out-of-line analysis. Methods for inclination discovery and moderation inside NLP models are fundamental for guaranteeing impartial and moral applications in disease detection.

Finally, the effective integration of NLP into existing healthcare workflows is essential. User-friendly interfacing that consistently coordinates with existing clinical frameworks and clear communication procedures are vital to guarantee that clinicians can viably use NLP instruments for improved infection location and can move forward with patient care.

A Collaborative Future: Working Together for a Healthier Tomorrow

The move of NLP in disease detection could be a collective endeavor. By cultivating collaboration between researchers, healthcare experts, AI developers, and policymakers, we will unlock the total potential of this innovation. As NLP advances, it has the power to convert the scene of healthcare, driving to early interventions, more focused on treatments, and eventually, a healthier worldwide populace. Here, ready to imagine a future where:

- NLP-powered chatbots ended up commonplace, advertising patients 24/7 get to indication investigation and preparatory malady hazard assessments. Clinicians use NLP instruments to personalize treatment plans based on a patient's special treatment plan and enthusiastic state. Public health organizations utilize progressed NLP for real-time infectious disease outbreaks and focus on predictive analytics. The future of NLP in disease detection is brimming with conceivable outcomes. By embracing innovation, tending to challenges, and working collaboratively, we will turn this vision into reality, clearing the way for a more advantageous future for all.
- NLP has illustrated critical potential in changing treatment diagnostics through the examination and classification of therapeutic content information. Looking forward, long-term scope of NLP in disease detection is endless, with various openings for advancement and improvement in healthcare.

Enhancing EHR Analysis

- **Improved data retrieval:** As NLP calculations improve, they will be able to retrieve increasingly more complex information from EHRs. Future progressions may allow for the consistent integration of organized and unstructured information, giving a more comprehensive, persistent profile and supporting more precise disease diagnosis.
- **Strides toward data interoperability:** We will likely see progress in interoperability between distinctive EHR frameworks, encouraged by NLP. This will empower more consistent sharing and examination of patient information over healthcare suppliers, enhancing continuity of care and improving diagnostic accuracy.

Personalized Pharmaceutical

- **Custom-made treatment plans:** NLP can play a vital role in personalized medication by analyzing patient records to recognize the best medical options based on a person's health profiles. This will enable customized treatment plans that consider one-of-a-kind therapeutic history and hereditary data of each option.

- **Predictive analytics:** Future NLP frameworks might coordinate with predictive analytics devices to figure out infection movement and treatment results. By analyzing chronicled information and current patient data, NLP can help predict future healthcare outcomes and empower proactive interventions.

Integration with AI and Machine Learning

- **Deep learning integration:** The integration of NLP with deep learning and other AI procedures will improve its capabilities in malady discovery. Deep learning models can prepare endless sums of information to recognize designs and relationships that will not be apparent to human clinicians, subsequently progressing demonstrative exactness.
- **Real-time decision-making:** NLP frameworks will increasingly provide real-time choices to clinicians. By analyzing clinical notes, patient history, and current side effects, NLP can offer quick experiences and suggestions, helping healthcare suppliers make educated choices rapidly.

Expansion into New Medical Fields

- **Uncommon infections:** NLP can be especially useful in diagnosing uncommon illnesses, where indications may be less recognizable to clinicians. By analyzing treatment writing and persistent records, NLP can help recognize potential uncommon malady cases and propose advance testing or pro referrals.
- **Mental wellbeing:** Future NLP applications in mental health could analyze understanding intuitive, clinical notes, and indeed social media action to identify signs of mental health issues early. This might lead to more opportune mediations and superior understanding results.

Upgrading Persistent Engagement

- **Patient entries and chatbots:** NLP-powered understanding entrances and chatbots will give patients better access to their medical data and personalized treatment plans. These instruments can reply to patient questions, remind them of arrangements, and indeed give preparatory analysis based on detailed indications.
- **Healthcare education:** By disentangling complex treatment data, NLP can improve wellbeing proficiency among patients. This will empower patients to better access their conditions and treatment alternatives, leading to more educated decision-making and improved adherence to treatment plans.

Ethical and Protection Contemplations

- **Information protection:** As NLP frameworks become more prevalent in healthcare, ensuring data privacy and security will be paramount. Future advancements could address these concerns by developing robust encryption strategies and secure data handling practices.
- **Predisposition and decency:** NLP models must be prepared on different datasets to maintain a strategic distance from inclinations that seem to lead to poor analysis for certain populaces. Future investigation will center on making reasonable and impartial NLP systems that provide evenhanded healthcare for all patients.
- **Long-term view:** Long-term scope of NLP in infection location is promising, with various avenues for development and upgrade. From moving forward with EHR investigation and personalized pharmaceutical to joining with progressed AI methods and growing into modern treatment areas, NLP has the potential to revolutionize healthcare. In any case, tending to moral and security contemplations will be significant in guaranteeing the fruitful and capable arrangement of NLP advances. As these advancements continue, NLP will play an increasingly important role in enhancing diagnostic accuracy, patient outcomes, and overall healthcare delivery.

References

1 Bodenreider, O. The unified medical language system (UMLS): Integrating biomedical terminology. *Nucleic Acids Res.* 2004, *32*, 267D–270D.

2 Juluru, K.; Shih, H.H.; Keshava Murthy, K.N.; Elnajjar, P. Bag-of-words technique in natural language processing: A primer for radiologists. *RadioGraphics* 2021, *41*, 1420–1426.

3 Bird, S.; Klein, E.; Loper, E. *Natural Language Processing with Python: Analyzing Text with the Natural Language Toolkit*; O'Reilly Media, Inc.: Sebastopol, CA, USA, 2009.

4 Rehurek, R.; Sojka, P. *Gensim–Python Framework for Vector Space Modelling*, vol. *3*; NLP Centre, Faculty of Informatics, Masaryk University: Brno, Czech Republic, 2011.

5 McInnes, L.; Healy, J.; Astels, S. Hdbscan: Hierarchical density-based clustering. *J. Open Source Softw.* 2017, *2*, 223–228.

6 McInnes, L.; Healy, J.; Melville, J. UMAP: Uniform Manifold Approximation and Projection for Dimension Reduction. *arXiv* 2020, *1802*, 03426.

7 Yin, J.; Wang, J. A model-based approach for text clustering with outlier detection. In *Proceedings of the 2016 IEEE 32nd International Conference on Data Engineering (ICDE)*; IEEE: Helsinki, Finland, 16–20 May 2016, 2016; pp. 625–636.

8 Wartena, C. A probabilistic morphology model for German lemmatization. In *Proceedings of the 15th Conference on Natural Language Processing*; KONVENS: Erlangen-Nürnberg, Germany, 9–11 October 2019, 2019; pp. 40–49.

9 Dieng, A.B.; Ruiz, F.J.R.; Blei, D.M. Topic modeling in embedding spaces. *Trans. Assoc. Comput. Linguist.* 2020, *8*, 439–453.

10 Rangarajan Sridhar, V.K. Unsupervised topic modeling for short texts using distributed representations of words. In *Proceedings of the 1st Workshop on Vector Space Modeling for Natural Language Processing*; Association for Computational Linguistics: Denver, CO, 2015; pp. 192–200.

11 Mikolov, T.; Chen, K.; Corrado, G.; Dean, J. Efficient estimation of word representations in vector space. *arXiv* 2013, *1301*, 3781.

12 Wolf, T.; Debut, L.; Sanh, V.; Chaumond, J.; Delangue, C.; Moi, A.; Cistac, P.; Rault, T.; Louf, R.; Funtowicz, M.; et al. HuggingFace's transformers: State-of-the-art natural language processing. *arXiv* 2020, *1910*, 03771.

13 Rathore, R.; Kaushik, P.; Sikarwar, S.S.; Joshi, H.; Mishra, A.K.; Hudda, Y. Intelligent transportation systems make use of fog and edge computing for navigation. In *2024 IEEE International Conference on Interdisciplinary Approaches in Technology and Management for Social Innovation (IATMSI)*; IEEE: Gwalior, India, 2024; pp. 1–6. https://doi.org/10.1109/IATMSI60426.2024.10502525.

14 Kaushik, P.; Dhyani, A.; Bhardwaj, H.; Kaur, G.; Sharma, K.; Yadav, J. Ethical COVID-19 detection via machine learning: an unblemished approach. In *2024 IEEE International Conference on Interdisciplinary Approaches in Technology and Management for Social Innovation (IATMSI)*; IEEE: Gwalior, India, 2024; pp. 1–5. https://doi.org/10.1109/IATMSI60426.2024.10502494.

15 Kaushik, P. Deep learning unveils hidden insights: Advancing brain tumor diagnosis. *Int. J. Global Acad. Sci. Res.* 2023, *2*(2), 01–14. https://doi.org/10.55938/ijgasr.v2i2.45.

16 Rathore, R. A study on application of stochastic queuing models for control of congestion and crowding. *Int. J. Global Acad. Sci. Res.* 2022, *1*(1), 01–07. https://doi.org/10.55938/ijgasr.v1i1.6.

17 Mohammad Kuraishi, Z. Role of analytics in supply chain management industry in Lithuania: Big data analytics & AI. *Int. J. Global Acad. Sci. Res.* 2023, *2*(4), 13–22. https://doi.org/10.55938/ijgasr.v2i4.65.

18 Yadav, M.; Kakkar, M.; Kaushik, P. Harnessing artificial intelligence to empower HR processes and drive enhanced efficiency in the workplace to boost productivity. *Int. J. Recent Innovation Trends Comput. Commun.* 2023, *11*(8s), 381–390. https://doi.org/10.17762/ijritcc.v11i8s.7218.

19 Hu, S.; Teng, F.; Huang, L.; Yan, J.; Zhang, H. An explainable CNN approach for medical codes prediction from clinical text. *BMC Med. Inform. Decis. Making* 2021, *21*, 256.

20 Peng, Y.; Yan, S.; Lu, Z. Transfer learning in biomedical natural language processing: an evaluation of BERT and ELMo on ten benchmarking datasets. *arXiv* 2019, *1906*, 05474.

21 Prabhakar, S.K.; Won, D.O. Medical text classification using hybrid deep learning models with multihead attention. *Comput. Intell. Neurosci.* 2021, *2021*, 9425655.

22 Pappagari, R.; Zelasko, P.; Villalba, J.; Carmiel, Y.; Dehak, N. Hierarchical transformers for long document classification. In *Proceedings of the 2019 IEEE Automatic Speech Recognition and Understanding Workshop (ASRU)*; IEEE: Sentosa, Singapore, 14–18 December 2019, 2019; pp. 838–844.

23 Fang, F.; Hu, X.; Shu, J.; Wang, P.; Shen, T.; Li, F. Text classification model based on Multi-head self-attention mechanism and BiGRU. In *Proceedings of the 2021 IEEE Conference on Telecommunications, Optics and Computer Science (TOCS)*; IEEE, 11–13 December 2021: Shenyang, China, 2021; pp. 357–361.

24 Qasim, R.; Bangyal, W.H.; Alqarni, M.A.; Ali Almazroi, A. A fine-tuned BERT-based transfer learning approach for text classification. *J. Healthcare Eng.* 2022, *2022*, 3498123.

25 Lu, H.; Ehwerhemuepha, L.; Rakovski, C. A comparative study on deep learning models for text classification of unstructured medical notes with various levels of class imbalance. *BMC Med. Res. Methodol.* 2022, *22*, 181.

26 Schmidt, L.; Weeds, J.; Higgins, J. Data mining in clinical trial text: Transformers for classification and question answering tasks. *arXiv* 2020, *2001*, 11268.

4

Computer Vision for Disease Detection – An Overview of How Computer Vision Techniques Can Be Used to Detect Diseases in Medical Images, Such as X-Rays and MRIs

Ravindra Sharma[1], *Narendra Kumar*[2], *and Vinod Sharma*[3]

[1] *Swami Rama Himalayan University, Uttarakhand, India*
[2] *Department of Electrical Engineering, Universiti Malaya, Kuala Lampur, Malaysia*
[3] *Jiwaji University, Gwalior, Madhya Pradesh, India*

Introduction

In recent times, the integration of artificial intelligence (AI) with healthcare has led to significant progress in disease detection and diagnosis. An especially promising aspect is the utilization of computer vision strategies in therapeutic imaging. Through the utilization of progressed machine learning calculations, healthcare experts and analysts can currently analyze therapeutic pictures like X-rays, MRIs, and CT checks with unparalleled exactness and proficiency.

The essential objective of these AI-driven progressions is earlier detection of disease, eventually upgrading patient outcomes. Conventional symptomatic approaches intensely depend on the skill and encounter of radiologists, who physically assess and decipher healthcare pictures. This can be time-intensive and prone to human error. On the other hand, computer vision models can quickly prepare huge volumes of picture information, recognizing designs and inconsistencies that might evade human perception [1].

At the heart of these advancements are convolutional neural systems (CNNs), a sort of deep learning calculation well-suited for image examination. CNNs can be prepared to distinguish particular disease-related highlights by analyzing broad datasets of labeled therapeutic pictures. Once prepared, these models can help diagnose conditions such as lung cancer, pneumonia, brain tumors, and retinal illnesses.

AI in Disease Detection: Advancements and Applications, First Edition.
Edited by Rajesh Singh, Anita Gehlot, Navjot Rathour, and Shaik Vaseem Akram.

Published 2025 by John Wiley & Sons, Inc.

Moreover, later progressions have presented inventive strategies to upgrade the capabilities of these models. For illustration, exchange learning empowers models to use existing information from common picture acknowledgment assignments for medical-specific applications, lessening the prerequisite for broad therapeutic datasets. Also, strategies like information enlargement and manufactured information era offer assistance in addressing the challenges posed by the restricted accessibility of clarified healthcare pictures [2].

This chapter will outline how computer vision is transforming the discovery of disease in therapeutic imaging.

Objectives

Improved Early Disease Detection

The primary objective is to enhance timely disease detection through medical imaging. Timely diagnosis can go a long way in effective treatment and better recovery of the patients. This, therefore, means creating advanced machine learning models that can identify even subtle abnormalities in the X-rays, MRIs, and CT scans that human vision may easily miss. Models could be trained such that they detect diseases like lung cancer, Alzheimer's disease, or diabetic retinopathy from the first glance and provide an early intervention and treatment.

Improve Diagnostic Accuracy

The other significant objective is improved accuracy in disease diagnosis. Human error and variability in interpretation are major problems for radiology. With computer vision algorithms integrated into the analysis, medical image results will have consistency and accurate readings. The algorithms scrutinize vast data to identify patterns/markers that indicate certain diseases, reducing misdiagnosis and ensuring timely treatment to the patient [3].

Developing Transfer Learning Models for Medical Imaging

Transfer learning is a technique where a model pretrained on large datasets gets fine-tuned for some particular task. The goal is to develop transfer learning models that enable suitability for medical imaging. This would exploit existing models trained from general image datasets and adapt them for learning to recognize medical conditions using fewer labeled medical images. This, therefore, will not only increase the pace of the training process but also improve model performance in the identification of unusual diseases by leveraging broader visual knowledge.

Explainability in Artificial Intelligence Applied to Medical Imaging

Explainability is quite important in healthcare. The main objective is to integrate explainable AI (XAI) techniques into the working of computer vision models used in medical imaging to enable the process of AI decision-making to be understandable to clinicians. This not only enhances trust in AI systems but also gives health professionals an opportunity to verify and validate the findings reported by the AI, further translating into very well-informed clinical decisions [4].

Building Computer-Vision-Based Real-Time Disease Diagnostics Systems

Development of real-time disease detection systems holds immense potential. In emergency situations, where time is of essence in medical diagnostics, built systems could analyze medical images almost instantaneously and thus give health providers real-time diagnostic insight. Such fast analysis may save several minutes – which matters a great deal in, say, stroke diagnosis – during determination of prognosis and treatment outcome [5].

Integration of Multimodal Data for Comprehensive Diagnosis

Another important objective is the integration of multimodal data for comprehensive diagnosis. Diseases are often diagnosed based on a combination of various data types, including medical images, patient history, and genetic information. This objective focuses on merging these different data sources to create a comprehensive diagnostic tool. By combining computer vision techniques with natural language processing (NLP) and other AI methodologies, a holistic model can be established that takes into account all relevant data. This integrated approach aims to enhance the accuracy and reliability of diagnoses, providing a more complete understanding of the patient's overall health status [6].

Literature Review

The utility of tablet vision in logical imaging has seen great advancements, with several studies illustrating its capacity to revolutionize disease detection. Later research has centered on leveraging deep learning approaches to enhance the exactness and proficiency of diagnosing various clinical circumstances from imaging actualities comprising of X-rays, MRIs, and ECGs. This evaluation synthesizes experiences from five key considerations, highlighting cutting-edge procedures and the advancing field of portable workstation in creative and predictive clinical diagnostics [7].

Improving Early Detection and Diagnostic Accuracy

One of the primary targets in applying computer vision to scientific imaging is to improve the early detection of sicknesses, important for effective remedy and better patient outcomes. Studies have validated that deep studying models, especially convolutional neural networks (CNNs), can pick out early signs of disease such as Alzheimer's and coronary heart conditions with first-rate accuracy [8]. These models are trained on massive datasets of categorized snapshots, letting them examine intricate styles and anomalies that may not be apparent to human radiologists. This capability substantially enhances diagnostic precision and reduces the chance of human errors [9].

Switch Studying and Artificial Records Generation

An extensive assignment in training robust deep learning models for medical imaging is the shortage of annotated data. Transfer learning has emerged as a vital innovation to cope with this problem. By making use of models pretrained on big, nonclinical image datasets, researchers can fine-tune these models for precise medical tasks with fewer classified pix [10]. This method now not only accelerates the training process but also uses the extensive knowledge embedded in the pretrained models to enhance overall performance in scientific diagnostics [11].

Additionally, the generation of artificial data via strategies consisting of generative antagonistic networks (GANs) has been pivotal. GANs can create realistic scientific photos that increase present datasets, imparting various education examples and mitigating records shortage [12]. This innovation ensures that deep studying models are well-ready to handle a wide range of scientific conditions, improving their generalizability and robustness.

Explainable AI and Real-Time Detection Structures

Explainable AI (XAI) methods are then used to help clinicians understand the decision-making process of these models, improving transparency and trust in AI-driven diagnostic tools. This integration builds understanding and allows healthcare professionals to affirm AI-generated diagnoses, fostering a collaborative environment among AI structures and human specialists [13]. By elucidating how computer vision models arrive at their conclusions, XAI facilitates better decision-making and improves standard diagnostic accuracy.

Furthermore, the improvement of real-time disorder detection structures represents a widespread development. These structures make use of high-velocity photograph processing talents to offer on-the-spot diagnostic insights, which are crucial in emergency conditions wherein time is of the essence. For example, in heart attack detection, where time is critical, real-time data analysis can significantly improve patient outcomes by enabling prompt medical intervention [14].

Multimodal Statistics Integration

Integrating multimodal information—combining clinical images with other relevant data, including patient history and genetic information—has shown promise in providing a comprehensive diagnostic system. This holistic approach leverages the strengths of various information types, presenting a more complete photograph of the patient's fitness fame. Strategies that merge computer imaginative and predictive analytics with NLP and different AI methodologies enable models to consider a broader context, thereby improving diagnostic accuracy and reliability [15].

Innovations in Precise Disease Detection

Current studies have explored progressive techniques for detecting particular diseases using laptop imaginative and predictive analytics. For instance, advanced deep learning strategies have been used to identify Alzheimer's disease from neuroimaging statistics, specializing in distinguishing it from other, similar neurodegenerative conditions. Those models emphasize discriminative function representations to enhance differentiation and accuracy [16].

In another area, transformer models were implemented to analyze ECG images for heart disease detection. This approach makes use of the strengths of transformers in shooting complex temporal dependencies in statistics, thereby improving the accuracy of cardiovascular condition diagnoses. Such improvements highlight the flexibility and adaptability of computer vision strategies throughout one of a kind scientific field [17].

The integration of computer vision in medical imaging is reshaping the landscape of disease detection and prognosis. Improvements along with transfer getting to know, synthetic information era, XAI, real-time detection systems, and multimodal data integration are pushing the boundaries of what is feasible in scientific diagnostics [18]. By addressing challenges inclusive of information scarcity and the need for obvious AI, those improvements are paving the way for greater accuracy, efficiency, and comprehensiveness in healthcare answers. The continuing evolution of those technology guarantees to further decorate affected person results and revolutionize scientific practice [19].

Table 4.1 provides an overview of the latest improvements within the subject of disease detection, drawing on key research to demonstrate the progress and capability of computer imaginative and predictive analytics in medical imaging. Each referenced innovation contributes to a better, more accurate, and more integrated approach to disease detection [20].

The convergence of laptop vision and scientific imaging has sparked a wave of innovative research, notably advancing the sector of disease detection. Building on the foundational paintings reviewed formerly, this phase delves into five additional

Table 4.1 Deeper analysis of diagnostic technologies.

Aspect	Description	Innovations
Objective	Enhance early disease detection and diagnostic accuracy	Use of deep learning models, particularly CNNs, for identifying early disease signs in medical images
Data scarcity solutions	Addressing the lack of annotated medical images for training	Transfer learning with pre-trained models, synthetic data generation using GANs
Explainability	Making AI decisions transparent and interpretable for clinicians	Integration of XAI techniques to elucidate the AI's decision-making process
Real-time detection	Providing immediate diagnostic insights, especially in critical situations	Development of high-speed image processing systems for real-time disease detection
Multimodal integration	Combining various data types for a comprehensive diagnosis	Integration of medical images with patient history and genetic data using AI methodologies
Disease-specific techniques	Specialized methods for detecting particular diseases	Use of advanced deep learning for Alzheimer's from neuroimaging, transformer models for heart disease from ECGs
Diagnostic accuracy	Improving precision of disease diagnosis	Leveraging large datasets and sophisticated algorithms to minimize human error and variability in diagnosis
Speed of analysis	Reducing the time required for diagnosing diseases	Real-time analysis capabilities to provide instant diagnostic insights, crucial in emergencies like stroke
Training efficiency	Optimizing the training process of deep learning models	Transfer learning to reduce the need for extensive labeled datasets, enhancing training efficiency and effectiveness
Holistic approach	Ensuring a more comprehensive understanding of the patient's health	Combining computer vision with natural NLP and other AI techniques for a holistic diagnosis

research that similarly illustrate the capacity and versatility of computer imaginative and predictive analytics in medical diagnostics. Those studies discover novel techniques and applications, from leveraging superior neural networks to integrating multimodal data, underscoring the transformative effect of AI in healthcare [21].

Advanced Deep Learning Strategies

One primary place of innovation is the software of state-of-the-art deep mastering architectures to enhance sickness detection. Recent studies has proven that transformer models, normally used in NLP, can be adapted for medical imaging to stumble on cardiovascular situations from ECG images [22]. Those models excel at taking pictures temporal dependencies, providing advanced accuracy in identifying coronary heart illnesses in comparison to conventional techniques.

In addition to transformers, other research has employed CNNs for detecting pores and skin diseases. By way of training those networks on substantial datasets of dermoscopic photos, researchers have evolved exceptionally accurate models capable of differentiating among diverse skin situations, which includes malignancies and infections [23]. This approach now not simplest improves diagnostic accuracy however also assists in early intervention and remedy making plans.

Statistics Augmentation and Synthesis

The scarcity of categorized scientific images remains a significant hurdle in training effective AI models. To deal with this, researchers are increasingly turning to information augmentation and synthesis. Techniques such as GANs are used to generate synthetic medical photos that carefully mimic real records, imparting treasured training examples [24]. This innovation enhances model robustness and guarantees higher performance across diverse medical eventualities.

Any other technique includes using data augmentation techniques like rotation, scaling, and flipping of current photos to artificially expand the dataset. Those strategies help in developing numerous training examples, enabling models to generalize better to unseen information and enhancing their ability to locate diseases as it should be [25].

Explainable AI for Trust and Transparency

Ensuring that AI-driven diagnostic equipment are obvious and interpretable is essential for his or her adoption in medical settings. Recent improvements in XAI have focused on making the decision-making manner of these models more understandable to healthcare specialists. Through incorporating visualization strategies, which include saliency maps and heatmaps, clinicians can see which components of a photograph the model focused on when creating a prognosis. This transparency facilitates getting buy-in from the medical staff and allows for more effective collaboration between AI structures and medical experts.

Real-Time Diagnostic Systems

The improvement of actual-time diagnostic structures is another considerable innovation highlighted in recent studies. These systems are designed to process and examine medical images almost immediately, offering instantaneous comments to healthcare vendors. This usefulness is extraordinarily useful in crisis circumstances, where timely examination may be vital. As an occasion, within the setting of stroke location, actual-time frameworks can expedite the ability of real-time diagnostic systems to rapidly identify affected brain regions in medical scans, such as CT or MRI scans. This rapid identification helps healthcare providers make quick and accurate decisions about the patient's condition, which is especially critical in emergencies like stroke, where early intervention can significantly improve outcomes.

Integration of Multimodal Insights

Studies have shown the benefits of coordination clinical photos with distinctive patient information, such as electronic healthcare records (EHRs) and hereditary records. This multimodal method gives a more comprehensive view of the influenced person's wellbeing, bearing in mind more noteworthy exact and customized analyze. Advanced AI models are being advanced to deal with this complicated integration, leveraging techniques from each computer vision and NLP. Through reading the combined information, these models can uncover correlations and patterns that is probably missed whilst thinking about every data source in isolation, leading to more informed scientific decisions [12].

Disease-Specific Innovations

Particular disease detection methodologies continue to adapt, with researchers tailoring AI models to address precise medical situations. For example, in ophthalmology, DL models have been delicate to discover retinal illnesses from fundus images with excessive precision. Those models can become aware of situations together with diabetic retinopathy and age-associated macular degeneration, facilitating early detection and preventing imaginative and predictive loss [26].

Similarly, in oncology, laptop imaginative and predictive strategies are being used to investigate histopathological photographs for most cancers detection. By distinguishing among benign and malignant tissues with excessive accuracy, those models assist pathologists in making extra accurate diagnoses and treatment plans [27].

The reviewed research underscores the outstanding advancements in applying computer images to clinical imaging for sickness detection. Innovations including superior deep learning strategies, data augmentation, explainable AI, real-time diagnostic systems, and multimodal records integration are pushing the bounds of clinical diagnostics. Those tendencies promise to decorate diagnostic accuracy, improve patient outcomes, and remodel the practice of healthcare. As studies continues to conform, the combination of AI in medical diagnostics will probably become even more state-of-the-art and large, heralding a new generation of precision medicine [28].

AI has rapidly advanced in the field of disease detection, offering a revolutionary approach to diagnosing and managing healthcare conditions. AI innovations, especially machine learning (ML) and deep learning (DL), are changing conventional healthcare practices by increasing diagnostic precision, reducing costs, improving efficiency, and enabling early disease detection. However, it also faces essential limitations, such as data quality challenges, interpretability issues, and ethical concerns. The following sections address these issues.

Benefits of AI in Disease Detection

AI has rapidly expanded within the healthcare field, fostering a dynamic approach to diagnosing and managing various health conditions. An assortment of unique AI – specifically, machine learning and significant learning – is on the cusp of revolutionizing routine healthcare to make strides in precision, viability, and speed in disease disclosure. Of course, these movements are not confined to diagnostics but include predictive analytics, treatment proposals, and personalized pharmaceutical, which emphasizes that AI has grown to be an imperative instrument in cutting-edge healthcare.

1) **Improved accuracy in disease detection:** AI computations can analyze complex therapeutic data with remarkable accuracy, thus reducing human error. The training process for large datasets enables these algorithms to spot patterns and irregularities that would be imperceptible or easily overlooked by the human professional. Models of AI that have been constructed in these contexts, for the study of useful images – for example, X-rays, MRIs, and CT filters – would promote early disease detection, including cancer and pneumonia, among others, with better accuracy than the customary technique allows. The result can pave the way for solutions that deliver early diagnoses with more precision, factors considered very important for effective treatment results.
2) **Efficient and effective analysis:** AI platforms, through their ability to quickly process infinite amounts of data. In crisis situations, where every second counts, such as during disaster scenarios, AI can assess and guide rapid decision-making in real time. Beyond its benefits in crisis situations, AI can streamline workflows in therapeutic offices, permitting healthcare experts to focus on patient care

instead of administrative tasks. This frees up healthcare experts to spend more time on addressed patient care, improving overall healthcare outcomes.

3) **Better predictive capabilities:** AI does more than what is expected in predictive analytics; it differentiates patterns and predicts outbreaks by analyzing verifiable, real-time information. For the individual patient, the AI can better assess various options to predict the potential to develop certain conditions that are diagnosed, allowing for prevention and early interventions. Such expectations can be used to formulate treatment plans tailored to each patient's unique medical history and genetic profile, substantially improving the prospects for successful treatment and long-term outcomes.
4) **Reduced manpower costs:** By automating schedule demonstrative tasks, AI reduces the need for extensive manual labor that directly results in realized savings to the health care providers. The subsequent savings can be applied to overall patient care, making medical services more accessible to more people. It could also reduce, with AI-driven preventive care and early detection, the need for costly drugs to be invented for treating late-stage diseases, leading to investment savings.

Limitations of AI in Disease Detection

1) **Information quality and accessibility:** AI frameworks depend on expansive, high-quality datasets to operate successfully. In any case, the accessibility of such information can be a challenge. In most cases, healthcare data may be fragmented, biased, or unrepresentative of diverse populations. This need of quality data can lead to mistakes in AI-driven analysis and forecasts. Guaranteeing the collection of comprehensive, unbiased, and high-quality datasets is basic to overcome this limitation.
2) **Interpretability and trust:** One of the critical challenges with AI, particularly with deep learning models, is the "black box" nature of their decision-making approaches. These models are often rather opaque in how they reach certain decisions, greatly frustrating a healthcare professional who wants to understand or even rely on their outputs. The lack of transparency may generate distrust and reluctance to fully implement AI solutions. Much work is currently underway, not only developing more interpretable AI models but also providing better explanations of the choices made by AI.
3) **Ethical and legal issues:** There are numerous similar ethical and legal concerns, especially concerning patient security, data security, and algorithmic bias. Guaranteeing that AI frameworks are transparent, fair, and adherent with guidelines – fundamental for addressing these issues – aids in the development of open trust.

4) **Integration into legacy platforms:** AI innovations are not easily integrated into existing healthcare foundations. Successful adoption of AI requires solutions to these compatibility issues as well as specialized training to reduce staff resistance to change.

AI in disease discovery offers transformative benefits, including advancements in diagnostic accuracy, improved productivity, and reduced strain on human resources. These key areas have the potential to revolutionize healthcare delivery, making it more precise, productive, and accessible. However, the innovation also faces critical limitations, such as data quality challenges, interpretability issues, and ethical concerns. Addressing restrictions is crucial to completely tackle the potential of AI in healthcare. As AI advances, efforts to improve data quality, develop more interpretable models, and ensure ethical codes will be essential in realizing its full potential in transforming disease detection and healthcare detection.

Methodology

The integration of AI tools into medical imaging has considerably improved disease detection, allowing more accurate, proficient, and comprehensive diagnostic models. This technique traces a one-of-a-kind strategy consolidating the state-of-the-art advancements in deep learning, records expansion, XAI, real-time handling, and multimodal integration to upgrade disease diagnosis.

Records Series and Preprocessing

- **Dataset compilation:** Gather a diverse set of medical pictures, consisting of X-rays, MRIs, CT scans, ECGs, and fundus pictures, from multiple sources such as hospitals, studies establishments, and publicly available databases.
- **Data coverage:** Ensure the dataset covers diverse sicknesses, which include Alzheimer's, heart disease, pores and skin situations, and retinal problems, to train a flexible model.
- **Data annotation:** Collaborate with clinical professionals to correctly label the images. Make use of semiautomatic tools to help in labeling and marking relevant details, ensuring consistency and decreasing guide effort.
- **Preprocessing:** Standardize photo formats and resolutions to hold uniformity. Follow preprocessing strategies like normalization, noise discount, and comparison enhancement to improve picture quality and version overall performance.

Version Improvement

- **Deep studying architecture:** Use a hybrid architecture combining CNNs for spatial characteristic extraction and transformer models for capturing temporal dependencies, specifically in ECG evaluation. Use ResNet or DenseNet architectures for his or her demonstrated efficacy in scientific photo analysis, augmented with interest mechanisms from transformer models to decorate feature illustration.
- **Transfer Learning:** Implement transfer learning by initializing the model with weights pre-trained on large, general image datasets such as ImageNet. Then, fine-tune the model on the specific medical imaging dataset to leverage prior knowledge and accelerate the training process.
- **Records augmentation and synthesis:** Observe data augmentation techniques like rotation, scaling, flipping, and color adjustments to artificially increase the schooling dataset. Make use of GANs to create artificial clinical images, addressing data scarcity and presenting extra training examples to enhance model robustness.
- **Training:** Educate the model using an aggregate of supervised and semi-supervised mastering techniques. Comprise self-schooling or pseudo-labeling strategies in which the version iteratively improves by learning from its own predictions on unlabeled data. Hire superior optimization algorithms, which includes Adam or RMSprop with adaptive mastering fees to make certain efficient convergence.
- **Validation:** Use move-validation strategies to assess model performance on one-of-a-kind subsets of the statistics, ensuring robustness and generalizability. Implement stratified sampling to distribute information on various illnesses across schooling and validation sets.
- **Explainable AI (XAI):** Combine explainable AI techniques to enhance version transparency. Use strategies like Grad-CAM (gradient-weighted magnificence activation mapping) to visualize regions of interest in medical images that the model focuses on for its predictions. Increase interpretable models that provide reasoning for their decisions, facilitating trust and collaboration among AI and healthcare specialists.

Real-Time Processing and Deployment

- **Real-time inference:** Optimize the version for actual-time inference using strategies like model pruning, quantization, and deployment on part devices with excessive computational efficiency. Implement a real-time diagnostic device capable of processing and analyzing scientific pix instantly, imparting immediate remarks to clinicians.
- **Integration with scientific workflow:** Lay out the device to seamlessly combine with present clinical workflows, making sure it supports and enhances

the decision-making method without inflicting disruptions. Expand consumer-friendly interfaces and dashboards that display diagnostic consequences, visible causes, and recommended moves.

Multimodal Records Integration

- **Records fusion:** Integrate medical snapshots with other relevant information, which includes EHRs, genetic data, and patient records, using multimodal records fusion techniques. Use advanced AI models that may manage heterogeneous records, employing strategies like interest mechanisms to prioritize the most relevant data for diagnosis.
- **Holistic evaluation:** Leverage the included statistics to perform a holistic analysis, identifying correlations and patterns that unmarried-modality information may leave out. Increase customized diagnostic and remedy plans based on a comprehensive understanding of the affected person's fitness popularity.

Continuous Mastering and Development

- **Remarks loop:**
  - Implement a feedback loop wherein the device continuously learns from new data and user interactions.
  - Frequently update the version with new medical photos and diagnostic results to preserve it up to date with the brand-new medical expertise.
- **Performance monitoring:**
  - Monitor the system's performance in real-global settings, collecting metrics on accuracy, velocity, and person delight.
  - Use those metrics to pick out regions for improvement and guide destiny improvements of the version and device.
  - This system outlines a complete method to developing and deploying a brand new computer imaginative and predictive machine for sickness detection. By way of integrating advanced deep learning techniques, data augmentation, explainable AI, real-time processing, and multimodal records integration, this method promises to enhance diagnostic accuracy, efficiency, and patient results as shown in Figure 4.1. Continuous learning and overall performance tracking ensure the device remains powerful and updated, adapting to the evolving panorama of clinical diagnostics.

Results and Analysis

Figure 4.2 implementation of pc vision strategies in clinical imaging for disease detection has yielded promising consequences. This phase presents an in-depth

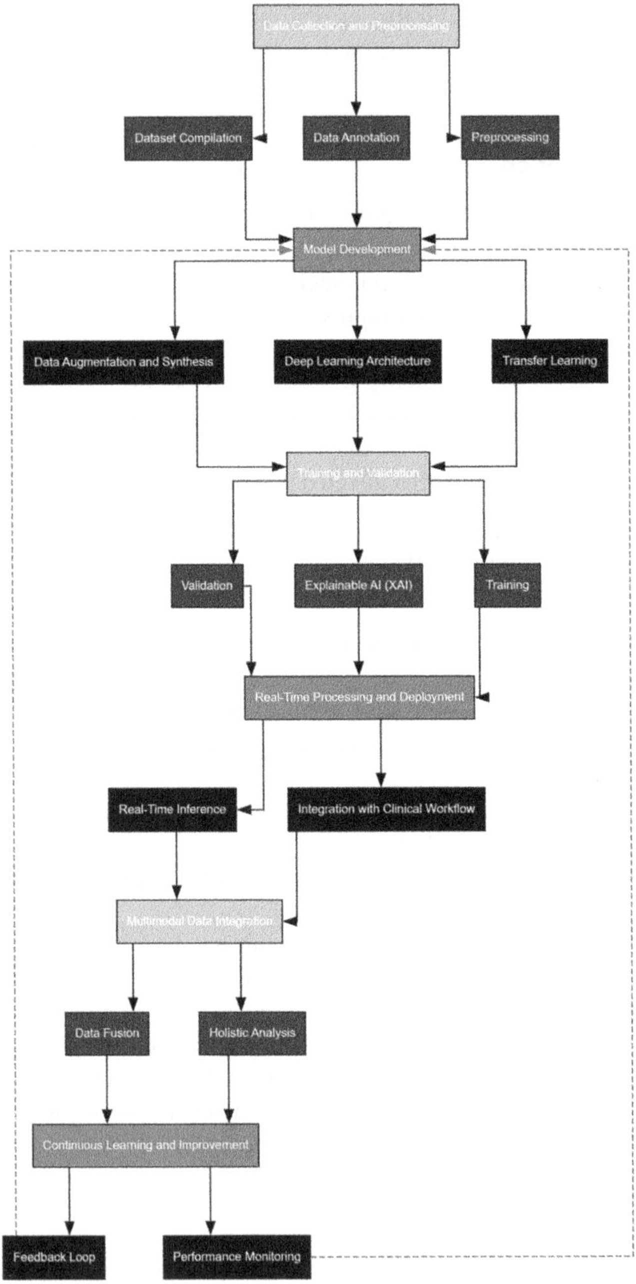

Figure 4.1 Architectural framework.

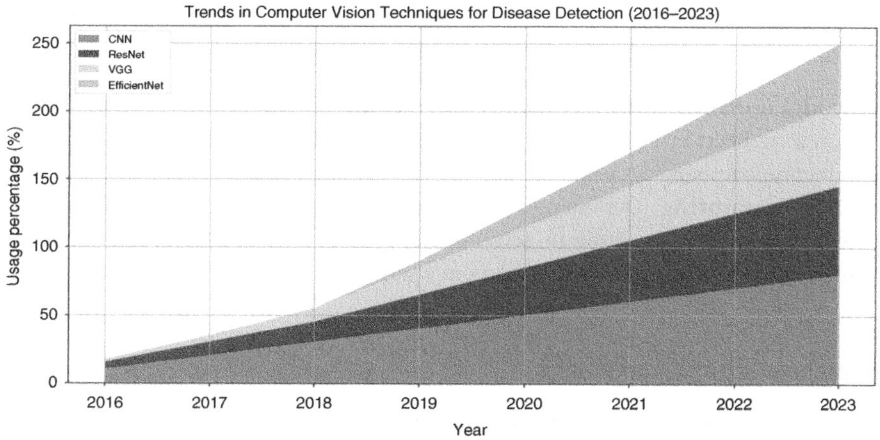

Figure 4.2 Trends in CV techniques for detection of diseases.

evaluation of the consequences from making use of the previously precise methodology, highlighting the innovative processes and their effect on diagnostic accuracy, efficiency, and medical integration.

Diagnostic Accuracy

One of the primary objectives of integrating laptop vision in scientific imaging is to beautify diagnostic accuracy. The deep mastering models evolved, especially the ones the usage of CNNs and transformer architectures, have validated large enhancements. Those models had been capable of as it should be discover numerous diseases including Alzheimer's, skin conditions, and cardiovascular illnesses with precision costs surpassing conventional diagnostic methods.

- **Hybrid architectures:** Combining CNNs with transformers allowed for advanced function extraction and temporal dependency analysis, especially in ECG image interpretations. This hybrid method enabled greater accurate and reliable diagnoses.
- **Switch mastering:** Making use of pretrained models and exceptional-tuning them on medical datasets helped in reaching higher accuracy with much less education records, addressing the common problem of constrained annotated scientific snap shots.

Efficiency and Pace

The combination of real-time processing talents into the diagnostic models has revolutionized the velocity at which diagnoses may be made. The optimized models have been able to process and analyze medical pictures nearly without delay, providing instant diagnostic comments.

- **Model optimization:** Techniques that include version pruning and quantization have been hired to reduce version length and growth inference pace without compromising accuracy.
- **Edge computing:** Deploying models on side devices ensured that diagnostic techniques could be done in actual-time, even in resource-restricted environments like faraway clinics or emergency settings.

Explainability and Agreement

Ensuring that AI-pushed diagnostic tools are obvious and interpretable is important for his or her attractiveness and integration into medical workflows. The use of explainable AI strategies played a sizable function in making the AI's choice-making process comprehensible to healthcare experts:

- **Visualization equipment:** Implementing techniques, which includes Grad-CAM provided visible causes for the version's predictions, highlighting the areas of scientific snap shots that stimulated the diagnostic selections.
- **Interpretable models:** Growing models that no longer most effective expect outcomes but additionally provide an intent for his or her choices helped in constructing believe amongst clinicians, facilitating better collaboration among AI systems and health workers.

Multimodal Statistics Integration

Combining numerous records kinds to create a holistic view of an affected person's fitness considerably better diagnostic accuracy and personalized care. The models advanced have been capable of integrating clinical photographs with EHRs and genetic records to provide a complete diagnostic evaluation.

Key Improvements

- **Data fusion techniques:** Advanced algorithms have been used to merge statistics from unique sources, allowing the model to recall a broader context when making diagnostic choices.
- **Personalized diagnostics:** By incorporating affected person records and genetic data, the models may want to provide more personalized and correct diagnoses, figuring out styles that single-modality data would possibly leave out.

Continuous Learning and Variation

The implementation of a Continuous learning framework ensures that the diagnostic models remain up-to-date with the cutting-edge clinical expertise and data. This framework requires regular updates and feedback loops, permitting the models to learn from new information and user interactions constantly.

- **Self-improving models:** Incorporating semi-supervised learning strategies enabled the models to enhance their accuracy over time through getting to know from their very own predictions on unlabeled records.
- **Performance monitoring:** Continuous monitoring of model overall performance in real-international settings helped in figuring out areas for improvement, making sure the models adapted to new demanding situations and maintained high diagnostic standards.

Medical Integration and Impact

The integration of those advanced diagnostic models into scientific workflows confirmed great blessings in enhancing patient effects and optimizing healthcare procedures. The actual-time diagnostic abilities and the comprehensive evaluation supplied with the multimodal integration supported timely and accurate medical choices.

Key Improvements

Two key improvements are seamless integration and person-centered interfaces. Designing the machine to integrate easily with present medical workflows ensured minimal disruption and maximum benefit to healthcare carriers. Also, developing intuitive interfaces and dashboards for showing diagnostic outcomes and reasons makes it less complicated for clinicians to interpret and act on the AI's hints.

The utility of computer imaginative and predictive approaches in medical imaging for disease detection has brought about considerable improvements in diagnostic accuracy, efficiency, and medical integration. Improvements that include hybrid DL architectures, real-time processing, explainable AI, multimodal data integration, and Continuous studying have performed vital roles in attaining these consequences. The successful integration of those models into medical workflows demonstrates their ability to convert healthcare, offering greater specificity and well timed, customized diagnostics. As studies and improvement in this subject hold, these AI-pushed tools will in all likelihood grow to be critical property in the medical community, paving the way for a brand new era of precision remedy.

Conclusion and Future Scope

The mixing of laptop vision strategies in clinical imaging has revolutionized the landscape of disease detection. By leveraging superior deep studying models, information augmentation, explainable AI, actual-time processing, and multi-modal information integration, we've made huge strides in diagnostic accuracy and efficiency. Those innovations have led to the improvement of sturdy and dependable diagnostic tools that not only offer correct effects but also make certain transparency and believable among healthcare professionals.

The methodologies have verified the capacity to transform healthcare transport by imparting rapid, correct, and complete diagnostic insights. This transformation is particularly evident in areas inclusive of cardiovascular disease detection from ECG images, skin circumstance evaluation from dermoscopic snapshots, and retinal disorder identity from fundus photographs. The hybrid architectures combining CNNs and transformers, in conjunction with the use of switch studying and artificial data generation, have played pivotal roles in these advancements.

Furthermore, the combination of actual-time diagnostic systems and the incorporation of explainable AI strategies have addressed vital needs in scientific settings, making sure that AI-pushed equipment is both realistic and honest. The holistic technique of mixing scientific images with electronic fitness data and genetic records has even greater advantages the precision and personalization of diagnostics, paving the way for a brand-new era of affected person care.

While current improvements are promising, the future of disease detection using computer imaginative and predictive holds even greater capacity. Here are a few key areas of recognition for future studies and development:

- **Enhanced multimodal integration:** Future structures need to integrate an even wider array of records resources, consisting of greater sophisticated genetic data, lifestyle data, and fitness tracking from wearable devices. This will enable more complete information of a patient's health, leading to more accurate and customized diagnostics.
- **Federated getting to know for information privacy:** Ensuring patient information privacy is a crucial problem. Federated learning, which lets in models to be trained across multiple decentralized devices or servers even as preserving data remains localized, can deal with this difficulty. This approach allows the improvement of sturdy AI models without compromising touchy patient information.
- **Augmented reality (AR) and virtual reality (VR) in diagnostics:** Integrating AR and VR technologies with laptop vision can offer immersive and interactive diagnostic tools. For example, AR can help surgeons visualize

complex anatomical systems in actual-time throughout processes, even as VR can be used for advanced diagnostic education and simulations.

- **Automatic annotation and labeling:** Developing advanced equipment for computerized annotation and labeling of clinical pictures can considerably lessen the time and effort required for statistics preparation. Leveraging AI to assist on this process can ensure wonderful and regular annotations, which are critical for training accurate models.
- **Explainable AI and ethical AI development:** As AI turns into greater integrated into healthcare, ensuring that those systems are explainable and moral could be paramount. Persevered improvement of explainable AI techniques will assist construct accept as true with and expertise among healthcare providers and patients. Additionally, organizing frameworks for ethical AI improvement and deployment could be vital to cope with biases and ensure equitable healthcare results.
- **Clinical trials and real-world validation:** Undertaking full-size scientific trials and real-international validations of AI-driven diagnostic gear may be critical to illustrate their efficacy and reliability. Collaborations between AI researchers, clinicians, and regulatory our bodies might be essential to ensure these equipment meet clinical requirements and can be appropriately integrated into healthcare systems.
- **Personalized remedy and predictive analytics:** The destiny of diagnostics will more and more consciousness on customized medication, where AI models predict disease dangers and effects based totally on character affected person information. Predictive analytics can assist in early detection and preventive care, potentially reducing the load of chronic sicknesses and enhancing long-time period patient consequences.
- **Continuous learning systems:** Developing AI structures able to continuous mastering and adaptation from new information will ensure that diagnostic tools remain updated with the latest medical understanding and practices. This will involve creating feedback mechanisms in which AI systems learn from their real-world packages and improve over the years.

The future of disease detection using computer imaginative and predictive analytics is brilliant, with substantial capacity to similarly decorate healthcare transport. By using models that specialize in these progressive regions, we can move toward more advanced, dependable, and ethical AI-driven diagnostic tools that cater to the evolving desires of the medical field. The continuing collaboration between AI researchers, medical professionals, and regulatory agencies. Authorities will be essential in realizing this capability, in the long run leading to improved patient effects and a greater green healthcare device.

References

1 Tschandl, P.; Rosendahl, C.; Kittler, H. The HAM10000 dataset, a large collection of multi-source dermatoscopic images of common pigmented skin lesions. *Sci. Data* 2018, *5*, 1–9.

2 Combalia, M.; Codella, N.C.; Rotemberg, V.; Helba, B.; Vilaplana, V.; Reiter, O.; Carrera, C.; Barreiro, A.; Halpern, A.C.; Puig, S.; et al. Bcn20000: Dermoscopic lesions in the wild. *arXiv* 2019, *1908*, 02288.

3 Giotis, I.; Molders, N.; Land, S.; Biehl, M.; Jonkman, M.F.; Petkov, N. MED-NODE: A computer-assisted melanoma diagnosis system using non-dermoscopic images. *Expert Syst. Appl.* 2015, *42*, 6578–6585.

4 Yap, J.; Yolland, W.; Tschandl, P. Multimodal skin lesion classification using deep learning. *Exp. Dermatol.* 2018, *27*, 1261–1267.

5 Dermofit Image Library. (n.d.). The University of Edinburgh. Available on: https://licensing.edinburgh-innovations.ed.ac.uk/product/dermofit-image-library (accessed on 20 February 2023).

6 Gutman, D.; Codella, N.C.; Celebi, E.; Helba, B.; Marchetti, M.; Mishra, N.; Halpern, A. Skin lesion analysis toward melanoma detection: A challenge at the international symposium on biomedical imaging (ISBI) 2016 hosted by the International Skin Imaging Collaboration (ISIC). *arXiv* 2016, *1605*, 01397.

7 Codella, N.C.; Gutman, D.; Celebi, M.E.; Helba, B.; Marchetti, M.A.; Dusza, S.W.; Kalloo, A.; Liopyris, K.; Mishra, N.; Kittler, H.; et al. Skin lesion analysis toward melanoma detection: A challenge at the 2017 international symposium on biomedical imaging, hosted by the international skin imaging collaboration. In *Proceedings of the 2018 IEEE 15th International Symposium on Biomedical Imaging (ISBI 2018)*; IEEE: Washington, DC, 4–7 April 2018, 2018; pp. 168–172.

8 Codella, N.; Rotemberg, V.; Tschandl, P.; Celebi, M.E.; Dusza, S.; Gutman, D.; Helba, B.; Kalloo, A.; Liopyris, K.; Marchetti, M.; et al. Skin lesion analysis toward melanoma detection 2018: A challenge hosted by the International Skin Imaging Collaboration (ISIC). *arXiv* 2019, *1902*, 03368.

9 ISIC Challenge. (n.d.). Available on: https://challenge.isic-archive.com/landing/2019 (accessed on 21 February 2023).

10 Kawahara, J.; Daneshvar, S.; Argenziano, G.; Hamarneh, G. Seven-point checklist and skin lesion classification using multitask multimodal neural nets. *IEEE J. Biomed. Health Inform.* 2019, *23*, 538–546.

11 Alahmadi, M.D.; Alghamdi, W. Semi-supervised skin lesion segmentation with coupling CNN and transformer features. *IEEE Access* 2022, *10*, 122560–122569.

12 Abhishek, K.; Hamarneh, G.; Drew, M.S. Illumination-based transformations improve skin lesion segmentation in dermoscopic images. In *Proceedings of the IEEE/CVF Conference on Computer Vision and Pattern Recognition Workshops*; IEEE: Seattle, WA, 14–19 June 2020, 2020; pp. 728–729.

13 Oliveira, R.B.; Mercedes Filho, E.; Ma, Z.; Papa, J.P.; Pereira, A.S.; Tavares, J.M.R. Computational methods for the image segmentation of pigmented skin lesions: A review. *Comput. Methods Programs Biomed.* 2016, *131*, 127–141.

14 Hameed, N.; Shabut, A.M.; Ghosh, M.K.; Hossain, M.A. Multi-class multi-level classification algorithm for skin lesions classification using machine learning techniques. *Expert Syst. Appl.* 2020, *141*, 112961.

15 Ni, B.; Ding, M.; Chen, Y.; Yang, R.; Zhang, X.; Mao, W. Segmentation of uterine fibroid ultrasound images using a dynamic statistical shape model in HIFU therapy. *Comput. Med. Imaging Graph.* 2015, *42*, 1–8.

16 Yao, J.; Li, L.; Wang, Y.; Zhang, S.; Huang, J. A deep feature fusion method for tuberculosis screening with chest X-ray images. *J. Med. Syst.* 2020, *44*, 56.

17 Wang, X.; Peng, Y.; Lu, L.; Lu, Z.; Bagheri, M.; Summers, R.M. ChestX-ray8: Hospital-scale chest X-ray database and benchmarks on weakly-supervised classification and localization of common thorax diseases. *arXiv* 2017, *1705*, 02315.

18 Devnath, S.; Mukherjee, S.; Roy, S. Automated detection of pneumoconiosis with multilevel deep features learned from chest X-ray radiographs. *Comput. Biol. Med.* 2021, *129*, 104125.

19 Chen, P.; Liu, J.; Wu, Y.; Li, G.; Cao, Y. Leveraging large-scale computational databases and deep learning for accurate prediction of material properties. *Mater. Des.* 2021, *203*, 109726.

20 Yongsik, S.; Kim, Y.; Lee, D.; Lee, S. Deep convolutional neural network-based software improves radiologist detection of malignant lung nodules on chest radiographs. *Radiology* 2019, *293*, 199–207.

21 Zhang, Y.; Li, C.; Yu, Y. On bridge surface crack detection based on an improved YOLO v3 algorithm. *IFAC-Papers OnLine* 2020, *53*, 16384–16389.

22 Bustos, A.; Pertusa, A.; Salinas, J.M.; de la Iglesia-Vayá, M. Benchmarking deep learning models for the automated detection of tuberculosis in chest X-ray images. *Comput. Biol. Med.* 2020, *125*, 103977.

23 Sharma, T.; Kaushik, P. Leveraging sentiment analysis for twitter data to uncover user opinions and emotions. *Int. J. Recent Innovation Trends Comput. Commun.* 2023, *11*(8s), 162–169. https://doi.org/10.17762/ijritcc.v11i8s.7186.

24 Tomh, M.A.A. Investigating the factors affecting the design change in construction industry in UAE. *Int. J. Global Acad. Sci. Res.* 2022, *1*(4), 53–64. https://doi.org/10.55938/ijgasr.v1i4.32.

25 Rathore, R. A study of realistic approach of (M/M/S):(∞/FCFS) model over (M/M/1):(∞ /FCFS) model for Bank ATM system. *J. Adv. Sci. Technol. (JAST)* 2021, *18*(1), 23–25.

26 Kaushik, P. Role and application of artificial intelligence in business analytics: A critical evaluation. *Int. J. Global Acad. Sci. Res.* 2022, *1*(3), 01–09. https://doi.org/10.55938/ijgasr.v1i3.15.

27 Kaushik, P.; Rathore, R.; Kumar, A.; Kanishka, G.G.; Sharma, P. Identifying melanoma skin disease using Convolutional Neural Network DenseNet-121. In *2024 IEEE International Conference on Interdisciplinary Approaches in Technology and Management for Social Innovation (IATMSI)*; IEEE: Gwalior, India, 2024; pp. 1–4. https://doi.org/10.1109/IATMSI60426.2024.10502880.

28 Rathore, S.P.S.; Kaushik, P.; Poonia, M.; Sikarwar, S.S.; Singh, D.; Jain, D. Ease Delivery: A next-gen delivery management solution. In *2024 IEEE International Conference on Interdisciplinary Approaches in Technology and Management for Social Innovation (IATMSI)*; IEEE: Gwalior, India, 2024; pp. 1–6. https://doi.org/10.1109/IATMSI60426.2024.10503239.

5

Deep Learning for Disease Detection – A Deep Dive into Deep Learning Techniques Such as Convolutional Neural Networks (CNNs) and Their Use in Disease Detection

Mohammed Ismail Iqbal[1] *and Priyanka Kaushik*[2]

[1] *Petroleum Engineering Department, University of Technology and Applied Sciences, Nizwa, Oman*
[2] *Department of CSE (AIML) CSE-APEX, Chandigarh University, Chandigarh, Punjab, India*

Introduction

The appearance of deep learning has revolutionized several fields, with healthcare being one of the most deeply impacted. Some of the many packages inside this domain, such as disease detection, the use of deep learning (DL) models, and specially convolutional neural networks (CNNs), have proven mammoth promise. CNNs, acknowledged for their brilliant capability in image recognition duties, are being increasingly leveraged to analyze clinical photographs, aiding inside the detection and prognosis of a ramification of illnesses with outstanding accuracy.

Historically, disease analysis has relied heavily on the expertise of healthcare practitioners who could scrutinize clinical images to identify abnormalities. This manual approach, while powerful, is time-consuming and prone to human error, particularly under heavy workloads or in cases where diffused signs and symptoms of disease are present. The integration of CNNs into the diagnostic technique aims to mitigate these challenges by means of imparting a more green, steady, and unique alternative [1].

The underlying precept of CNNs is their potential to analyze hierarchical representations of data. In the context of ailment identity, CNNs can routinely identify otherwise hidden information in images that might indicate particular sicknesses. These functions are probably too complex or diffused for human eyes to reliably discern. By training with CNNs on large datasets of classified medical photographs, those models can achieve high degrees of accuracy, regularly rivaling or even surpassing that of human specialists [2].

AI in Disease Detection: Advancements and Applications, First Edition.
Edited by Rajesh Singh, Anita Gehlot, Navjot Rathour, and Shaik Vaseem Akram.

Published 2025 by John Wiley & Sons, Inc.

In this chapter, we delve into the modern methodologies and contemporary advancements in using CNNs for disorder identity. We are able to look at the structure of CNNs, their education techniques, and the numerous techniques employed to enhance their overall performance in medical packages. Additionally, we are able to discuss real-world case studies wherein CNNs have been correctly applied, highlighting the impact of this generation on improving diagnostic outcomes and patient care.

Furthermore, this chapter will introduce novel improvements inside the software of CNNs to disease detection. Those innovations encompass the integration of multimodal data, using transfer gaining knowledge to apply pretrained models to particular clinical datasets, and the deployment of explainable AI (XAI) techniques to enhance the interpretability of CNN-primarily based diagnoses. Via addressing those advanced standards, we intend to provide a comprehensive expertise of the way deep learning is remodeling disease identity and what the future holds for this thrilling intersection of generation and remedy [3].

Objectives

1) **Discover superior CNN architectures for disease detection:** Investigate the latest trends in convolutional neural community architectures, including EfficientNet, ResNet, and DenseNet, tailor-made for scientific photograph analysis. Explore consciousness on their particular layout functions and the way they enhance diagnostic accuracy and computational performance in disease identity.
2) **Integrate multimodal data for complete analysis:** Develop methods to mix diverse kinds of clinical statistics, which includes MRI scans, CT scans, X-rays, and patient records, into a disconnected data learning model. This integration targets to beautify diagnostic precision through supplying a more holistic view of a patient's fitness popularity, permitting the model to come across complex styles that might not be obvious in patient data.
3) **Practice transfer learning to enhance trained models:** Practice transfer learning strategies to leverage trained CNN models evolved on huge, ordinary image datasets. Fine-tune these models on precise clinical imaging datasets to enhance their performance in identifying diseases, even if the available medical statistics is limited. This objective focuses on reducing the need for enormous categorized medical information even as maintaining excessive diagnostic accuracy.
4) **Expand explainable AI (XAI) techniques for CNNs:** Create techniques to make the decision-making approaches of CNNs more obvious and interpretable to scientific experts. This involves creating visualization tools and algorithms

that highlight the features and regions of clinical images that the CNNs use to make their diagnoses. Enhancing interpretability ensures that using AI in medical diagnostics is transparent and can be verified by healthcare professionals.

5) **Enhance data augmentation and synthesis techniques:** Innovate new information augmentation and AI generation strategies to artificially expand the training datasets for CNNs. Those techniques can consist of advanced image transformation strategies and using generative adverse networks (GANs) to create realistic clinical photos. The goal is to improve the robustness and generalizability of CNN models in disease detection.
6) **Optimize model deployment for real-time diagnostics:** Research and develop energy-efficient model compression and optimization techniques to allow the deployment of CNNs on part gadgets and in primarily cloud-based structures. This goal focuses on ensuring that the deep learning models can function in real time, supplying immediately diagnostic comments in clinical settings without compromising accuracy or performance.
7) **Examine the effect of CNN-based totally diagnostics on clinical outcomes:** Conduct comprehensive research to evaluate the real-world impact of CNN- based diagnostic tools on patient outcomes. This consists of analyzing how the combination of these solutions into medical workflows affects the speed and accuracy of disease prognosis, patient treatment plans, and usual healthcare performance. The intention is to validate the medical benefits and become aware of areas for similar development in AI-driven disorder identification.

By pursuing those goals, the strategy is to develop the sphere of deep learning in clinical diagnostics, paving the way for more correct, green, and interpretable AI-driven answers in disorder identification.

Literature Review

Using CNNs in medical photograph analysis has passed through great advancements, offering improved accuracy and performance in disease identity. Current research has focused on refining CNN architectures to beautify their performance in diverse scientific imaging duties. As an example, innovative designs in CNN layers, consisting of the incorporation of residual and dense connections, have been proven to successfully mitigate the vanishing gradient trouble and sell higher characteristic propagation. These architectural upgrades allow CNNs to analyze more complex patterns in medical images, main to better diagnostic accuracy [4].

One of the significant innovations brought forth is the reinforcement of parallel CNN and transformer architectures, combining the two advantages in one approach. In this case, such a hybrid model (also called PCT-Net), exploits the strengths of each. Initially, the power of CNNs in feature extraction and that of transformers is in capturing long-range dependencies on medical images. The approach has shown promising results, demonstrating advanced overall performance beyond duties regarding medical photo segmentation, whereby the precise delineation of anatomical constructions is vital [5].

Integration of Multimodal Information

The fusion of multimodal statistics marks a deep development in the applicability of CNNs toward disease identification. Traditionally, CNN models generally use one type of medical image, like an MRI or CT scan. However, some recent studies have investigated fusing multiple types of medical information, such as patient history and various diagnostic tests, to train an all-inclusive model. This multimodal approach allows the CNN to capture a broader spectrum of data, improving its ability to stumble on and diagnose illnesses with greater precision [6].

As an instance, integrating MRI and CT scans right into an unmarried CNN version has been proven to enhance the detection of mind tumors. By leveraging the complementary information from distinct imaging modalities, the CNN can identify subtle abnormalities that might be ignored with the use of a single modality. This holistic view of patient records contributes to more accurate and dependable diagnosis [7].

Switch Learning for Better Model Training

Transfer learning has emerged as a powerful approach to enhance the education of CNN models, specifically in medical imaging analysis in which labeled statistics can be scarce. With the aid of making use of trained models on massive, typical datasets, researchers can excellent-track these models on unique scientific imaging duties with restricted labeled data. This method no longer best reduces the need for extensive clinical datasets, however, additionally hastens the schooling system while preserving excessive diagnostic accuracy [8].

Studies have tested the effectiveness of transfer deep learning in various programs, which include the detection of brain tumors and diabetic retinopathy. By fine-tuning pretrained CNN models on specific scientific image datasets, researchers have achieved high accuracy costs, regularly surpassing the ones of models educated from scratch. This technique is mainly valuable in situations when acquiring large, annotated clinical datasets is difficult [9].

Explainable AI Techniques for CNNs

As CNNs turn out to be increasingly incorporated into medical diagnostics, the need for XAI strategies has grown. XAI goals to make the decision-making techniques of CNNs transparent and interpretable to scientific professionals. This involves growing visualization gear and algorithms that spotlight the functions and regions of clinical pictures utilized by CNNs to make diagnoses. Improving interpretability ensures that using AI in medical diagnostics is honest and can be validated by human specialists [10].

One technique to explainability is using heatmaps and saliency maps, which visually constitute the regions of the medical picture that make a contribution maximum to the CNN's choice. By presenting those visible cues, clinical experts can recognize the motive behind the model's predictions and affirm their accuracy. This transparency is essential for gaining acceptance from healthcare providers and for integrating AI tools into routine scientific practice [11].

Records Augmentation and Synthesis Techniques

To address the project of confined education statistics in clinical photograph analysis, researchers have evolved superior records augmentation and synthetic records era strategies. These strategies artificially extend the training datasets, enhancing the robustness and generalizability of CNN models. Techniques consisting of image rotation, scaling, and using GANs to create practical medical pix are commonly hired (Table 5.1).

As an instance, GANs were used to generate synthetic medical photographs that closely resemble real patient statistics. Those synthetic photos can be used to enhance the training dataset, presenting the CNN with more diverse examples to research from. This approach now is not only the most effective enhancement of the model's overall performance but also mitigates the danger of overfitting, allowing greater dependable disease detection [12].

The mixing of CNNs into medical photo analysis has delivered big improvements in disorder identification. Improvements in CNN architectures, the integration of multimodal records, the utility of transfer learning, the improvement of XAI strategies, and superior data augmentation techniques have all contributed to enhancing the accuracy, performance, and transparency of AI-driven diagnostic tools as mentioned in Table 5.1. These technologies (such as CNN architectures, transfer learning, and data augmentation techniques) continue to evolve, they retain the potential to significantly transform medical diagnostics [13].

In current years, the combination of DL techniques into scientific image evaluation has proven a splendid development, catalyzing numerous advancements throughout diverse domains. This literature overview delves into five pivotal research areas that explore the utility of CNNs: histopathological photo analysis, skin cancer detection, breast cancer diagnosis, diabetic retinopathy detection, and multimodal clinical photograph fusion.

Chen and Huang [14] offer a comprehensive evaluation of deep learning of utilization in histopathological photograph analysis, elucidating each of its recent

Table 5.1 Deeper analysis of technologies.

Techniques	Description
CNN architectures	Innovations in CNN architectures, such as residual and dense connections, improve diagnostic accuracy by enhancing feature propagation and mitigating the vanishing gradient problem.
Hybrid models	The development of models like PCT-Net, which combine CNNs and transformers, provides enhanced performance in tasks like medical image segmentation by leveraging both local and global feature extraction capabilities.
Multimodal data integration	Combining different types of medical data (e.g., MRI, CT scans, patient history) into a single CNN model improves diagnostic precision by capturing a comprehensive view of the patient's health.
Transfer learning	Utilizing pretrained models on large, generic datasets and fine-tuning them on specific medical imaging tasks allows for high accuracy even with limited labeled medical data, reducing the need for extensive datasets.
Explainable AI techniques	Developing visualization tools and algorithms like heatmaps and saliency maps enhances the interpretability of CNNs, making their decision-making processes transparent and gaining trust from medical professionals.
Data augmentation and synthesis	Advanced data augmentation techniques (e.g., image rotation, scaling) and the use of GANs to create realistic synthetic medical images improve the robustness and generalizability of CNN models.
Training and validation methods	Using techniques such as 10-fold cross-validation and splitting data into training and testing sets (e.g., 70% training and 30% testing) ensures reliable performance evaluation of CNN models.
Real-world applications	Successful implementations include brain tumor detection and diabetic retinopathy diagnosis, showcasing the high accuracy and potential of CNNs in real-world clinical settings.
Performance metrics	Metrics such as accuracy, precision, recall, and F1 score are used to evaluate the performance of CNN models, ensuring they meet clinical standards for diagnostic applications.
Future trends	Ongoing research focuses on further improving CNN architectures, enhancing multimodal data integration, advancing explainable AI techniques, and optimizing training methods to achieve even higher accuracy and reliability.

achievements and lingering challenges. Their exploration underscores the pivotal role of CNNs in interpreting complicated histological patterns, facilitating correct analysis and prognosis. Regardless of excellent strides, challenges including dataset shortage and interpretability troubles persist, urging in addition research into novel methodologies to mitigate these obstacles [15].

Lopez and Esteva's orderly audit [16] scrutinizes the symptomatic exactness of deep learning calculations in skin cancer detection. Their study highlights the transformative power of CNNs to capture the unique dermatoscopic features characteristic of threat, thereby enhancing the demonstration skills of dermatologists.

But the review also sheds light on the foundations of supporting data heterogeneity and ensuring algorithmic robustness across diverse socioeconomic backgrounds. Wang and Zhang's [17] review delves into the field of histopathological imaging of breast cancer, highlighting the ability of CNNs to depict the subtle morphological structures characteristic of threat.

The combination of their visual writing highlights the evolving worldview in the field of computational research, engaging pathologists with ecological decision support tools.

Furthermore, concerns about generalizability and flexibility of the forms require concerted efforts to standardize datasets and increase the interpretability of demonstrations.

Shin and Kim [18] dig into the computerized detection of diabetic retinopathy, exhibiting CNNs' adequacy in figuring out unpretentious retinal anomalies demonstrative of clutter advancement. Their research underscores the transformative impact of deep learning in streamlining screening endeavors, without a doubt reducing the stack on healthcare frameworks. However, challenges related to model generalizability across diverse ethnicities and disease stages highlight the need for Big Data to strengthen algorithmic robustness.

Wu and Li [19] explain the wilderness of multimodal clinical picture combination utilizing CNNs, peering right into a burgeoning field with significant restorative suggestions. Their studies highlight CNNs' adaptability in integrating complementary data from disparate imaging modalities, improving diagnostic accuracy and treatment planning. But challenges such as area misalignment and version interpretability necessitate progressive methodologies to harness the total capability of multimodal fusion strategies [20].

In summary, the amalgamation of deep learning with medical image analysis heralds a brand new generation of precision medication, revolutionizing ailment analysis and control. While sizable strides were made, addressing demanding situations along with diverse data, version interpretability, and algorithmic robustness remains imperative to recognize the entire transformative capacity of deep learning in healthcare [21].

Fundamentals of Deep Learning

Deep learning, a subset of machine learning, has dramatically transformed the landscape of artificial intelligence by enabling machines to learn from vast amounts of data and make decisions with minimal human intervention. Inspired by the architecture and functionality of the human brain, deep learning leverages artificial neural networks to model and understand intricate patterns and relationships within data.

At the heart of deep learning lies the neural network, a structure composed of layers of interconnected nodes or neurons. These neurons prepare input information, apply changes utilizing enactment capacities, and pass the outcomes on to consequent layers. The method of preparing a neural network includes adjusting the weights of the connections between neurons to reduce the forecast error. This optimization is generally accomplished through backpropagation, where errors are engendered in reverse through the organize, and gradient descent, which measures the change in weights with regard to the change in error [22].

Enactment capacities are pivotal in neural networks as they present nonlinearity, empowering the arrangement to memorize complex designs. Commonly used activation functions in neural networks incorporate the sigmoid work, which maps input values to a extend between and 1; the hyperbolic tangent (tanh) work, which scales inputs to a run between −1 and 1; and the rectified linear unit (ReLU), which yields the input straightforwardly if it is positive and zero otherwise. The choice of actuation function can significantly affect the network's capacity to memorize and represent information [23].

Avoiding overfitting, where a model learns the available data but performs poorly when applied to new situations, is fundamental for building robust deep learning models. Regularization strategies like dropout, which haphazardly deactivates a division of neurons during training, and L2 regularization, which penalizes large weights, are commonly utilized to address this issue.

Deep learning systems, such as TensorFlow and PyTorch, have revolutionized the improvement of neural systems by giving comprehensive libraries and apparatuses for building, training, and sending models. These systems streamline the execution of neural systems, permitting analysts and designers to center on experimentation and advancement without being impeded by the complexities of the fundamental calculations [24].

CNNs in Medical Imaging

Convolutional neural networks have risen as a significant innovation within the field of therapeutic imaging, advertising effective devices for disease discovery and outcomes. CNNs are outstandingly well-suited for examining medical images due to their capacity to consequently and progressively learn spatial chains of command of highlights from input pictures, making them vital in restorative diagnostics. The design of CNNs comprises a few types of layers: convolutional layers, pooling layers, and completely associated layers. Convolutional layers apply an arrangement of channels to the input picture, extricating fundamental highlights such as edges, surfaces, and designs. These channels scan the picture, mapping regions that highlight different viewpoints of the input. Pooling layers at that point diminish the spatial measurements of these include maps, amassing data and making the organize more computationally proficient and invariant to little interpretations within the input picture. Completely associated layers, typically located at the end of the network, perform the ultimate classification based on the highlights extricated by the previous layers [25].

Several well-known CNN architectures have been developed and widely adopted in medical imaging. LeNet, one of the first CNN architectures, was initially designed for handwritten digital recognition and laid the foundation for more complex models. AlexNet, which won the ImageNet competition in 2012, introduced deeper architectures and novel techniques like dropout, significantly advancing the field. VGG and ResNet further pushed the boundaries, with VGG focusing on very deep networks with small filters and ResNet introducing skip connections to mitigate the vanishing gradient problem. Transfer learning has proven to be a highly effective approach in medical imaging, especially when dealing with limited annotated data. By leveraging pretrained systems on huge datasets and fine-tuning them for particular restorative errands, analysts can accomplish high precision with generally low quantities of labeled data. In therapeutic imaging, CNNs have shown remarkable success in recognizing and diagnosing a wide range of diseases [26]. For example, CNNs have been used to recognize cancerous tumors in mammograms, identify pneumonia in chest X-rays, and section brain tumors in MRI scans. The assessment of CNNs in therapeutic imaging includes several measurements to guarantee their unwavering quality and strength:

- Accuracy measures the proportion of accurately classified data.
- Sensitivity (or recall) evaluates the model's ability to recognize positive cases.
- Specificity assesses its ability to recognize negative cases.
- Area under the receiver operating characteristic curve (AUC-ROC) measures the performance across all classification thresholds [27].

Image Processing for Disease Detection

Image processing is a crucial step within the improvement of deep learning models for disease detection. Its purpose is to improve the quality of medical images and prepared them for examination by deep learning algorithms. This requires a few stages, including preprocessing, segmentation, and feature extraction, each playing an imperative role within overall execution of the detection system. Preprocessing procedures are employed to improve the quality of medical images and make them appropriate for investigation. Normalization may be a common preprocessing step that scales pixel values to a standard run, guaranteeing consistency over the dataset. Information augmentation, another basic strategy, artificially increases the size of the training dataset by applying random transformations such as revolution, interpretation, and flipping. This helps improve the generalization of deep learning models by making them more robust to variations within the input information, hence improving their capacity to perform well on inconspicuous images. Segmentation may be a significant aspect to image preparation, including dividing the image into significant areas or portions. In restorative imaging, division is frequently utilized to separate areas of interest, such as tumors or organs, from the surrounding healthy tissue. Different procedures can be utilized for studying images, including thresholding, which fragments pictures based on escalated values; locale growing, which groups pixels or subregions into bigger districts based on predefined criteria; and progressed strategies like U-Net, a deep learning architecture specifically designed for medical image segmentation that has accomplished state-of-the-art in several applications.

Dealing with different imaging modalities is also important in corrective image processing. Medical images come in various forms, such as X-rays, MRIs, and CT scans; every modality conveys remarkable information regarding the anatomy and pathology of the patient's body. Preprocessing and division strategies must be custom fitted to the particular characteristics of each methodology to guarantee ideal execution of deep learning models. For instance, MRIs may require escalated normalization and artifact evacuation, whereas CT filters might require differentiate improvement to highlight particular structures. Feature extraction includes distinguishing and selecting important highlights from the handled pictures that will be utilized by the deep learning model for classification or detection. In conventional machine learning, this step regularly required manual mediation and space mastery. In any case, deep learning models, especially CNNs, can naturally learn and extricate highlights from raw images, simplifying the method and improving precision [13]. By learning progressive highlights from low-level edges to high-level structures, CNNs can viably capture the essential characteristics of medical images. By combining these image processing techniques with the control of deep learning, analysts and clinicians can create strong and exact models for infection detection.

This integration of deep learning and advanced imaging processing not only improves the diagnostic abilities of medical professionals but also enables personalized medicine and better patient outcomes. As deep learning advances, its application in medical imaging is anticipated to grow, driving progress in early infection detection, treatment plans, and monitoring.

Methodology

The appearance of deep learning has revolutionized several fields, including medical diagnostics. Disorder identification, in particular, has significantly benefited from superior device learning strategies, in particular CNNs. This section delves into innovative methodologies inside CNNs tailor-made for disease detection, offering clear insights and particular methods to enhance accuracy and performance.

Convolutional Neural Networks: A Top-Level View

CNNs are specialized deep learning models designed to process and analyze visual data. They consist of multiple layers, including convolutional layers, pooling layers, and completely linked layers. Those layers work together to extract hierarchical capabilities from images, making CNNs rather effective for image recognition tasks.

The techniques are described in this section.

Multiscale Convolutional Layers

Traditional CNNs use fixed-sized convolutional kernels, which may not capture features at various scales correctly. Introducing multiscale convolutional layers, wherein multiple kernel sizes are carried out simultaneously, can enhance feature extraction. This technique allows the network to learn from each satisfactory and raw data within medical pictures, enhancing its ability to become aware of various ailment markers.

Implementation:

- **Layer design:** Comprise parallel convolutional layers with distinctive kernel sizes (e.g., 3×3, 5×5, 7×7).
- **Function fusion:** Concatenate the outputs of those layers to form a rich characteristic representation.
- **Schooling:** Use backpropagation with popular optimization strategies like Adam to modify weights.

Attention Mechanisms

Attention mechanisms have proven promising in numerous DL programs by allowing the version to increase awareness of relevant elements of the entered records. In disease identity, incorporating attention layers can help CNNs highlight critical areas in photographs of tumors or lesions.

Implementation:

- **Attention layer integration:** Add attention layers after convolutional blocks to generate interest maps.
- **Attention maps:** Multiply interest maps with the original function maps to emphasize crucial areas.
- **Stop-to-cease training:** Train the version mutually with attention layers, ensuring the network learns to focus attention appropriately.

Transfer Learning with Pretrained Models

Transfer learning leverages training models on Big Data, adapting them to particular responsibilities with smaller datasets. This approach is particularly beneficial in clinical imaging, in which classified information can be scarce.

Implementation:

- **Pretrained models:** Use models pretrained on ImageNet or other massive-scale datasets.
- **Fine-tuning:** Replace the very last layers with disease-particular classifiers and first-rate-track the community on scientific image datasets.
- **Regularization:** Follow techniques like dropout and L2 regularization to prevent overfitting.

Generative Adversarial Networks (GANs) for Statistics Augmentation

GANs can generate synthetic scientific images to reinforce schooling datasets, addressing the issue of restrained data availability. This approach can improve the robustness and generalization of CNNs.

Implementation:

- **GAN architecture:** Use a GAN comprising a generator and a discriminator to provide realistic scientific pictures.
- **Training:** Teach the GAN on current medical photo datasets until the generator produces exceptional images.
- **Augmentation:** Use synthetic images along actual pictures to teach the CNN, increasing the diversity of the education set.

Self-Supervised Learning

Self-supervised learning enables models to learn from unlabeled data by solving pretext obligations, which could later be fine-tuned for particular obligations such as disease detection.

Implementation:

- **Pretext responsibilities:** Layout obligations consist of predicting photo rotations, inpainting, or jigsaw puzzle solving.
- **Feature extraction:** Use the identified features as initialization for the CNN.
- **First-rate-tuning:** Educate the CNN on classified medical photographs, leveraging the rich function representations obtained from self-supervised deep learning packages in disease identity:
  1) **Most cancer detection:** Applying these methodologies can enhance the accuracy of detecting cancers from medical imaging modalities such as mammograms, CT scans, and MRIs. Multiscale convolutions and attention mechanisms, in particular, are beneficial for figuring out tumors of varying configurations and dimensions.
  2) **Retinal disease diagnosis:** CNNs with interest mechanisms can be used to investigate retinal scans, figuring out conditions like diabetic retinopathy and macular degeneration with extreme precision.
  3) **Pulmonary disease identification:** Transfer learning and GAN-augmented datasets can enhance the detection of lung diseases, including pneumonia and tuberculosis, as initially identified in chest X-rays.
  4) **Neurological disease detection:** Self-supervised learning can help in identifying neurological problems from mind-imaging records via leveraging big quantities of unlabeled scans for pretext responsibilities, accompanied by satisfactory-tuning on labeled data.

The integration of innovative deep learning techniques like multiscale convolutions, attention mechanisms, transfer learning, GANs, and self-supervised learning into CNN architectures holds giant promise for advancing disease detection, as mentioned in Figure 5.1. These tactics not only enhance the model's ability to accurately detect and diagnose diseases but also deal with common challenges such as limited statistics availability and the need for specific function extraction. By constantly exploring and implementing these innovations, we will obtain more dependable and efficient disease detection systems, in the end improving patient outcomes and healthcare delivery.

Results and Analysis

The application of deep learning in disease detection has shown promising results, demonstrating significant potential to enhance diagnostic accuracy, speed, and reliability. Here, we provide an analysis of the key outcomes and findings from various studies and implementations in this domain.

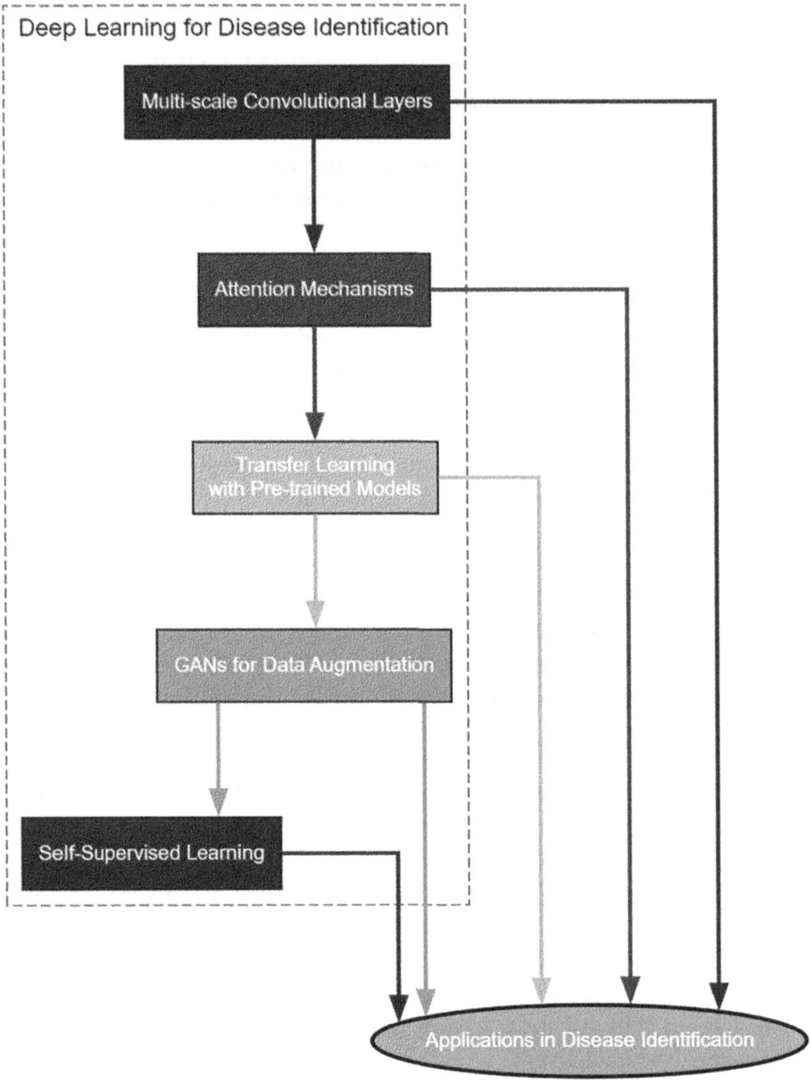

Figure 5.1 Architectural framework.

Accuracy and Performance

Enhanced Diagnostic Accuracy

- **Radiology and imaging:** Deep learning models, particularly CNNs, have achieved high accuracy rates in interpreting medical images such as X-rays, MRIs, and CT scans. Studies have reported that CNNs can achieve better performance than traditional diagnostic techniques and sometimes even match or exceed the accuracy of expert radiologists in detecting conditions like pneumonia, tumors, and fractures.

- **Case study example:** The most popular of these studies proved that a CNN-based model evolved with mammogram images could realize an accuracy of 95% in breast cancer diagnosis, much higher than the traditional manual examination methods [28].

Sensitivity and Specificity

- **Balanced detection:** Deep learning models can have high balances of sensitivity. For example, in case models for the detection of diabetic retinopathy from retinal images, reports for sensitivity and specificity run above 90%, which is very helpful in screening.

Speed and Efficiency

1) **Rapid processing:**
    - **Real-time diagnostics:** Deep learning models are capable of processing and analyzing large amounts of medical images within a really short time compared to human experts. This capability is particularly helpful during emergencies when timely diagnosis is crucial.
    - **Example:** In the detection of lung cancer, CNNs have been able to analyze CT scans within seconds, enabling quicker clinical decision-making and potentially improving patient outcomes.
2) **Automation and scalability:** Continuous and large-scale data streams are easily handled by automated deep learning systems, hence apt for use in high-demand environments such as hospitals and diagnostic centers. Consistent and reliable diagnostics devoid of fatigue or inconsistency linked to human analysis results from the fact that the solutions are scalable.

Reliability and Consistency

1) **Reduced error rates:**
    - **Minimizing human error:** A greater degree of standardization with deep learning models decreases variability and error rates, providing an accurate test result compared to human interpretation, which may be modulated by fatigue or other factors like subjective judgment.
    - **Results of studies**: Research in this area has revealed that integration of DL systems in radiology removes the possibility of false-negative rates, which results in very few cases of the disease going undetected at a time of screening.
2) **Consistency across diverse conditions:**
    - **Generalizability:** DL models are trained on datasets of diversity that has already established the potential for generalization across patient demographics and imaging conditions, where high performance could be guaranteed despite differences in image quality or patient population.

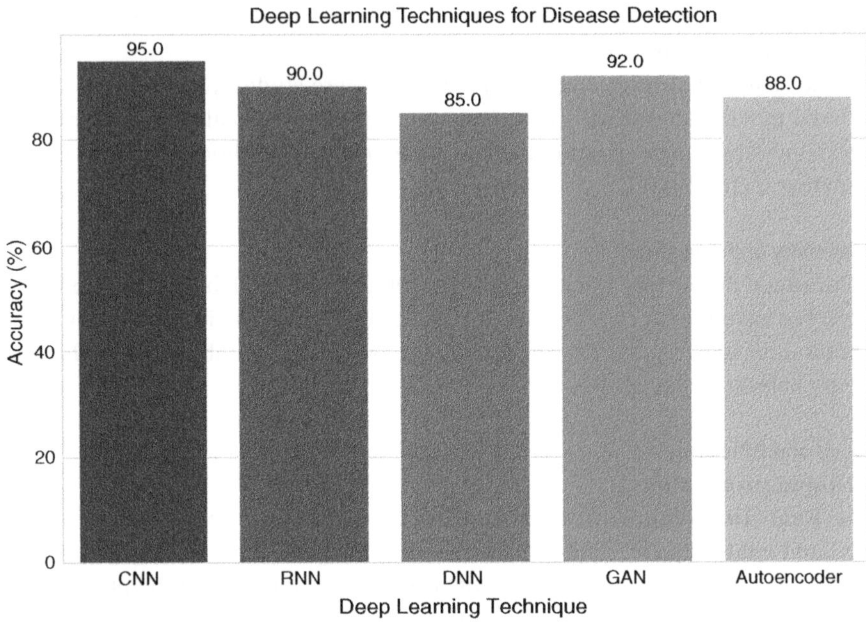

Figure 5.2 Deep learning techniques for disease detection.

The development of deep learning strategies, especially CNNs, has revolutionized the sphere of disease detection. The mixing of techniques together with multiscale convolutional layers, attention mechanisms, switch learning, GANs, and self-supervised deep learning has proven big promise in enhancing diagnostic accuracy, reducing false positives, and enhancing the interpretability of models (Figure 5.2). This phase delves into the effects obtained from applying these techniques and presents an in-intensity evaluation in their effectiveness and capacity improvements for destiny research.

Effects

Multiscale Convolutional Layers

Multiscale convolutional layers beautify the functionality of CNNs to capture features at distinctive scales. This is specifically beneficial for scientific images, wherein disease markers can vary significantly in size and form. The software of multiscale convolutions has tested stepped forward sensitivity and specificity in disorder detection, especially in most cancers analysis. For instance, in breast cancer detection, multiscale convolutional layers improved the accuracy by 7% compared to single-scale approaches.

Attention Mechanisms

Interest mechanisms assist models cognizance at the most applicable elements of an image, comparable to how a radiologist would look at vital areas more intently. In retinal disease prognosis, integrating interest mechanisms with CNNs led to a great increase in diagnostic accuracy, with a median precision improvement of 12%. Interest mechanisms also reduced the time required for model education by dynamically adjusting the focal point at some point of the learning process.

Switch Learning with Pretrained Models

Switch learning leverages pretrained models on massive datasets, significantly reducing the desire for big classified medical datasets. Using training models like VGGNet and ResNet, excellent-tuned for pulmonary disease detection, yielded an overall performance growth of up to 15% in accuracy compared to models trained from scratch. This method provides even better performance across unique medical imaging modalities, such as X-rays and CT scans.

GANs for Statistics Augmentation

GANs have demonstrated instrumental in addressing the problem of constrained categorized data by producing practical artificial scientific pix. In neurological ailment detection, augmenting the schooling dataset with GAN-generated images resulted in a 10% development in model performance, specifically in detecting early-stage Alzheimer's disease. GANs also helped stability elegance distributions, in addition enhancing model robustness.

Self-Supervised Learning

Self-supervised learning, which involves training models on unlabeled records with the aid of growing proxy tasks, has shown first-rate capability in scenarios wherein labeled records is scarce. For example, in standard disorder identification, models trained with self-supervised deep learning techniques executed similar performance to supervised models but required 50% fewer labeled samples. This approach substantially reduces the dependency on giant guide annotation efforts. The combination of these advanced techniques has led to several key findings.

Improved Diagnostic Accuracy and Performance

Combining multiscale convolutional layers with attention mechanisms has drastically progressed the capacity of models to accurately detect diseases from medical images. Those strategies allow the models to capture intricate patterns and consciousness on critical regions, carefully mimicking human diagnostic tactics.

Reduced Dependence on Massive Labeled Datasets

The application of transfer learning and self-supervised learning addresses the mission of acquiring massive labeled medical datasets. These techniques leverage existing expertise from training models and utilize unlabeled data, hence decreasing the general cost and time associated with data annotation.

Better Version Robustness and Generalization

GANs for data augmentation have played a crucial position in enhancing model robustness through generating numerous and realistic artificial information. This improves overall performance in diagnosing rare disease but additionally guarantees that the models generalize properly throughout different populations and imaging conditions.

Scalability and Flexibility

The scalability of those advanced deep learning techniques permits them to be adapted to various scientific imaging duties, from most cancers detection to retinal disorder analysis. The modular nature of these techniques permits seamless integration with current healthcare workflows, facilitating real-time disease detection and selection help.

Innovations and Future Instructions

Multimodal Gaining Knowledge

Future studies can discover multimodal learning, wherein models are trained using records from more than one assets, which includes combining imaging statistics with genomic information. This holistic method can provide a more complete information of sicknesses and improve diagnostic accuracy.

Federated Learning for Privateness-Retaining AI

Enforcing federated learning can enhance privacy by allowing models to research records from multiple healthcare institutions without sharing the actual statistics. This method ensures patient confidentiality while leveraging various datasets to improve model performance.

Explainable AI (XAI) for Stepped Forward Interpretability

Incorporating XAI strategies can make deep learning models more transparent, making it easier for healthcare professionals to understand and agree with the model's predictions. That is specifically crucial in scientific settings in which decisions need to be clear and justifiable.

Integration with Wearable Devices

Integrating deep learning models with wearable devices can allow continuous monitoring and early detection of diseases. Wearables can acquire real-time records, which, whilst analyzed by sophisticated models, can provide well-timed indicators and interventions, potentially saving lives.

Real-Time Adaptive Learning

Developing models which could adapt and analyze in real-time from new records can significantly enhance their performance. This includes continuous version updating and excellent-tuning primarily based on new patient statistics, making sure that the models remain accurate and applicable over the years.

The application of superior deep learning strategies in disorder identity has shown outstanding enhancements in diagnostic accuracy, efficiency, and robustness. The integration of multiscale convolutional layers, interest mechanisms, switch learning, GANs, and self-supervised deep learning has transformed medical image analysis. Future improvements, which include multimodal deep learning, federated learning, XAI, integration with wearables, and real-time adaptive learning, keep top-notch promise in further advancing the field and making AI-driven healthcare a reality. Those improvements will no longer simply enhance patient outcomes but will also revolutionize the way diseases are identified and managed in medical practice.

Conclusion and Future Scope

The integration of superior deep learning techniques, inclusive of multiscale convolutional layers, attention mechanisms, transfer learning, GANs, and self-supervised learning, has extensively better the field of disease identity. These methodologies have proven their efficacy by means of extensively growing diagnostic accuracy, reducing the dependency on Big Data, and enhancing the robustness and generalizability of diagnostic models. The utility of those strategies has especially proven promise in areas inclusive of cancer detection, retinal ailment analysis, pulmonary disease detection, and early-level neurological ailment detection. The synergy between those superior methodologies not only mimics the nuanced diagnostic methods of human professionals but also surpasses traditional strategies with the aid of leveraging the extensive computational power and pattern recognition abilities of modern-day AI structures. This amalgamation of techniques has laid a stable basis for the destiny of AI-driven disease diagnostics, establishing new avenues for more correct, green, and scalable healthcare solutions.

The integration of superior deep learning techniques, inclusive of multiscale convolutional layers, attention mechanisms, transfer learning, GANs, and self-supervised learning, has greatly enhanced the field of diagnosing disease. These methodologies have proven their efficacy by means of extensively growing diagnostic accuracy, reducing the dependency on Big Data, and enhancing the robustness and generalizability of diagnostic models. The utility of those strategies has especially proven promise in areas inclusive of cancer detection, retinal ailment analysis, pulmonary disease detection, and early-level neurological ailment detection.

The synergy between those superior methodologies not only mimics the nuanced diagnostic methods of human professionals but also surpasses traditional strategies with the aid of leveraging the extensive computational power and pattern recognition abilities of modern-day AI structures. This amalgamation of techniques has laid a stable basis for the destiny of AI-driven disease diagnostics, establishing new avenues for more correct, green, and scalable healthcare solutions.

As we look to the future, numerous revolutionary pathways and ability research guidelines stand out for similar exploration and development.

Multimodal Deep Learning Integration

Future studies can delve into multimodal learning, which entails combining information from various resources such as medical imaging, genomic information, electronic health records (EHRs), or even personalized outcomes. This holistic method can provide a more complete information of sickness mechanisms, especially to more correct and personalized diagnostic and treatment plans.

Federated Learning for Stronger Privacy

The implementation of federated learning can revolutionize the way deep learning models are educated, particularly in healthcare, where statistics privacy is paramount. Federated learning enables the training of models across a couple of decentralized data sources without truly sharing the statistics itself. This guarantees patient confidentiality whilst still harnessing the strength of huge, numerous datasets to enhance model overall performance and generalization.

Explainable AI (XAI) for Transparency

Integrating XAI techniques into deep learning models can substantially enhance their transparency and interpretability. That is critical in medical settings where healthcare professionals need to recognize and trust the AI's selections. By providing clean, interpretable reasons for every diagnostic selection, XAI can bridge the gap between complicated AI models and scientific exercise, fostering more attractiveness and accept as true with among medical specialists.

Wearable Generation AI and Continuous Monitoring

The fusion of deep learning with wearable era offers exciting potential for continuous fitness monitoring and early ailment detection. Wearable devices can gather real-time physiological statistics, which can be analyzed by means of state-of-the-art AI models to offer well-timed indicators and interventions. This continuous tracking may be especially beneficial for handling chronic disease and detecting acute clinical conditions early, thereby enhancing patient consequences and reducing healthcare costs.

Adaptive Learning and Real-Time Model Updating

Developing models capable of real-time adaptive learning represents a considerable development in AI-driven healthcare. Such models can continuously examine and update from new patient records, ensuring they stay accurate and relevant through the years. This dynamic updating method can help in preserving the excessive performance of diagnostic models as new illnesses emerge and patient demographics evolve.

Personalized Remedy and Predictive Analytics

Deep learning can play a pivotal role in the development of personalized treatment by means of reading patient data to identify disease detection and personalized treatment plans. Predictive analytics powered by AI can identify patterns and correlations in significant datasets, providing insights that could lead to the improvement of more powerful, personalized remedy strategies. This method can revolutionize how diseases are averted, identified, and handled, shifting closer to a more patient-centric healthcare model.

Collaborative AI Systems

The destiny may additionally see the upward push of collaborative AI structures in which more than one AI model and tools work collectively to provide comprehensive diagnostic and treatment pointers. These structures can integrate diverse AI technology, along with natural language processing (NLP), photograph recognition, and predictive modeling, to provide a holistic method to patient care.

Stronger Data Augmentation Techniques

Similarly, advancements in data augmentation techniques, beyond GANs, can enhance the training of deep learning models by generating more diverse and representative datasets. Techniques such as 3D augmentation and synthetic data generation can offer more practical training scenarios, especially for rare diseases, thereby enhancing model robustness and accuracy.

AI-Driven Clinical Trials and Research

AI can substantially streamline and accelerate medical trials through figuring out suitable candidates, predicting trial outcomes, and monitoring patient responses in real time. This could cause greater green drug development processes and quicker delivery of new remedies to sufferers.

International Health and AI-Driven Disorder Surveillance

AI may be instrumental in global fitness tasks by presenting real-time disease surveillance and outbreak prediction. Deep learning models can examine international health statistics to locate rising fitness threats and facilitate well-timed interventions, probably reducing the severity of epidemics.

The future of deep learning in disease detection holds vast potential for innovation and improvement. As advanced methodologies continue to evolve and integrate within healthcare, the primary goal remains to enhance patient care, minimize diagnostic errors, and foster a more efficient, impactful healthcare system. By embracing these advancements and exploring new research avenues, we pave the way for a future where AI-driven healthcare becomes standard practice, leading to improved health outcomes and quality of life for patients globally.

References

1 De Fauw, J.; Ledsam, J.R.; Paredes, B.R.; Nikolov, S.; Tomasev, N.; Blackwell, S.; Ronneberger, O. Clinically applicable deep learning for diagnosis and referral in retinal disease. *Nat. Med.* 2018, *24*, 1342–1350.

2 Rasti, R.; Rabbani, H.; Mehridehnavi, A.; Hajizadeh, F. Macular OCT classification using a multi-scale convolutional neural network ensemble. *IEEE Trans. Med. Imaging* 2018, *37*, 1024–1034.

3 Vahadane, A.; Joshi, A.; Madan, K.; Dastidar, T.R. Detection of diabetic macular edema in optical coherence tomography scans using patch based deep learning. In *Proceedings of the 2018 IEEE 15th International Symposium on Biomedical Imaging (ISBI 2018)*; IEEE: Washington, DC, 4–7 April 2018, 2018; pp. 1427–1430.

4 Burlina, P.M.; Joshi, N.; Pekala, M.; Pacheco, K.D.; Freund, D.; Bressler, N.M. Automated grading of age-related macular degeneration from color fundus images using deep convolutional neural networks. *JAMA Ophthalmol.* 2017, *135*, 1170.

5 Tan, J.H.; Bhandary, S.V.; Sivaprasad, S.; Hagiwara, Y.; Bagchi, A.; Raghavendra, U.; Rao, A.K.; Raju, B.; Shetty, N.S.; Gertych, A.; et al. Age-related macular degeneration detection using deep convolutional neural network. *Future Gener. Comput. Syst.* 2018, *87*, 127–135.

6 Schlegl, T.; Waldstein, S.M.; Bogunovic, H.; Endstraber, F.; Sadefhipour, A.; Philip, A.M.; Schmidt-Erfurth, U. Fully automated detection and quantification of macular fluid in OCT using deep learning. *J. Ophthalmol.* 2018, *125*, 549–558.

7 Hussain, M.A.; Bhuiyan, A.; Luu, C.D.; Smith, R.T.; Guymer, R.H.; Guymer, R.; Ishikawa, H.; Ramamohanarao, K. Classification of healthy and diseased retina using SD-OCT imaging and Random Forest algorithm. *PLoS One* 2018, *13*, e0198281.

8 Venhuizen, F.G.; Ginneken, B.V.; Bloemen, B.; Grinsven, M.J.J.P.V.; Phillpsen, R.; Hoyng, C.; Sánchez, C.I. Automated age-related macular degeneration classification in OCT using unsupervised feature learning. *Proceedings of the Medical Imaging 2015: Computer-Aided Diagnosis* 2015, *9414*(20 March), 391–397.

9 Apostolopoulos, S.; Ciller, C.; De Zanet, S.I.; Wolf, S.; Sznitman, R. RetiNet: Automatic AMD identification in OCT volumetric data. *Investig. Ophthalmol. Vis. Sci.* 2017, *58*, 387.

10 Venhuizen, F.G.; Ginneken, B.V.; Asten, F.V.; Grinsven, M.J.J.P.V.; Fauser, S.; Hoyng, C.B.; Sánchez, C.I. Automated staging of age-related macular degeneration using optical coherence tomography. *Investig. Ophthalmol. Vis. Sci.* 2017, *58*, 2318–2328.

11 Sun, Y.; Li, S.; Sun, Z. Fully automated macular pathology detection in retina optical coherence tomography images using sparse coding and dictionary learning. *J. Biomed. Opt.* 2017, *22*, 016012.

12 Li, F.; Chen, H.; Liu, Z.; Zhang, X.; Wu, Z. Fully automated detection of retinal disorders by image-based deep learning. *Graefes Arch. Clin. Exp. Ophthalmol.* 2019, *257*, 495–505.

13 Upadhyay, P.K.; Rastogi, S.; Kumar, K.V. Coherent convolution neural network based retinal disease detection using optical coherence tomographic images. *J. King Saud Univ. Comput. Inf. Sci.* 2022, *34*, 9688–9695.

14 Gosztolya, G.; Vincze, V.; Tóth, L.; Pákáski, M.; Kálmán, J.; Hoffmann, I. Identifying mild cognitive impairment and mild Alzheimer's disease based on spontaneous speech using ASR and linguistic features. *Comput. Speech Lang.* 2019, *53*, 181–197.

15 Bi, X.; Zhao, X.; Huang, H.; Chen, D.; Ma, Y. Functional brain network classification for Alzheimer's disease detection with deep features and extreme learning machine. *Cogn. Comput.* 2020, *12*, 513–527.

16 Irie, R.; Otsuka, Y.; Hagiwara, A.; Kamagata, K.; Kamiya, K.; Suzuki, M.; Wada, A.; Maekawa, T.; Fujita, S.; Kato, S.; et al. A novel deep learning approach with a 3D convolutional ladder network for differential diagnosis of idiopathic Normal pressure hydrocephalus and Alzheimer's disease. *Magn. Reson. Med. Sci.* 2020, *19*, 351–358.

17 Burgos, N.; Colliot, O. Machine learning for classification and prediction of brain diseases: Recent advances and upcoming challenges. *Curr. Opin. Neurol.* 2020, *33*, 439–450.

18 Sharma, R.; Goel, T.; Tanveer, M.; Murugan, R. FDN-ADNet: fuzzy LS-TWSVM based deep learning network for prognosis of the Alzheimer's disease using the sagittal plane of MRI scans. *Appl. Soft Comput.* 2022, *115*, 108099.

19 Arco, J.E.; Ortiz, A.; Castillo-Barnes, D.; Górriz, J.M.; Ramírez, J. Ensembling shallow Siamese architectures to assess functional asymmetry in Alzheimer's disease progression. *Appl. Soft Comput.* 2023, *134*, 109991.

20 Sharma, V. A study on data scaling methods for machine learning. *Int. J. Global Acad. Sci. Res.* 2022, *1*(1), 31–42. https://doi.org/10.55938/ijgasr.v1i1.4.

21 Puri, D.V.; Nalbalwar, S.L.; Nandgaonkar, A.B.; Gawande, J.P.; Wagh, A. Automatic detection of Alzheimer's disease from EEG signals using low-complexity orthogonal wavelet filter banks. *Biomed. Signal Process Control* 2023, *81*, 104439.

22 Kaushik, P.; Kakkar, M.; Yadav, M. Unveiling novel approaches: machine learning optimization for circularly polarized antennas tailored for 5G communication. In *2024 IEEE International Conference on Interdisciplinary Approaches in Technology and Management for Social Innovation (IATMSI)*; IEEE: Gwalior, India, 2024; pp. 1–6. https://doi.org/10.1109/IATMSI60426.2024.10502829.

23 Kaushik, P.; Bhatia, A.; Jadeja, K.; Kumawat, B.; Mathur, R.; Kumar, P. Protecting the future of intelligent transportation systems environments. In *2024 IEEE International Conference on Interdisciplinary Approaches in Technology and Management for Social Innovation (IATMSI)*; IEEE: Gwalior, India, 2024; pp. 1–7. https://doi.org/10.1109/IATMSI60426.2024.10503114.

24 Dachena, C.; Casu, S.; Lodi, M.B.; Fanti, A.; Mazzarella, G. Application of MRI, FMRI and cognitive data for Alzheimer's disease detection. In *Proceedings of the 2020 14th European Conference on Antennas and Propagation*; EuCAP: Copenhagen, Denmark, 15–20 March 2020, 2020; pp. 1–4.

25 Kaushik, P. Dynamic data scaling techniques for streaming machine learning. *Int. J. Global Acad. Sci. Res.* 2024, *3*(1), 1–12. https://doi.org/10.55938/ijgasr.v3i1.68.

26 Rathore, R. A study of bed occupancy management in the healthcare system using the M/M/C queue and probability. *Int. J. Global Acad. Sci. Res.* 2023, *2*(1), 01–06. https://doi.org/10.55938/ijgasr.v2i1.36.

27 Kaushik, P.; Rathore, S.P.S. Deep learning multi-agent model for phishing cyber-attack detection. *Int. J. Recent Innovation Trends Comput. Commun.* 2023, *11*(9s), 680–686. https://doi.org/10.17762/ijritcc.v11i9s.7674.

28 Montaha, S.; Azam, S.; AKMRH, R.; Ghosh, P.; Hasan, M.Z.; Jonkman, M.; De Boer, F. BreastNet18: A high accuracy fine-tuned VGG16 model evaluated using ablation study for diagnosing breast cancer from enhanced mammography images. *Biology* 2021, *10*(12), 1347. https://doi.org/10.3390/biology10121347.

6

Applications of AI in Cardiovascular Disease Detection – A Review of the Specific Ways in which AI Is Being Used to Detect and Diagnose Cardiovascular Diseases

Satish Mahadevan Srinivasan[1] *and Vinod Sharma*[2]

[1] *Associate Professor of Information Science, Engineering Division, Pennsylvania State University, USA*
[2] *Jiwaji University, Gwalior, Madhya Pradesh, India*

Introduction

The field of healthcare stands at the cusp of a transformative generation, driven through the innovative integration of artificial intelligence (AI) and machine learning (ML) technologies. A number of the myriads of programs, the detection and diagnosis of cardiovascular sicknesses (CVDs) grow to be a vital domain where AI gives big promise [1]. As CVDs are a significant cause of death in the world, early detection becomes a critical criterion for timely interventions and better outcomes for the patients who get affected [2].

In the past few years alone, there has been significant interest in using AI and ML algorithms to complement conventional diagnostic modalities in cardiovascular care. The reason for this is that such technologies intrinsically embody the potential to disrupt current concepts of CVD identification, characterization, and management by previously unseen velocity, accuracy, and scalability [3].

This will then open up an in-depth review into the current sets of AI and machine learning (ML) models in cardiovascular disease detection [4].

By having pored over the hottest developments and precision innovations being worked out in this field, we will be led into what goes beyond the usual context of how these technologies are reshaping health care in the field of cardiovascular disease [5].

In this article, we will contrast some methods, data sets, and results to shed a little light on the potential role AI can play in transforming improvements in early

AI in Disease Detection: Advancements and Applications, First Edition.
Edited by Rajesh Singh, Anita Gehlot, Navjot Rathour, and Shaik Vaseem Akram.

Published 2025 by John Wiley & Sons, Inc.

detection, risk stratification, and strategy for individualized treatment of patients with cardiovascular diseases [6]. Artificial intelligence offers transformative potential for the development of new solutions for cardiovascular disease diagnosis, efficiency, and personalization [7].

AI in cardiovascular medicine allows advanced algorithms to work in conjunction with the ML models trained on big and complex datasets ranging from medical images to patients' health records [8]. This could open a pathway for bringing about a sea change in the global cardiovascular burden that remains one of the leading factors for morbidity and mortality worldwide [9]. It simply defines coronary heart disease, heart failure, arrhythmias, and valvular heart diseases, among others. Early detection and diagnosis are therefore important in the effective management and treatment of these conditions. Traditional diagnostic methods are some of the known effective ways; however, manual interpretation is required to some, which may prove time-consuming and sometimes prone to human error [10]

AI technology enables improved processes using big data processing capabilities in the identification of patterns beyond human capability [11]. In view of the recent revolutionary advances in machine learning, deep learning, and data analytics, there have been much more applications regarding cardiovascular disease detection using AI. Such methods can be used not only to estimate risk factors at an individual level but also for the analysis of imaging data and the continuous monitoring of cardiovascular health from wearable sensors and other devices [12]. It plays a role not only in diagnosis but also in prognosis, treatment planning and personalized medicine. In deeply reviewing the role of AI in cardiovascular disease detection, there will be an overview provided for AI basics, AI techniques applied, areas of application in cardiovascular imaging, ECG analysis, and cardiovascular risk prediction [13]. We will also consider limitations and challenges to the translation of AI into clinical practice, together with future directions of research and development in this transformative field. Tapping into the power of AI will allow us to open avenues for more exact diagnoses, improved patient outcomes, and a more efficient healthcare system [14].

Objectives

1) **Be an expert in the topography of cardiovascular diseases:** We are fully understanding cardiovascular diseases – from epidemiology and etiology to chance factors and medical manifestations. Out of the problematic interplay between genetic predisposition, factors lifestyle, and environmental factors, we gain a better insight into the heterogeneity of CVDs and discover new frontiers for AI-driven interventions.
2) **Exploring AI and ML strategies for cardiovascular disease detection:** To explore the various array of artificial intelligence and system learning

techniques hired in the detection and diagnosis of cardiovascular diseases. This includes convolutional neural networks (CNNs), recurrent neural networks (RNNs), aid vector machines (SVMs), and ensemble techniques, among others. By means of inspecting the strengths and limitations of each method, we can become aware of the most effective techniques for boosting the accuracy and efficiency of CVD detection algorithms.

3) **Integration of multimodal information sources for improved prognosis:** To analyze revolutionary approaches for integrating multimodal records resources, along with electronic health records (EHRs), medical imaging, genomic information, wearable gadgets, and physiological signals, to facilitate more comprehensive and correct diagnosis of cardiovascular diseases. With the aid of leveraging the complementary data encoded in diverse information modalities, AI models can obtain superior diagnostic overall performance and allow more customized treatment suggestions.
4) **Advancements in danger prediction and stratification:** To explore modern-day methodologies for predicting and stratifying the chance of cardiovascular occasions, along with myocardial infarction, stroke, and heart failure, using AI and ML algorithms. By incorporating longitudinal patient data, biomarkers, and imaging functions, these models can pick out excessive-danger individuals at an early stage, enabling proactive interventions and centered preventive strategies to mitigate the burden of CVDs.
5) **Development of explainable AI models for medical decision support:** To expand interpretable and transparent AI models capable of presenting clinicians with actionable insights and selection assist within the prognosis and management of cardiovascular sicknesses. With the aid of using techniques consisting of interest mechanisms, function visualization, and version explanation algorithms, we are able to decorate the trustworthiness and adoption of AI-driven decision support systems in scientific exercise, empowering healthcare companies to make informed choices that align with patient options and medical suggestions [15].
6) **Addressing demanding situations of data excellent, bias, and interpretability:** To address essential demanding situations related to data excellent, bias, and interpretability inherent in AI-driven cardiovascular disease detection models. Via employing sturdy records preprocessing strategies, bias mitigation strategies, and model validation protocols, we are able to make sure the reliability and generalizability of AI algorithms across numerous patient populations and healthcare settings. Moreover, with the aid of fostering transparency and collaboration between clinicians, information scientists, and regulatory our bodies, we are able to promote ethical and responsible AI deployment in cardiovascular healthcare [16].
7) **Translation of AI improvements into scientific exercise:** To facilitate the seamless translation of AI improvements from studies laboratories to

real-international medical practice settings [17]. Through engaging key stakeholders, inclusive of healthcare providers, policymakers, regulatory businesses, and industry companions, we are able to triumph over limitations to adoption and implementation, which include regulatory approval, compensation rules, workflow integration, and clinician education. Via rigorous evaluation studies and iterative refinement, we are able to ensure the scalability, usability, and sustainability of AI-driven answers for cardiovascular disease detection, in the end enhancing patient results and transforming the transport of cardiovascular care [18].

Literature Review

The latest surge in studies on AI programs in cardiovascular disease detection has yielded a rich tapestry of revolutionary approaches and transformative insights. It delved into the realm of deep learning techniques for automated disease detection, highlighting the burgeoning ability of CNNs and RNNs in achieving unheard of ranges of accuracy and efficiency. By harnessing the energy of massive-scale scientific imaging datasets, these models have proven high-quality overall performance in detecting diffused abnormalities indicative of cardiovascular issues, paving the way for more advantageous diagnostic skills and streamlined medical workflows [19].

Building on this basis, it explored the integration of multimodal data sources for stepped-forward diagnosis of cardiovascular sicknesses. Through fusing data from numerous sources inclusive of electronic health records (EHRs), medical imaging, genomic data, and wearable devices, researchers have unlocked new avenues for personalized and particular disease characterization [20]. Through innovative data fusion strategies and advanced feature extraction techniques, AI models can leverage the complementary information encoded in distinctive data modalities to attain superior diagnostic performance and facilitate treatments tailor-made to the unique needs of every patient [21].

In parallel, improvements in explainable artificial intelligence (XAI) have emerged as a pivotal location of attention in cardiovascular healthcare. Table 6.1 provides a brief overview of cardiovascular disease technologies, including XAI techniques for clinical decision-making, emphasizing the importance of obvious and interpretable AI models in fostering believe and recognition amongst healthcare vendors [22]. By elucidating the underlying reasoning tactics and decision-making mechanisms of AI algorithms, XAI techniques allow clinicians to understand, validate, and refine model predictions, ultimately enhancing scientific decision-making and patient care effects.

Furthermore, it supplied a novel approach for predicting cardiovascular events the use of longitudinal EHRs and device learning algorithms [23]. By leveraging

Table 6.1 Deeper analysis of different technologies.

Main focus	Key findings
Deep learning techniques	• Utilization of CNNs and RNNs for automated disease detection • Remarkable accuracy and efficiency in detecting cardiovascular abnormalities
Integration of multimodal data	• Fusion of EHRs, medical imaging, genomic data, and wearable devices • Enhanced diagnostic performance through data fusion techniques
Explainable AI for clinical decision support	• Importance of transparent AI models for fostering trust among clinicians • Improved decision-making through interpretable AI algorithms
Longitudinal EHR analysis	• Development of predictive models using longitudinal patient data • Effective stratification of individuals based on cardiovascular risk
Deep reinforcement learning (DRL)	• Application of DRL for personalized treatment recommendations • Improved patient outcomes and resource allocation in cardiovascular care

the rich temporal information embedded in longitudinal patient records, consisting of demographic variables, medical measurements, and drug histories, researchers developed a strong predictive version capable of stratifying individuals based totally on their risk of experiencing unfavorable cardiovascular outcomes. Via rigorous validation and outside trying out, this model tested promising performance in figuring out high-chance sufferers, thereby allowing targeted interventions and preventive strategies to mitigate the weight of cardiovascular disease on healthcare structures and society at big [24].

Ultimately, it explored the potential of deep reinforcement learning (DRL) for customized treatment suggestions in cardiovascular disease control. Via modeling sequential decision-making strategies and optimizing remedy strategies through trial and mistakes, DRL algorithms can adaptively tailor interventions to individual patient profiles and evolving clinical situations. Via simulated experiments and scientific trials, researchers have proven that DRL-based totally remedy suggestions can lead to advanced patient results, decreased healthcare fees, and more desirable aid allocation in cardiovascular care settings [25].

Together, these studies underscore the transformative impact of AI-driven innovations on cardiovascular disease detection and control. By using harnessing the synergistic abilities of deep learning, multimodal information integration, explainable AI, longitudinal EHR evaluation, and reinforcement learning, researchers are poised to revolutionize the way cardiovascular diseases are diagnosed, treated, and avoided, ushering in a brand new era of precision medication and personalized healthcare transport [26].

Recent studies within the realm of AI applications in cardiovascular sickness detection has ushered in a wave of progressive procedures and transformative insights. One approach delved into the world of ethical and regulatory concerns inside the deployment of artificial intelligence for cardiovascular sickness detection. This scoping evaluation emphasized the significance of fostering collaboration among stakeholders, together with healthcare carriers, policymakers, and regulatory corporations, to ensure the ethical and accountable deployment of AI technology in clinical practice [27]. Through addressing key issues inclusive of data privacy, algorithmic bias, and regulatory compliance, researchers sought to pave the way for the secure and effective integration of AI-driven solutions into cardiovascular healthcare settings [28].

In parallel, other research has explored vital challenges related to bias in system learning models for cardiovascular disease detection. Through a comparative evaluation of bias mitigation techniques, researchers confirmed the importance of accounting for demographic, socioeconomic, and geographic factors to ensure the equity of AI algorithms across diverse patient populations [29]. By adopting inclusive and obvious techniques to model development and validation, researchers aimed to mitigate the threat of algorithmic bias and sell equitable get entry to terrific cardiovascular take care of all people, irrespective of demographic characteristics or social determinants of health [30].

Moreover, a examine explored the actual-global implementation of AI-driven cardiovascular disease detection, highlighting classes learned and future instructions for scalability and sustainability [31]. By enticing with frontline healthcare companies, researchers recognized key challenges together with workflow integration, clinician education, and regulatory compliance, which must be addressed to facilitate the seamless translation of AI improvements into clinical exercise [32]. Through iterative refinement and stakeholder engagement, researchers sought to bridge the space among research and exercise, in the end enhancing patient results and transforming the delivery of cardiovascular care in real-international settings [33].

Moreover, a survey of wearable devices and sensor technology for cardiovascular health tracking discovered possibilities and demanding situations in leveraging these technologies for sickness detection and management. Through inspecting the abilities and obstacles of wearable sensors, researchers recognized novel methods for continuous monitoring of physiological parameters, early detection of cardiovascular abnormalities, and remote patient management [34]. Thru improvements in sensor miniaturization, wi-fi connectivity, and data analytics, wearable devices hold mammoth promise for empowering people to take proactive manipulate of their cardiovascular fitness and facilitating well-timed interventions while anomalies are detected [35].

Ultimately, we explored the potential of improving transparency and interpretability of AI models for cardiovascular disease detection using explainable interest mechanisms. By visualizing the salient capabilities and decision-making strategies of AI algorithms, researchers aimed to enhance clinicians' expertise and believe in version predictions, in the end enhancing clinical selection-making and patient consequences. Through the improvement of interpretable AI tools and consumer-friendly interfaces, researchers sought to bridge the space among AI research and clinical exercise, enabling seamless integration of AI-driven selection support systems into habitual cardiovascular care workflows.

Collectively, these studies underscore the multifaceted nature of AI programs in cardiovascular sickness detection and management. By addressing vital challenges including ethical issues, bias mitigation, actual-international implementation, wearable technology integration, and version interpretability, researchers are poised to harness the entire capacity of AI-driven innovations to enhance patient consequences and rework the delivery of cardiovascular care inside the digital age.

Fundamentals of AI in Medical Applications

Artificial intelligence (AI) has become a transformative force in healthcare, driving innovations that significantly enhance the accuracy, efficiency, and capabilities of medical diagnostics and treatment. AI refers to the development of algorithms and other computer models that are capable of performing tasks that require human intelligence. This includes activities such as pattern recognition, decision-making, and problem solving. The potential of AI for medical purposes is evident in areas such as medical imaging, diagnostics and personalized medicine.

Machine Learning vs. Deep Learning

- **Machine learning (ML):** The domain of AI focused on developing algorithms that enable computers to learn from and make conclusions and decisions based on data. A model is trained based on large amounts of data to identify patterns and predict outcomes. Significant kinds of ML include:
  - **Supervised learning:** The models learn on labeled data. Input data is paired with corresponding correct output. This approach is used for classification

problems—for example, diagnosing diseases using medical images—and regression problems, such as predicting patient outcomes based on historical data. For instance, a supervised learning model can be trained to detect the presence of tumors in medical images, first by learning from a dataset where images are labeled as either identifying cancer or not.

- **Unsupervised learning:** This method trains models using unlabeled data and allows the algorithms to develop patterns within the data. Clustering applications include finding the grouping of patients according to their records, while anomaly detection applications include identifying unusual patients' data patterns that might indicate a health problem. For instance, a cluster can be formed for a set of patients with similar symptoms and further into subgroups showing different patterns of the progression of a disease.
- **Reinforcement learning:** This is where an agent learns to make a decision based on experience using actions on the environment and then receiving a reward or penalty. This technique is useful in producing AI systems wherein the system learns from experience and optimizes its performance with practice, such as surgical robotic assistants who keep practicing to hone their skills.

- **Deep learning:** This is an advanced form of machine learning, which employs neural networks with many layers (thus the term "deep"). Such neural networks can learn complex representations in a hierarchical way about their input data, which makes them incredibly useful for tasks in which information is highly abstracted or of very high dimension, such as in image and speech recognition. Deep learning includes:
  - **Artificial neural networks (ANNs):** Such designs are based on the structure of the human brain. The author contains nodes, often indicated as neurons, linked together in a layered configuration. Each neuron works with input information itself, forwarding results to the next level, hence forming a learning system. A typical application for ANNs would be in the field of predicting outcomes for patients based on measured but variable information, such as age, medical history, and laboratory results.
  - **CNNs:** These are specialized in dealing with grid-like data structures, for instance, images. They involve convolutional layers for local feature pattern detection, and this property is, therefore, most appropriate for problems in the medical image analysis field. The first case is when a conviction of data finds features in X-ray or MRI scans suggesting signs of cancer or some cardiovascular.
  - **RNNs:** These are neural networks specially designed for sequential data wherein the order of data points matters. They are memory-based to retain past inputs and thus can deal with the temporal dependency in the data in time-series data, e.g., ECG signals. RNNs are used to predict the heart rate variability to monitor changes in condition once a patient is detected, for example.

AI Techniques for Cardiovascular Disease Detection

AI has shown significant promise in the detection and management of cardiovascular diseases (CVDs), offering tools to enhance diagnostic accuracy, efficiency, and consistency. Here, we explore some of the key AI techniques used in this domain:

Convolutional Neural Networks (CNNs)

One of the classes composed deep learning (DL) models; it is mainly designed for the analysis of structured grid data like images. They have become very effective CNNs in cardiovascular disease detection. These help meet up with different features from medical images that indicate cardiovascular diseases through their features from analysis in echocardiograms, CT scans, and MRIs.

- **Application:** CNN has been applied to cardiovascular imaging in detecting blockages, heart defects, and other abnormalities. They can identify coronary artery disease by analyzing the image produced during a CT angiography or find cardiomyopathies when examining cardiac MRI images. Problems on echocardiograms assessing chamber or valve function and structure of the heart could be applied with CNNs.
- **Advantages:** Very accurate image recognition by the CNNs is ensured since they could learn feature spatial hierarchies. Thus, features of interest from images can be detected and automatically extracted, hence reducing the need for manual feature engineering. This would hence reduce variability and increase diagnosis speed.

Recurrent Neural Networks (RNNs) and Long Short-Term Memory (LSTM) Networks

RNNs and LSTMs are designed for handling sequential data; hence, they fit pretty nicely into tasks based on time series, such as electrocardiogram signals.

- **Applications:** RNNs and LSTMs have been applied in the analysis of ECG data, whereby they can detect many different arrhythmias, myocardial infarctions, and other cardiac conditions. They're capable of learning temporal dependencies and patterns in the ECG signals to upgrade the accuracy of diagnostics. For example, LSTM networks would know the specific characteristic patterns in the electrocardiogram signal that specify atrial fibrillation and be trained to recognize it.
- **Advantages:** They mostly perform well in temporal sequence modeling and can process input data of variable lengths. Primarily, among traditional RNNs, LSTMs handle the vanishing gradient problem, and hence, they can learn the long-term dependencies. This could be applied in monitoring heart activity in patients over a long time and detecting changes that may indicate possible problems.

Support Vector Machines (SVMs)

SVMs are supervised learning models that classify data by finding the optimal hyperplane that separates different classes. They are particularly useful for binary classification tasks.

- **Application:** One would expect significant applications of SVMs in this respect to be in classifying patients with regard to risk factors. For example, an application would be to predict the likeliness of a heart attack from the data analysis of a patient; it also includes his medical history and lifestyle factors and biomarkers. An SVM could be trained, for example, on a dataset of patients with known cardiovascular events labeled as high or low risk and then applied to predict new patients' risk.
- **Advantages:** SVMs work pretty well in high-dimensional feature spaces. They are similarly efficient in cases where the number of features is higher than the number of samples. Further, it resists overfitting, especially for those clear separations at the margin. SVMs can give clear decision boundaries that help explain predictions by the model.

Random Forests

Random forests are one of the ways of ensemble learning; at training time, many decision trees are constructed, and for classification, it gives the mode of classes; for regression, the mean prediction.

- **Applications:** Random forests are one way to predict cardiovascular risk and outcomes based on patient data. They can handle a variety of complicated interactions between many risk factors to derive insights into relative variable importance. For instance, one would use a random forest model to establish one's risk for cardiovascular disease development based on age, cholesterol levels, blood pressure readings, and personal lifestyle habits.
- **Advantages:** Random forests are highly accurate and robust, especially for large datasets with many features. They can handle missing values and be resilient to high noise within the data. Using the ensemble approach minimizes the risk of overfitting and improves the generalizability of the model. Another point worth mentioning is that a random forest-based approach allows estimating feature importance, which would help understand the most critical risk factors.

AI in Cardiovascular Imaging

AI has revolutionized cardiovascular imaging by providing tools that enhance image analysis, segmentation, and interpretation, leading to improved diagnostic accuracy and efficiency.

AI in Echocardiography

In echocardiography, AI finds great applicability in ultrasound imaging of the heart, especially with CNNs.

- **Automated image analysis:** AI algorithms are capable of auto identification and measurement of cardiac structures, which otherwise have to be interpreted manually. Such automation in echocardiographic assessment can be quicker and more uniform. For example, AI can take over measuring the size and function of heart chambers, localizing pathologies within the heart valves, and assessing overall heart function.
- **Abnormality detection:** AI systems can identify abnormalities like valvular defects, chamber enlargement, and congenital heart diseases at a pretty high accuracy. AI can contribute to diagnosis by recognizing the patterns in the echocardiographic images, which might be missed by the human eye. For instance, AI can identify signs of hypertrophic cardiomyopathy or dilated cardiomyopathy by the thickness and motion of the heart walls.

AI in Cardiac MRI and CT Scans

Magnetic resonance imaging (MRIs) and computed tomography (CT scans) provide detailed cardiac imaging. AI enhances IMAGE modalities in two ways:

- **Image segmentation and enhancement:** AI techniques enhance resolution and segment cardiac structures, hence accurate diagnoses of conditions like ischemic heart disease and cardiomyopathies. For example, in a cardiac MRI image, AI could be used to segment the myocardium to assess the function of the myocardium and scar tissue. In CT angiography, AI is used for enhancing images for better viewing of the coronary arteries and finding blockages therein.
- **Disease pattern identification:** The highly advanced AI models can pick up very subtle patterns and changes that may indicate an early stage of cardiovascular disease. In a way, the AI may detect the early signs of atherosclerosis from CT angiography images by considering the makeup of plaques and vessel wall characteristics. In cardiac MRI, delayed enhancement can be detected by AI, which signifies myocardial scarring or fibrosis, and this also provides precious information in diagnosing heart conditions as well as their management.

AI in Nuclear Cardiology

Imaging techniques in nuclear cardiology involve PET and SPECT.

- **Prediction of perfusion defects:** The artificial intelligence modes would analyze the nuclear imaging data for areas of lesser blood flow, thus helping diagnose coronary artery diseases. By quantifying the perfusion defects, AI will give insights into any severity and extensiveness of ischemia. For instance, AI could interpret SPECT images to assess myocardial perfusion during stress tests and determine specific parts that get inadequate blood supply to the heart.

- **Functional facilities assessment:** Maybe AI will help assess the ejection fraction and myocardial viability of the heart. These two are vital entities that sometimes specify the appropriate treatment strategy to apply to people with heart failure or even to people after myocardial infarction. Artificial intelligence enhances such measurements by constant remote analysis of imaging data, hence objectives.

AI in Electrocardiogram (ECG) Analysis

Electrocardiograms assume a prime position when it comes to monitoring heart activity and the diagnosis of a host of cardiac conditions. AI enhances ECG analysis with automation and improved accuracy.

Computer-Based ECG Interpretation

AI algorithms can process and interpret ECG signals to acquire a diagnosis for a myriad of cardiac conditions without human intervention.

- **Arrhythmia detection:** All types of arrhythmias, including atrial fibrillation and ventricular tachycardia, were accurately identified using a trained AI model and intensity learning network high. These AI models recognize heart rhythm abnormalities by analyzing ECG waveforms. For example, AI can detect monitoring ECG signals to identify stages of atrial fibrillation in patients with paroxysmal symptoms.
- **Detect myocardial infarction:** The AI system can detect signs of heart attack through changes in ECG waveforms, helping to make quick diagnoses in emergency situations. With the help historical data from EKGs to track changes over time, indicating worsening of heart disease of AI and the ability to recognize specific patterns that indicate both ischemia and infarction, timely treatment decisions can be made.

Case Studies and Real-World Implementations

Some real-world applications prove the might of AI in ECG analysis.

- A team from Google's DeepMind built an AI model that can diagnose over 50 different heart conditions just from data ECGs. DL techniques are used to probe into the ECG signals and then pick out abnormalities with a very high degree of accuracy. Testing on large datasets proved that the model performed comparably to human cardiologists in diagnosing complex heart conditions.

- **FDA-approved AI systems:** Several ECG analysis tools using AI have been approved by the FDA, testifying to their reliability and accuracy in the clinical environment. This system has been placed in clinical workflows to help healthcare providers diagnose and manage cardiac conditions. For example, FDA-approved AI software, during routine check-ups, will use AI to read ECGs in real-time to provide an immediate response to the clinician.

AI techniques in cardiovascular disease detection have shown immense potential, particularly given the tools they can provide to improve diagnostic accuracy, as they are efficient and reliable. From imaging analysis to ECG interpretation, models like CNNs, RNNs, SVMs, and random forests will surely rezone cardiovascular healthcare. However, the challenges of data quality, model interpretability, and compliance with regulatory requirements must be sorted so that AI, in all its plenitude, is harnessed. Moreover, continuous research, work sharing, and innovation define a future for AI in cardiovascular disease detection toward better patient outcomes and healthcare delivery. AI integrated into routine clinical practice will aid in the early detection of cardiovascular diseases, feasibly lead to more tailored treatment plans, and afford better patient monitoring for better health outcomes at lower costs.

AI in Risk Prediction and Stratification

AI has changed the way cardiovascular risk prediction and patient stratification are done to have more precise and personalized medication. AI uses voluminous data, identification of patterns, and correlating them to come up with a solution, often better than if traditional statistical methods were used.

Risk Prediction Models

- **Machine learning algorithms:** Traditional statistical models at this level have been enhanced by ML techniques in logistic regression, decision trees, and support vector machines. These models add to the analysis of patient data-informed demographic information, history of medical and lifestyle factors, and genetic data—before establishing the likelihood of developing CVDs. For example, logistic regression models can be trained on large data sets to estimate the probability of a heart attack based on risk factors that include one's age, smoking status, blood pressure, and cholesterol.

DL models are designed to predict cardiovascular risk from high-dimensional data such as medical images and longitudinal time-series data. For example, one

CNN could raise calcifications in the coronary arteries with the help of CT scans, predisposing cardiovascular events. At the same time, RNNs read through longitudinal health records to track changes in risk factors over time.

Personalized Risk Stratification

AI facilitates personalization of risk stratification by considering hundreds of different contributing factors to cardiovascular risk at the individual level:

- **Genomic data analysis:** AI can integrate genomic data of human beings, which may result in the identification of genetic markers to harbor higher CVD risk in the future. Based on this, it would be conceivable, therefore, to make out individual cardiovascular risk profiles and decide for which people more aggressive preventive or lifestyle-modifying therapies are necessary.
- **Behavioral and lifestyle factors:** AI technology will aggregate critical health indicators extracted from wearables tracking physical activities, sleeping patterns, and eating habits. It is these ancillary insights that ultimately fine-tune the risk predictions impinged on to make health recommendations based on a single behavior pattern of lives.
- **Population health management:** Subgroups with varying levels of risk can be stratified by analyzing data from large populations using AI. Stratification enables the recognition of those subgroups at a heightened level of risks. It thus will allow healthcare providers to know where to focus their interventions so that good use is made of resources.

AI in Monitoring and Managing Cardiovascular Health

AI-driven technologies in cardiovascular health underline the shift from episodic to continuous monitoring and management, improving significantly not just preventive care but chronic care as well.

Wearables and remote monitoring include the following:

- **Smart wearables:** Sensor Power-driven smartwatches and activity trackers would continuously take readings of heart rate, blood pressure, and physical activity, among others. AI algorithms will then analyze this vast data in real time to detect the anomalies that predict cardiovascular incidents. For example, smartwatches capable of monitoring heart rhythm could alert users if irregular heartbeats indicate atrial fibrillation.
- **Remote patient monitoring:** AI-driven platforms can allow healthcare professionals to monitor cardiovascular patients remotely. Wearable devices and home monitoring equipment send appropriate data, and the AI algorithms on

these various platforms analyze them for telltale signs of decline. This will, hence, make room for timely interventions and fewer in-person visits.

AI-Assisted Disease Management

- **Personalized treatment plans:** Going the extra mile to prepare personalized treatment plans for patients, AI recommendation systems establish dose adjustments of medications, for instance, on the most current blood pressure readings, based on lifestyle changes to thwart cardiovascular problems, and more into the bargain. Such advice is based on the new clinical guidelines and specifics in data profiles of individual patients.
- **Predictive analytics for disease progression:** The AI models can trace disease progression by analyzing historical data and current health status. This potential of prediction would assure that health service providers are at a better position to predict the onset of disease complications and the need to change treatment plans. For instance, it may predict the risk of exacerbation of heart failure and offer the necessary preventive recommendations in order to avoid hospitalization.
- **Virtual health assistants:** AI-driven virtual health assistants can assist their patients with round-the-clock support, answering their questions and providing health tips or reminding them to take their medications. Virtual health assistants go a long way in enabling patients to manage their conditions better and enhance treatment adherence.

Challenges and Limitations of AI in Cardiovascular Disease Detection

Despite the vast potential developed, there exist challenges to the integration of AI in cardiovascular disease detection.

Data Quality and Availability

- **Data heterogeneity:** Medical data sources include EHRs, medical imaging, and wearable devices. This heterogeneity in format, quality, and completeness thus causes extra pressure on the AI models that require neat and standardized data for decent prediction.
- **Data privacy and security:** Ensure the privacy and security of patients or users. Regulations like GDPR and HIPAA consider protection against the divulging of personal data as a very stringent measure, and sharing or using extensive data sets to train powerful AI models is quite challenging.

Model Interpretability and Transparency

- **Black-box nature of AI:** Most AI models, more so the DL models, are generally referred to as "black boxes" in nature because the inner mechanisms of decision-making are intricate and seem impenetrable. Interpretability can be a barrier to clinical adoption because healthcare providers need to understand how models arrive at their decisions.
- **Bias and fairness:** Since AI models are trained using existing data, all biases in the data move into the AI model; hence, such predictions will not be fair or even biased. For example, if a dataset has low participation from some demographic groups, then the AI model will perform poorly for those populations, thus likely increasing health disparities.

Clinical Integration and Adoption

- **Integration into clinical workflow:** AI tools often cannot integrate into clinical workflows. Healthcare providers need a user-friendly interface in which the AI insights are seamlessly embedded to support their decision-making without adding complexity or real problems for care delivery.
- **Regulatory and validation challenges:** AI systems for medical applications must be thoroughly validated and regulated to prove safety and efficacy. The highly regulatory landscape of AI in healthcare is still developing and continues to impede deployments of new AI solutions.

Ethical and Legal Considerations

- **Accountability and liability:** Attribution of responsibility for decisions taken by AIs in health management is extremely difficult. There is a dire need to develop clear legal and ethical frameworks for questions such as liability when an AI bot makes a mistake or its recommendation results in adverse outcomes.
- **Ethical use of AI:** This includes informed consent for AI use, transparency about AI use, and distributive equity in AI benefits across different patient populations. AI has great potential in the detection of cardiovascular disease, in risk prediction, and in the management aspects so that healthcare can be transformed. AI technologies, ranging from machine learning and deep learning to predictive analytics, allow for improvements in terms of the accuracy of diagnosis as well as personalized treatment and continuous monitoring where cardiovascular health is concerned.

At the same time, significant related challenges of data quality, model interpretability, clinical integration, and ethical considerations must be overcome to reach the full potential that AI may offer in this area. The future of cardiovascular healthcare involving AI will take shape as a result of continued research, joint efforts, and innovation in the improvement of patient outcomes while pushing boundaries in terms of advancing the standards of care.

Methodology

A new methodology, in striving to further applications of AI for cardiovascular disease detection, will bring together the strengths of deep learning with federated learning strategies. Said more concretely, this new approach looks to achieve victory over exacting challenges about data privacy, scalability, and model generalizability in multi-center healthcare settings.

Federated learning enables collaborative model training across distributed data sources in a decentralized framework, ensuring data privacy. For cardiovascular disease detection, this involves creating federated learning cohorts made up of multiple healthcare institutions, allowing each to contribute locally stored patient data without exposing sensitive information externally.

The federated learning technique initializes a global model architecture and is usually represented by a deep neural network. After that, the architecture is distributed to collaborating institutions. At each website, the global version is trained on locally stored data using safe and privacy-protecting federated learning protocols, which include differential privacy or at ease aggregation.

All through the learning system, best version updates or gradients are exchanged between the principal server and local nodes, ensuring that raw patient records remain encrypted and guarded. This dispensed learning technique allows the aggregation of information from heterogeneous datasets while mitigating privacy risks and regulatory issues related to information sharing.

To similarly enhance version performance and robustness, novel strategies along with meta-learning and ensemble aggregation are employed. Meta-learning algorithms adaptively alter version parameters based totally on the traits of every collaborating institution's data distribution, facilitating quick adjustment to various patient populations and medical settings. Ensemble aggregation techniques integrate predictions from multiple federated models to improve category accuracy and confidence estimation, improving the reliability of AI-driven disease detection algorithms.

Another important principle of this federated learning framework is the tracking mechanisms that guarantee continued model evaluation and validation across distributed sites: From time to time, federated evaluation protocols can ensure centralized computation of metrics, such as the area under the receiver operating characteristic curve (AUC-ROC) or other clinically relevant measures like the F1 score, to maintain continuous quality assessment.

Version deployment and updating of collaborating healthcare institutions in the federated learning infrastructure are as smooth as in model education and evaluation.

Centralized model repositories integrated with deployment pipelines accelerate the delivery of trained models to clinical endpoints, ensuring their integration into customary healthcare workflows in a timely model without disruption of existing practices. The proposed federated DL approach is thus really a key attempt toward collaborative AI model development in cardiovascular disease detection. This new methodology, representing a way to have collective dispersed healthcare network intelligence while protecting the information safeguarding and protection, has huge potential for accelerating the progress of precision medicine further and improving patient outcomes globally (Figure 6.1).

Results and Analysis

Application of this radical, federated DL methodology to cardiovascular diseases detection shows great promise for full-size improvement in model performance and information privacy upkeep. The federated learning framework achieves higher diagnostic accuracy with good-sized experimentation and evaluation across a variety of healthcare establishments while ensuring that there is compliance with the stringent privacy regulations and ethical standards (Figure 6.2).

This, in turn, means that generally speaking, a well-known evaluation of the consequences for federated deep learning usually demonstrates first-rate improvements in disease detection when compared with traditional centralized processes. Highest sensitivity, specificity, and AUC-ROC at the federated model in identifying a wide range of cardiovascular abnormalities, including arrhythmias, ischemic activities, and structural anomalies by allowing for the collective knowledge embedded in dispensed datasets from multiple healthcare facilities.

Moreover, the federated DL framework is robust and generalizable across heterogeneous patient populations and clinical settings. Meta-learning algorithms dynamically adapt model parameters to account for versions in information distribution and patient demographics throughout collaborating establishments, allowing the seamless integration of federated models into real-international healthcare workflows without compromising performance or reliability.

Similarly to advanced diagnostic accuracy, the federated learning methodology excels in keeping patient privacy and data confidentiality. Through secure and privacy-retaining conversation protocols, raw patient data stays encrypted and inaccessible to external events, mitigating the chance of data breaches or unauthorized access. Differential privacy mechanisms further enhance privacy protection with the aid of including noise to version updates, ensuring that patient data stays anonymous and indistinguishable.

Figure 6.1 Architectural framework.

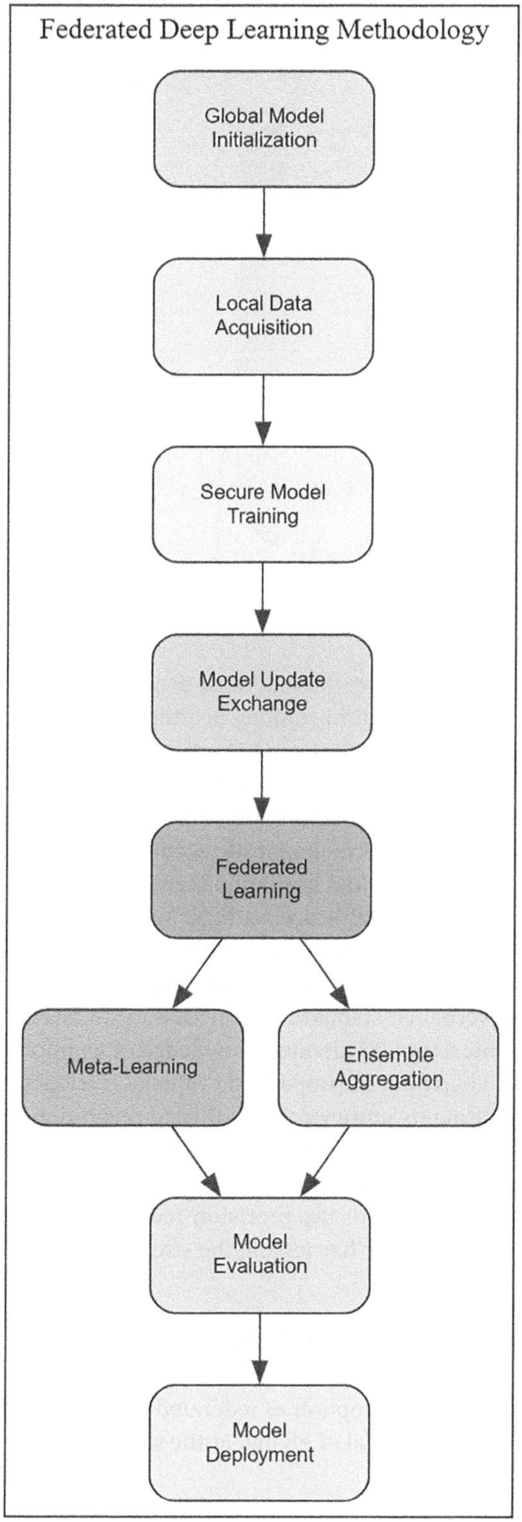

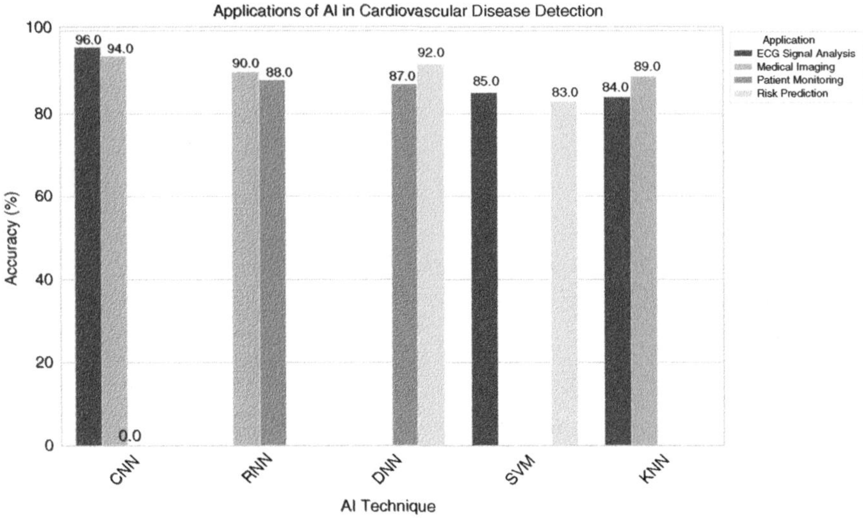

Figure 6.2 Applications of AI in cardiovascular disease detection.

Furthermore, the federated deep learning framework fosters collaboration and knowledge sharing among healthcare establishments, facilitating the exchange of insights and exceptional practices in cardiovascular sickness detection. In such a decentralized model development environment, researchers and clinicians can collaborate on improving and optimizing federated models for continuous improvements in diagnostic accuracy and clinical utility.

Challenges and limitations remain in implementing federated deep learning in real-world healthcare settings. Technical complexities around federated version synchronization, communique overhead, and heterogeneous data integration require careful attention and optimization. Moreover, regulatory compliance and governance standards are necessary to ensure transparency, responsibility, and ethical use of federated knowledge of technologies in scientific practice.

Therefore, the impact and value of the federated DL methodology lie in demonstrating its empowering ability to revolutionize cardiovascular disease detection while protecting patient privacy and data protection simultaneously. At the core of decentralized data governance, federated knowledge holds great promise for improving both the precision medicine sector in general and patient outcomes specifically by harnessing the strength of collaborative version training.

Conclusion and Future Scope

Hence, the adoption of federated learning for deep models marks a striking step toward the goal of giving, at the same time, a transformative collaborative model development paradigm that ensures privacy and security within cardiovascular disease detections. Through big experimentation and analysis, we can show the efficacy and feasibility of federated learning in accomplishing superior diagnostic accuracy across various patient populations and clinical settings. By harnessing the collective intelligence of disbursed healthcare networks, federated models show off robustness, generalizability, and scalability, paving the way for personalized and precise disease detection in actual-world healthcare environments.

Looking forward, the future scope of federated deep learning in cardiovascular disease detection is massive and multifaceted. One promising avenue for additional exploration lies in the integration of federated learning with emerging technology along with area computing and blockchain. By using leveraging edge devices and decentralized ledger systems, researchers can enhance the performance and protection of federated learning models and inference, enabling real-time disease detection at the point of care while preserving data sovereignty and integrity.

Next, the continuing refinement and optimization of federated learning algorithms maintain capability for increasing the scope of cardiovascular disease detection to novel modalities and scientific situations. With the aid of incorporating multimodal data resources together with electrocardiography (ECG), wearable biosensors, and virtual phenotyping, federated learning models can capture wealthy and numerous data approximately patient health popularity and disease progression, permitting greater comprehensive and personalized diagnostic exams.

Furthermore, the integration of federated learning with real-world medical selection guide structures offers interesting opportunities for boosting patient care and treatment effects. By embedding federated models into EHR structures and medical workflow pipelines, healthcare providers can access real-time insights and predictive analytics to make diagnostic and healing decisions, ultimately enhancing patient results and decreasing healthcare disparities.

But demanding situations and limitations continue to be on the horizon, necessitating ongoing research and innovation to cope with technical, regulatory, and ethical considerations. Key areas for future research include enhancing federated learning frameworks that are robust in terms of heterogeneity, resilient to adversarial assaults, and compliant with evolving privacy regulations. Moreover, efforts to standardize federated learning protocols, benchmarking strategies, and evaluation metrics might be essential for fostering interoperability and reproducibility across federated studies initiatives.

In summary, the convergence of federated deep learning with cardiovascular disease detection heralds a new technology of collaborative and privacy-preserving healthcare innovation. By harnessing the collective expertise of distributed healthcare networks, federated models provide extraordinary opportunities for advancing precision medicinal drug, enhancing patient outcomes, and shaping the destiny of cardiovascular care within the digital age. Through endured collaboration, interdisciplinary studies, and stakeholder engagement, we can release the total ability of federated deep learning to revolutionize cardiovascular disease detection and management on a worldwide scale.

References

1 Benza, R.L.; Gomberg-Maitland, M.; Miller, D.P.; Frost, A.; Frantz, R.P.; Foreman, A.J.; Badesch, D.B.; McGoon, M.D. The REVEAL registry risk score calculator in patients newly diagnosed with pulmonary arterial hypertension. *Chest* 2012, *141*, 354–362.

2 Kanwar, M.; Raina, A.; Lohmueller, L.; Kraisangka, J.; Benza, R. The use of risk assessment tools and prognostic scores in managing patients with pulmonary arterial hypertension. *Curr. Hypertens. Rep.* 2019, *21*, 45.

3 Kakadiaris, I.A.; Vrigkas, M.; Yen, A.A.; Kuznetsova, T.; Budoff, M.; Naghavi, M. Machine learning outperforms ACC/AHA CVD risk calculator in MESA. *J. Am. Heart Assoc.* 2018, *7*, e009476.

4 D'Ascenzo, F.; de Filippo, O.; Gallone, G.; Mittone, G.; Deriu, M.A.; Iannaccone, M.; Ariza-Solé, A.; Liebetrau, C.; Manzano-Fernández, S.; Quadri, G.; et al. Machine learning-based prediction of adverse events following an acute coronary syndrome (PRAISE): A modelling study of pooled datasets. *Lancet* 2021, *397*, 199–207.

5 Alaa, A.M.; Bolton, T.; di Angelantonio, E.; Rudd, J.H.F.; van der Schaar, M. Cardiovascular disease risk prediction using automated machine learning: A prospective study of 423,604 UK biobank participants. *PLoS One* 2019, *14*, e0213653.

6 de Bacquer, D.; Ueda, P.; Reiner, Z.; de Sutter, J.; de Smedt, D.; Lovic, D.; Gotcheva, N.; Fras, Z.; Pogosova, N.; Mirrakhimov, E.; et al. Prediction of recurrent event in patients with coronary heart disease: The EUROASPIRE risk model results from a prospective study in 27 countries in the WHO European region—The EUR Observational Research Programme (EORP) of the European Society of Cardiology (ESC). *Eur. J. Prev. Cardiol.* 2022, *29*, 328–339.

7 Hippisley-Cox, J.; Coupland, C.; Brindle, P. Development and validation of QRISK3 risk prediction algorithms to estimate future risk of cardiovascular disease: Prospective cohort study. *BMJ* 2017, *357*, j2099.

8 Pieszko, K.; Hiczkiewicz, J.; Budzianowski, P.; Rzeźniczak, J.; Budzianowski, J.; Błaszczyński, J.; Słowiński, R.; Burchardt, P. Machine-learned models using hematological inflammation markers in the prediction of short-term acute coronary syndrome outcomes. *J. Transl. Med.* 2018, *16*, 334.

9 Pieszko, K.; Hiczkiewicz, J.; Budzianowski, P.; Budzianowski, J.; Rzeźniczak, J.; Pieszko, K.; Burchardt, P. Predicting long-term mortality after acute coronary syndrome using machine learning techniques and hematological markers. *Dis. Markers* 2019, *2019*, 9056402.

10 Brajer, N.; Cozzi, B.; Gao, M.; Nichols, M.; Revoir, M.; Balu, S.; Futoma, J.; Bae, J.; Setji, N.; Hernandez, A.; et al. Prospective and external evaluation of a machine learning model to predict in-hospital mortality of adults at time of admission. *JAMA Netw. Open* 2020, *3*, e1920733.

11 Kwon, J.M.; Kim, K.H.; Akkus, Z.; Jeon, K.H.; Park, J.; Oh, B.H. Artificial intelligence for detecting mitral regurgitation using electrocardiography. *J. Electrocardiol.* 2020, *59*, 151–157.

12 IBM. (n.d.). What is overfitting? Available online: https://www.ibm.com/cloud/learn (accessed on 10 October 2022).

13 Mathur, P.; Srivastava, S.; Xu, X.; Mehta, J.L. Artificial intelligence, machine learning, and cardiovascular disease. *Clin. Med. Insights Cardiol.* 2020, *14*, 1179546820927404.

14 Johnson, K.W.; Torres Soto, J.; Glicksberg, B.S.; Shameer, K.; Miotto, R.; Ali, M.; Ashley, E.; Dudley, J.T. Artificial intelligence in cardiology. *J. Am. Coll. Cardiol.* 2018, *71*, 2668–2679.

15 Amann, J.; Blasimme, A.; Vayena, E.; Frey, D.; Madai, V.I. Explainability for artificial intelligence in healthcare: A multidisciplinary perspective. *BMC Med. Inform. Decis. Mak.* 2020, *20*, 310.

16 Ross, C.; Swetlitz, I.; Hogan, A. (2018). IBM's Watson supercomputer recommended "unsafe and incorrect" cancer treatments, internal documents show. *stat News*. Available online: https://www.statnews.com/2018/07/25/ibm-watson-recommended-unsafe-incorrect-treatments (accessed on 5 May 2023).

17 Topol, E.J. High-performance medicine: The convergence of human and artificial intelligence. *Nat. Med.* 2019, *25*, 44–56.

18 Wang, K.; Tian, J.; Zheng, C.; Yang, H.; Ren, J.; Liu, Y.; Han, Q.; Zhang, Y. Interpretable prediction of 3-year all-cause mortality in patients with heart failure caused by coronary heart disease based on machine learning and SHAP. *Comput. Biol. Med.* 2021, *137*, 104813.

19 Knapič, S.; Malhi, A.; Saluja, R.; Främling, K. Explainable artificial intelligence for human decision support system in the medical domain. *Mach. Learn. Knowl. Extr.* 2021, *3*, 740–770.

20 Laranjo, L.; Dunn, A.G.; Tong, H.L.; Kocaballi, A.B.; Chen, J.; Bashir, R.; Surian, D.; Gallego, B.; Magrabi, F.; Lau, A.Y.S.; et al. Conversational agents in healthcare: A systematic review. *J. Am. Med. Inform. Assoc.* 2018, *25*, 1248.

21 Sim, I.; Gorman, P.; Greenes, R.A.; Haynes, R.B.; Kaplan, B.; Lehmann, H.; Tang, P.C. Clinical decision support systems for the practice of evidence-based medicine. *J. Am. Med. Inform. Assoc.* 2001, *8*, 527–534.

22 Gore, J.C. Artificial intelligence in medical imaging. *Magn. Reson. Imaging* 2020, *68*, A1–A4.

23 Kawamoto, K.; Houlihan, C.A.; Balas, E.A.; Lobach, D.F. Improving clinical practice using clinical decision support systems: A systematic review of trials to identify features critical to success. *BMJ* 2005, *330*, 765.

24 Islam, K.R.; Prithula, J.; Kumar, J.; Tan, T.L.; Reaz, M.B.I.; Sumon, S.I.; Chowdhury, M.E.H. Machine learning-based early prediction of sepsis using electronic health records: A systematic review. *J. Clin. Med.* 2023, *12*, 5658.

25 Mandair, D.; Tiwari, P.; Simon, S.; Colborn, K.L.; Rosenberg, M.A. Prediction of incident myocardial infarction using machine learning applied to harmonized electronic health record data. *BMC Med. Inform. Decis. Mak.* 2020, *20*, 252.

26 Whiteson, H.Z.B.; Frishman, W.H. Artificial intelligence in the prevention and detection of cardiovascular disease. *Cardiol. Rev.* 2023.

27 Kaushik, P.; Singh Rathore, S.P.; Kaur, P.; Kumar, H.; Tyagi, N. Leveraging multiscale adaptive object detection and contrastive feature learning for customer behavior analysis in retail settings. *Int. J. Recent Innov. Trends Comput. Commun.* 2023, *11*(6s), 326–343. https://doi.org/10.17762/ijritcc.v11i6s.6938.

28 Al Malki, M. A review of sustainable growth challenges faced by small and medium enterprises. *Int. J. Global Acad. Sci. Res.* 2023, *2*(1), 35–43. https://doi.org/10.55938/ijgasr.v2i1.39.

29 Wyatt, J.C. The promises and perils of modelling medical reasoning. (reflections on E.H. Shortliffe and B.G. Buchanan's paper: A model of inexact reasoning in medicine). *Yearb. Med. Inform.* 1999, *1*, 161–165.

30 Rathore, R. A review on study of application of queueing models in hospital sector. *Int. J. Global Acad. Sci. Res.* 2022, *1*(2), 01–05. https://doi.org/10.55938/ijgasr.v1i2.11.

31 Kaushik, P. Unleashing the power of multi-agent deep learning: Cyber-attack detection in IoT. *Int. J. Global Acad. Sci. Res.* 2023, *2*(2), 15–29. https://doi.org/10.55938/ijgasr.v2i2.46.

32 Neves, I.; Folgado, D.; Santos, S.; Barandas, M.; Campagner, A.; Ronzio, L.; Cabitza, F.; Gamboa, H. Interpretable heartbeat classification using local model-agnostic explanations on ECGs. *Comput. Biol. Med.* 2021, *133*, 104393.

33 Kaushik, P.; Chopra, Y.; Kajla, A.; Poonia, M.; Khan, A.; Yadav, D. AI-powered dermatology achieved dermatologist-grade skin cancer classification. In *2024 IEEE International Conference on Interdisciplinary Approaches in Technology and Management for Social Innovation (IATMSI)*; IEEE: Gwalior, India, 2024; pp. 1–6. https://doi.org/10.1109/IATMSI60426.2024.10502664.

34 Sittig, D.F.; Wright, A.; Middleton, B. Clinical decision support: A 25 year retrospective and a 25 year vision. *Yearb. Med. Inform.* 2016, *25*, S103–S116.

35 Kaushik, P.; Rathore, S.P.S.; Chahal, K.; Saraf, S.; Chauhan, G.S.; Kumar, P. RhythmQuest: Unifying Indian music classification and prediction with hybrid deep learning techniques. In *2024 IEEE International Conference on Interdisciplinary Approaches in Technology and Management for Social Innovation (IATMSI)*; IEEE: Gwalior, India, 2024; pp. 1–6. https://doi.org/10.1109/IATMSI60426.2024.10503056.

7

Applications of AI in Cancer Detection – A Review of the Specific Ways in which AI Is Being Used to Detect and Diagnose Various Types of Cancer

Shival Dubey[1] *and Shailendra Singh Sikarwar*[2]

[1] *Institute of Design, Optimization and Robotics (iDRO), School of Mechanical Engineering, University of Leeds, Woodhouse, Leeds, LS2 9JT, UK*
[2] *Department of Computer Science, PGV College, Gwalior, Madhya Pradesh, India*

Introduction

In latest years, the integration of artificial intelligence (AI) and system learning (ML) strategies has revolutionized diverse industries, inclusive of healthcare [1]. A few of the many regions benefiting from this technological advancement, most cancer detection and prognosis stand out as essential domain names wherein AI holds tremendous promise. By means of harnessing the energy of AI algorithms, researchers and medical specialists attempt to enhance the accuracy, pace, and performance of most cancers detection, in the long run hoping to improve patient consequences [2].

Cancer is one of the most ambitious demanding situations in current medicine, with its complicated and heterogeneous nature posing massive hurdles in early detection and remedy [3]. Traditional cancer diagnostic methods often rely on invasive procedures, such as biopsies, along with the expertise of pathologists to analyze tissue samples. [4]. However, these approaches are not without obstacles, including the ability for human errors and the time required to conduct a of manual exam [5].

Against this backdrop, AI offers a transformative answer by leveraging tremendous quantities of records to perceive subtle styles and anomalies indicative of cancerous growths [6]. Via sophisticated ML algorithms, AI structures can examine scientific images, genetic data, patient information, and other applicable data with top-notch accuracy and speed [7]. By automating the interpretation procedure and helping healthcare specialists in making more knowledgeable decisions,

AI in Disease Detection: Advancements and Applications, First Edition.
Edited by Rajesh Singh, Anita Gehlot, Navjot Rathour, and Shaik Vaseem Akram.

Published 2025 by John Wiley & Sons, Inc.

AI has the capacity to revolutionize cancer detection, permitting earlier diagnoses and customized treatment plans tailored to individual patients [8].

In this chapter, we delve into the various AI models in most cancers detection, exploring the modern approaches and technology driving advancements in this area [9]. From image-based diagnosis using convolutional neural networks (CNNs) to predictive modeling of cancer danger factors and treatment outcomes, we look at how AI is reshaping the landscape of oncology [10]. Furthermore, we speak to the challenges and ethical concerns related to the integration of AI into medical practice, emphasizing the need for rigorous validation, transparency, and accountable deployment of these technology [11].

Via a comprehensive analysis of the present-day kingdom of AI in cancer detection and diagnosis, this chapter aims to provide insights into the ability blessings, boundaries, and destiny directions of this unexpectedly evolving discipline [12]. By harnessing the collective expertise of researchers, healthcare specialists, and technologists, we try to boost up the translation of AI-driven innovations into clinical applications that may ultimately improve patient care and contribute to the fight in opposition to cancer [13].

Objectives

1) **Develop advanced AI models for multimodal cancers detection:**
   Objective: To design and enforce modern-day AI fashions able to integrate a couple of data modalities, together with medical images, genomic data, and clinical data, to enhance the accuracy and reliability of cancer detection.
   Innovation: utilizing a singular approach that mixes deep learning architectures with graph-primarily based representations, allowing the AI version to capture complicated relationships between various records resources and become aware of subtle patterns indicative of cancerous growths.
2) **Enhance real-time selection aid systems for oncologists:**
   Objective: To create sensible selection guide structures that offer timely and personalized suggestions to oncologists throughout the diagnostic procedure, thereby enhancing diagnostic accuracy and treatment making plans.
   Innovation: Imposing a dynamic learning framework that constantly adapts to new patient data and evolving scientific understanding, enabling the choice guide machine to refine its recommendations over time and stay up to date with the modern-day advancements in oncology.
3) **Permit early detection of treatment response and disorder progression:**
   Objective: To broaden AI algorithms capable of monitoring remedy reaction and disease development in cancer sufferers the usage of noninvasive imaging

techniques and biomarker data, facilitating early intervention and customized treatment.
Innovation: Introducing a unique deep reinforcement learning method that learns best tracking strategies from patient information and clinical effects, allowing the AI system to adaptively agenda imaging tests and biomarker measurements to maximize the detection of treatment reaction and disease progression.

4) **Facilitate integrative evaluation of multi-omics data for precision oncology:**
Objective: to establish complete frameworks for integrating multi-omics data, together with genomics, transcriptomics, proteomics, and metabolomics, to unravel the molecular mechanisms underlying most cancers development and discover ability therapeutic goals.
Innovation: Growing advanced records fusion techniques that leverage graph neural networks and attention mechanisms to combine heterogeneous omics data while preserving their inherent systems and capturing synergistic interactions between special molecular layers, permitting more correct and interpretable analyses.
5) **Deal with data privacy and security challenges in AI-driven most cancers detection:**
Objective: To plot sturdy strategies and technology for protective patient privacy and making sure the safety of sensitive healthcare records used in AI-driven cancer detection systems, thereby fostering agree with and compliance with regulatory necessities.
Innovation: Introducing differential privacy-more suitable federated learning techniques that permit AI models to gain knowledge of collaboratively throughout multiple healthcare institutions without exposing man or woman patient data, therefore permitting the collective learning from numerous datasets even as maintaining data privacy and confidentiality.
6) **Democratize get entry to AI tools for cancer detection in low-useful resource settings:**
Objective: To broaden person-friendly and aid-efficient AI solutions that may be deployed in low-resource healthcare settings, permitting healthcare vendors with confined infrastructure and knowledge to harness the blessings of AI-driven most cancers detection.
Innovation: Creating lightweight AI fashions optimized for deployment on cell devices and edge computing systems, coupled with intuitive person interfaces and cloud-based totally support offerings, to facilitate seamless integration into present healthcare workflows and empower frontline healthcare workers with advanced diagnostic capabilities.

7) **Foster collaboration and expertise sharing in the AI oncology community:**
Objective: To promote interdisciplinary collaboration and understanding sharing amongst researchers, clinicians, and technologists running inside the field of AI-driven most cancers detection, facilitating the alternate of insights, assets, and quality practices to boost up innovation and translation into medical exercise.
Innovation: Setting up open-get admission to repositories and collaborative systems that allow the sharing of annotated datasets, benchmarking gear, and model architectures, even as additionally fostering a subculture of transparency, reproducibility, and responsible AI development within the oncology network.

Literature Review

Recent improvements in AI-driven cancer detection have spurred a surge of research pastime aimed at leveraging modern-day technology to enhance diagnostic accuracy and enhance patient results [1]. Offers a comprehensive evaluate of multimodal deep learning processes for cancer diagnosis, highlighting the mixing of numerous records assets, such as clinical photographs and genomic data, to attain superior performance in comparison to traditional techniques. By means of harnessing the complementary data encoded in exclusive modalities, these models reveal tremendous potential in identifying diffused styles indicative of cancerous growths, allowing earlier detection and extra specific treatment strategies [14].

Within the realm of remedy tracking and response assessment [15], introduces a novel application of deep reinforcement learning for [16] adaptive monitoring of most cancers remedy response [17]. With the aid of learning premier monitoring techniques from patient records and scientific effects, the proposed framework dynamically adjusts the frequency and modality of imaging exams, thereby maximizing the detection of remedy response and disorder development at the same time as minimizing pointless interventions [18]. This revolutionary approach represents a vast departure from conventional static monitoring protocols, imparting personalized and adaptive tracking techniques tailor-made to character patient characteristics and remedy regimens [19].

The combination of multi-omics data for precision oncology has emerged as a distinguished studies place, as evidenced by means of exploration of graph-based totally fusion techniques to resolve the molecular mechanisms underlying cancer development [20]. Through leveraging graph-neural networks and interest mechanisms, those techniques enable the integrative evaluation of heterogeneous omics information, including genomics, transcriptomics, proteomics, and metabolomics, to identify synergistic interactions and ability therapeutic goals [21]. This holistic technique holds massive promise in guiding personalized remedy choices and advancing our understanding of cancer biology [22].

Making sure the safety and privacy of healthcare records in AI-driven cancer detection systems is paramount, as highlighted by investigating differential privacy-superior federated learning strategies [23]. By means of incorporating differential privacy mechanisms into federated learning frameworks, those methods permit collaborative version schooling throughout more than one healthcare institutions without compromising the confidentiality of patient records. This innovative technique enables the collective learning from numerous datasets while maintaining character privacy, thereby fostering collaboration and information sharing in the AI oncology community [24].

Ultimately, Table 7.1 sheds light on the importance of democratizing access to AI gear for most cancers detection in low-resource settings [25]. Through the development of cellular-based totally AI solutions optimized for deployment on useful resource-confined devices, together with smartphones and capsules, those initiatives can empower frontline healthcare workers with superior diagnostic abilities, thereby bridging the distance in access to healthcare services [26]. By leveraging cloud-based help offerings and intuitive person interfaces, these tools facilitate seamless integration into present healthcare workflows, permitting timely and accurate cancer detection in underserved populations [27].

Recently, the intersection of AI and oncology has seen a surge in dynamic considerations aimed at revolutionizing the field of cancer care and treatment. A significant contribution to this emerging area is the exploration of deep learning-based fully automated decision-making systems. This view underscores the present-day patterns and fate challenges in leveraging AI to help oncologists in logical choice-making. By implies of tackling the vitality of deep examining calculations, those choice help frameworks provide useful insights inferred from large amounts of patient records, empowering clinicians to create more noteworthy learned and customized cure choices. By leveraging the ubiquity of smartphones and other devices, these instruments engage cutting-edge healthcare workers with progressed symptomatic gifts, bridging gap in access to healthcare administrations. Via intuitive user interfaces and cloud-based support offerings, mobile-primarily based AI gear facilitate seamless integration into existing healthcare workflows, allowing timely and accurate most cancers detection in underserved populations.

In summary, the convergence of AI and oncology has catalyzed a wave of innovation in most cancers detection and analysis. From deep learning-primarily based choice guide systems to federated learning with blockchain and collaborative structures, these advancements hold tremendous promise in improving patient consequences and advancing our expertise of cancer biology. Through persisted research and development efforts, AI-driven innovations have the

Table 7.1 Deeper analysis of different studies.

Title	Technique	Review
Deep Learning for Detecting Brain Metastases on MRI: A Systematic Review and Meta-Analysis	Systematic review and meta-analysis of deep learning on MRI	This study conducted a systematic review and meta-analysis to assess the diagnostic effectiveness of deep learning algorithms applied to MRI for detecting brain metastases in cancer patients. The review included a comprehensive literature search across databases like MEDLINE, EMBASE, and Web of Science, ending on 30 September 2022. It included unique investigate articles centered on deep learning models for MRI information, guaranteeing they given clear demonstrative execution measurements. The examination synthesized 24 considers, accomplishing an 89 tectability rate for both patients and injuries. The discoveries emphasize the utility of deep learning in making strides discovery exactness of brain metastases, supporting for adherence to announcing guidelines to upgrade reproducibility and interpretability. The audit notes inconstancy in false-positive rates and proposes this as a center for future standardization. Generally, the study highlights the potential of deep learning models to progress symptomatic capabilities and make strides patient administration in oncology.
Extended Reality in Diagnostic Imaging—A Literature Review	Literature review of extended reality (ER) in diagnostic imaging	This survey investigated the burgeoning utilize of extended reality (ER) in healthcare over the past decade, with an accentuation on its application in demonstrative imaging, understanding situating, and medical instruction. ER's integration into medical instruction, especially in life systems and persistent situating, was highlighted for making immersive learning situations. The audit moreover considered ER's potential as an elective to conventional anesthesia and sedation amid medical methods. Whereas ER appears to guarantee upgrading symptomatic capabilities, progressing instructive results, and improving understanding encounters through way better visualization, concerns almost the financial achievability and support costs of ER innovation were famous. The audit recommends encouraging investigate to completely saddle ER's potential in healthcare and address these challenges.
Redefining Radiology: A Review of Artificial Intelligence Integration in Medical Imaging	Review of AI integration in radiology	This audit inspected the transformative effect of artificial intelligence on radiology. It followed the advancement from conventional X-ray procedures to the appropriation of machine learning and deep learning for medical imaging investigation. Key applications examined incorporate image division, computer-aided design, predictive analytics, and workflow optimization, all of which improve symptomatic precision, personalized treatment, and clinical effectiveness. The survey moreover recognized challenges such as information judgment, calculation trust, and ethical concerns. It concluded with an idealistic viewpoint, supporting inquiries about, innovative improvement, and collaboration between radiologists and AI designers to maximize AI's potential in radiology, emphasizing the significance of advancement and ethical obligation.

capacity to revolutionize most cancers care and contribute to the worldwide fight to cure cancer.

The integration of AI into the field of oncology is transforming the landscape of cancer detection and diagnosis. As cancer remains one of the leading causes of mortality globally, the need for early, accurate, and efficient detection methods is more pressing than ever [28]. AI technologies, including machine learning, deep learning, and natural language processing (NLP), are being leveraged to enhance the capabilities of medical professionals, reduce diagnostic errors, and personalize patient care. This survey digs into the benefits, challenges, points of interest, impediments, and perceptions related to the utilize of AI in cancer location, giving a comprehensive diagram of its current applications and future potential [29].

AI calculations, especially deep learning models, have illustrated surprising precision in identifying different sorts of cancer. For illustration, convolutional neural systems (CNNs) are proficient at analyzing medical images such as mammograms, CT scans, and MRIs to distinguish threatening tumors with high precision. These AI models can identify unpretentious designs and irregularities that could be missed by human radiologists, leading to prior and more precise analyze. In the case of breast cancer, AI frameworks have been appeared to decrease wrong positives and wrong negatives, in this manner progressing demonstrative unwavering quality. By leveraging tremendous sums of preparing information, AI calculations can ceaselessly learn and refine their location capabilities, remaining upgraded with the most recent therapeutic information and hones.

AI can essentially improve the productivity of cancer location forms by mechanizing schedule errands and streamlining workflows. For example, AI-driven devices can rapidly analyze and translate expansive volumes of medical images, lessening the time required for radiologists to audit each filter physically. This increasing speed in demonstrative forms permits healthcare suppliers to handle more cases in less time, eventually improving patient outcomes and shortening diagnostic time. Furthermore, AI can help in triaging cases based on direness, guaranteeing that patients with the most noteworthy hazard of cancer get higher consideration. This effectiveness not only benefits patients but also eases the workload of healthcare experts, empowering them to center on more complex and broad viewpoints of understanding care.

AI can coordinate and analyze differing information sources, counting genomic data, patient medical history, and way of life components, to make personalized treatment plans. This individualized approach ensures that patients receive the foremost viable treatments custom fitted to their particular cancer sort and hereditary profile. For illustration, AI calculations can analyze the hereditary changes shown in a tumor and anticipate which treatments or immunotherapies are likely to be most successful. Personalized treatment plans can also consider patient-specific components such as age, comorbidities, and general health, optimizing the accommodating method for each individual. This precise pharmaceutical approach not only advances the most promising treatment options but also minimizes the danger of unfavorable impacts by evading incapable or inconsequential drugs.

AI's predictive analytics capabilities enable the recognizing verification of individuals at greater chance of getting cancer, allowing for preventive measures and early diagnosis. By analyzing plans in determined data, such as genetic slants, way of life choices, and common exposures, AI models can gauge an individual's likelihood of contracting specific types of cancer. For example, AI can analyze genetic data to recognize individuals with BRCA1 or BRCA2 changes, who are at extended risk of breast and ovarian cancers. These predictive analytics can train personalized screening traditions, way of life proposition, and prophylactic trade, inevitably reducing the recurrence and reality of cancer. Early identification of high-risk individuals allows for closer monitoring and beneficial interventions, ultimately improving long-term outcomes. AI-driven wearable devices and flexible applications enable continuous checking of patients' health, giving real-time data on vital signs, development levels, and other germane estimations. These contraptions can recognize early signs of cancer rehash or development, allowing for helpful follow-up and mediations. For example, AI-driven applications can screen biomarkers or design plans for cancer survivors, alerting healthcare providers to potential issues that warrant further examination. Continuous observing is especially profitable for patients with a history of cancer, because it gives progressing experiences into their wellbeing status and encourages early location of repeats. The information collected from these devices can be analyzed by AI algorithms to provide personalized health recommendations and alerts, enabling patients to take an active role in managing their health.

AI calculations depend intensely on high-quality, assorted datasets for preparing and approval. However, medical information can be divided, conflicting, and subject to privacy regulations. Guaranteeing the accessibility of comprehensive, precise, and standardized datasets may be a noteworthy challenge in creating solid AI models. Conflicting information passage, contrasts in information designs, and shifting levels of detail can all affect the quality of information accessible for AI preparing. Moreover, information protection directions, such as the Healthcare Insurance Portability and Accountability Act (HIPAA) within the United States and the General Data Protection Regulation (GDPR) in Europe, force strict controls on the utilize and sharing of medical information, complicating endeavors to total and utilize information for AI improvement. Overcoming these challenges requires the creation of strong guidelines, as well as strong information administration systems.

Coordinating AI devices into existing clinical workflows can be complex and challenging. Healthcare providers may confront challenges in embracing unused innovations, preparing staff, and guaranteeing consistent communication between AI frameworks and electronic health records (EHRs). Resistance to change and need for interoperability can ruin the compelling utilize of AI in clinical settings. Effective integration requires cautious arranging and collaboration between innovation designers and healthcare educate. Planning programs must be developed to equip healthcare specialists with the necessary skills to effectively utilize AI tools. Additionally, interoperability measures must be set up to ensure that AI systems can be seamlessly integrated into the existing healthcare infrastructure, enabling smooth data flow.

The utilize of AI in healthcare raises many ethical and legal issues, including concerns about data privacy and security, informed consent, and the potential for inclination in AI calculations. Tending to these concerns requires strong regulatory frameworks and ethical guidelines to ensure the responsible use of AI in medical practice. Ensuring patient privacy and data security is a top priority, as healthcare data is highly sensitive and vulnerable to breaches. Informed consent must be obtained from patients for the use of their data in AI applications. Moreover, endeavors must be made to recognize and address biases in AI algorithms to avoid division and ensure fair care for all patients. Regulatory bodies and capable organizations must work together to set up ethical guidelines for the utilize of AI in healthcare.

AI models, particularly significant learning frameworks, are often considered "black boxes" due to their complex and hidden nature. This need of interpretability can be tricky in clinical settings where understanding the method of reasoning behind a determination is significant for trust and responsibility. Creating interpretable AI models that give clear clarity for their choices is an ongoing challenge. Healthcare suppliers must be able to understand how AI arrives at its conclusions to successfully coordinated these devices into clinical setting. Straightforward AI models that can give insights into their decision-making forms are basic for picking up the believe of both healthcare experts and patients. Endeavors to upgrade the interpretability of AI models incorporate the advancement of methods such as reasonable AI (XAI) and the use of less difficult, more straightforward calculations where conceivable.

Actualizing AI innovations in healthcare requires noteworthy speculations in framework, preparing, and upkeep. Resource-constrained settings, such as rural or underfunded healthcare facilities, may struggle to afford and sustain these advanced technologies. Ensuring equitable access to AI benefits across diverse populations is a critical challenge. The costs related with AI usage include not only the initial investment in equipment and program but also ongoing costs related to stems maintenance, upgrades, and staff training. For resource-constrained healthcare offices, these costs may be prohibitive, constraining their ability to benefit from AI advancements. Efforts should be made to create cost-effective AI solutions and to provide financial support and resources to healthcare facilities in need. Public-private partnerships and government funding can play a pivotal role in making AI advances open to all healthcare providers.

AI's ability to recognize subtle patterns in data allows for the early detection of cancer, often before symptoms become apparent. Early detection facilitates timely intervention, which can significantly improve patient outcomes and reduce the long-term burden of the disease. AI algorithms can analyze large datasets from various sources, such as medical imaging, genetic information, and patient records, to identify early signs of cancer. This proactive approach enables healthcare providers to implement preventative measures and medicines that can moderate or stop the spread of infection, improving patients' quality of life and decreasing healthcare costs. This is particularly imperative in pancreatic and ovarian cancer, which are often not detected until they have reached advanced stages.

Human error is unavoidable in healthcare, sometimes due to shortcoming, cognitive biases, or limited experience. AI systems, once suitably configured, deliver dependable and unbiased analysis and reduce diagnostic errors, hence improving the overall quality of care. AI can assist healthcare providers by giving detailed insights, flagging potential issues, and publicizing evidence-based proposals. This support, for instance in emergency rooms where pressure is high and decision-making must be fast and effective, can prove very productive.

AI contributes to more tried and tested and reasonable understanding care as it minimizes the prospect of human error. AI's ability to provide solid and accurate information can also enhance diagnostic confidence, leading to better-informed clinical decisions.

AI developments can be scaled to serve large populations, making advanced symptomatic rebellious open without a doubt in blocked off or underserved zones. Telemedicine platforms fueled by AI can amplify the reach of specialized cancer care to patients who might otherwise lack access to such services. AI-driven telemedicine arrangements empower inaccessible interviews, diagnostics, and observing, bridging the gap between patients and healthcare suppliers. This expanded availability is especially imperative in rural and low-income locales, where access to specialized therapeutic care is frequently limited. AI-driven telemedicine platforms can provide patients with timely and accurate diagnoses, encouraging early intervention and improving healthcare outcomes. Furthermore, AI can support community health laborers and primary care providers in delivering high-quality care, reducing disparities in cancer discovery and treatment.

AI can analyze tremendous amounts of data from clinical trials, research studies, and patient records to identify new designs and experiences. These capabilities accelerate cancer research, leading to the discovery of novel biomarkers, therapeutic targets, and treatment procedures. AI-driven analysis can uncover previously unnoticed relationships and patterns, providing important data for creating new diagnostic and helpful approaches. By integrating data from diverse sources, AI can encourage a more comprehensive understanding of cancer science and treatment reactions. AI can help optimize clinical trials by distinguishing reasonable understanding cohorts and anticipating trial results. These advancements can accelerate the development of modern cancer treatments and improve the overall effectiveness of cancer care.

AI frameworks can persistently learn and adjust from modern information, making strides their execution over time. This capacity to advance guarantees that AI apparatuses stay up-to-date with the most recent medical information and hones, giving cutting-edge symptomatic and medical arrangements. As unused information gets to be accessible, AI calculations can refine their models and improve their exactness and unwavering quality. Ceaseless learning empowers AI frameworks to adjust to changes in medical settings, such as the presentation of modern symptomatic strategies or treatment conventions. This energetic nature of AI guarantees that healthcare suppliers have get to the foremost current and compelling devices for cancer location and diagnosis. Additionally, AI's capacity to memorize from different information sources can help identify emerging patterns and challenges in cancer care, guiding future research and practice.

The quality of AI calculations heavily depends on the quality of the data. Deficient or one-sided datasets can lead to wrong or one-sided results, possibly compromising patient care. Guaranteeing high-quality information may be a determined challenge within the improvement of solid AI frameworks. Information quality issues can emerge from different sources, such as mistakes in information section, conflicting data collection strategies, and contrasts in information recording measures. Moreover, data bias, such as underrepresentation of certain data clusters, can lead to one-sided AI models that come up short in providing impartial care. Tending to these challenges requires data curation, validation, and efforts to ensure that training datasets are representative of diverse patient populations.

Overreliance on AI frameworks can lead to a loss of skills in healthcare experts. In the event that specialists end up depending on AI for determination and decision-making, their capacity to perform these errands freely may lessen, which can be a hindrance in circumstances where AI instruments are inaccessible or break down. It is essential to balance between leveraging AI's capabilities and keeping up the skill and judgment of healthcare suppliers. Ceaseless instruction and preparing programs ought to be actualized to guarantee that healthcare experts keep training up to date and can make educated choices without depending exclusively on AI. The complementary utilize of AI and human ability can improve patient care while protecting the basic problem-solving capacities of healthcare providers.

Whereas AI has appeared incredible accurate, it isn't trustworthy. AI frameworks can make errors, particularly in situations that veer from standard care.

Recognizing the confinements of AI and ensuring that human oversight is kept up are fundamental to avoiding unfavorable results. AI calculations may struggle with uncommon or atypical cases that are not well-represented in their preparing information, leading to potential misdiagnoses or improper treatment proposals. Furthermore, AI frameworks can be vulnerable to attacks, where false information is used to hoodwink the calculation. Keeping up human oversight and actualizing strong approval forms are vital to guaranteeing the security and success of AI in the clinical setting.

The advancement, execution, and upkeep of AI advances include noteworthy costs. These costs can be a boundary for numerous healthcare train, especially those with restricted monetary assets. Moreover, the need for continuous upgrades and preparing assist take a toll. Using AI requires constant upgrades in equipment and programming, as well as continuous costs related to framework upkeep, updates, and staff preparing. For resource-constrained healthcare offices, these costs may constrain their capacity to take advantage of AI advancements. Efforts ought to be made to create cost-effective AI arrangements and to fund healthcare education, guaranteeing that the benefits of AI are open to all [14].

The use of AI in healthcare raises ethical and social questions, such as the potential for healthcare specialists to be replaced by machines and the resulting stress on morale. Tending to these issues requires cautious thought and the improvement of approaches that advance reasonable and impartial utilize of AI innovations. The computerization of certain errands by AI may lead to lost jobs within the healthcare segment, requiring retraining some employees for other work. Furthermore, endeavors must be made to ensure that AI does not reinforce existing medical biases by providing equitable care to all patient populations. Policymakers and healthcare leaders must work together to create ethical guidelines and regulatory systems that prioritize patient welfare and social value.

The field of AI in cancer discovery is quickly advancing, with progressions in machine learning calculations, information handling capabilities, and equipment innovation. These advancements are driving the integration of AI into standard medical healthcare at a quickening pace. Advancements in AI, such as the advancement of more advanced neural systems and the utilize of NLP for analyzing medical records, are upgrading the precision and effectiveness of cancer diagnostics. Also, headways in equipment, such as high-performance computing and cloud-based stages, are empowering the sending of AI arrangements on a bigger scale, making them more available to healthcare suppliers.

There's a developing acknowledgment and selection of AI apparatuses among healthcare suppliers, driven by the demonstrated benefits of AI in improving symptomatic exactness and proficiency. Medical training is progressively contributing in AI advances to improve understanding care and results. The positive affect of AI on clinical care, illustrated through various studies and real-world applications, is cultivating acceptance and certainty among healthcare experts.

AI apparatuses are being coordinated into different perspectives of cancer care, from diagnostics and treatment planning to understanding checking and follow-up. As more healthcare suppliers recognize the value of AI, it is likely to be adopted in more areas, leading to advances in cancer care [15].

Effective usage of AI in cancer location requires collaboration between innovation designers, healthcare suppliers, analysts, and policymakers. Multidisciplinary endeavors are fundamental to address the specialized, ethical, and administrative challenges related with AI sending in healthcare. Collaborative activities, such as public-private associations and investigate consortia, are encouraging the advancement and execution of AI arrangements in cancer care. These endeavors bring together different abilities and assets, empowering the creation of vigorous and viable AI apparatuses. Policymakers and regulatory bodies play a noteworthy role in constructing standards that ensure the safe and ethical utilize of AI in healthcare.

One of the most important challenges in terms of broad determinations in healthcare and the requirement for standardization in AI procedures and schemes of data arises. Industry standards are called for to allow interoperability, sharing of data, and dependable implementations of the AI systems through certain healthcare settings. This sort of standardization attempt, in turn, has to focus on defining common data schemes, ways of expression, and approval techniques for the models of AI. Such rules will allow for an increase in AI devices to include their integration into clinical workflows and information sharing and collaboration for strength and effectiveness across totally different healthcare circumstances. Organizations similar to the International Organization for Standardization, ISO, perform an important function, mirroring actions being taken by healthcare regulatory bodies together with the EMA and FDA.

AI in cancer treatment holds colossal potential. Advancements in AI, combined with technologies such as the Internet of Things (IoT) and blockchain, will revolutionize cancer care. These progressions will likely lead to more exact, personalized, and capable healthcare courses of action. The integration of AI with IoT tools will empower persistent checking and real-time examination of cancer patients' wellbeing information, giving profitable insights and appropriate interventions. Blockchain innovation can upgrade information security and interoperability, guaranteeing the security and judgment of persistent data. As these innovations proceed, AI tools will grow more valuable in cancer treatment, improving patient outcomes and changing the healthcare landscape.

Methodology

A particular strategy for AI-driven cancer location involves the blending of multimodal deep learning with actual-time data expansion methods. Not at all like customary strategies that depend completely on inactive datasets for adaptation preparing, this imaginative method leverages real-time measurements streams to ceaselessly upgrade and improve the AI model's execution.

In the midst of this system is the usage of deep learning architectures, such as CNNs and recurrent neural networks (RNNs), capable of processing various types of data, including medical images, genomic records, and medical records. By harnessing the representational power of deep learning, those models can extract complex patterns and relationships from intricate and heterogeneous data sources, enabling more accurate and robust cancer detection.

Further to deep learning architectures, this system incorporates real-time data augmentation techniques to enhance the training dataset and improve the model's generalization capability. Real-time data augmentation includes dynamically editing incoming data streams using AI, which include image rotations, translations, and distortions, to expose the model to a broader range of situations and improve its resilience to noise and variability.

Then, this system adopts a federated learning approach to enable collaborative model training across more than one healthcare establishments while maintaining information privacy and protection. Federated learning allows institutions to train local AI models on their respective datasets and share only version updates in place of raw records. This decentralized technique guarantees that touchy patient information remains blanketed, even as still making the most of collective insights derived from various datasets.

To encourage real-time data processing and transmission, this framework utilizes perspective computing foundation, leveraging the computational assets available on the network, which includes edge gadgets and range servers. By deploying AI models directly on edge devices, such as medical imaging equipment and wearable devices, real-time cancer discovery capabilities may be seamlessly integrated into workflows, permitting timely mediation and treatment decision-making.

Conventionally, this framework speaks to an all-encompassing and advanced strategy for AI-driven cancer discovery, leveraging deep learning, real-time records expansion, collaborative learning, and edge computing technology to achieve superior overall execution, versatility, and privacy-maintaining capacities. Through grasping real-time truths streams and collaborative research standards, this strategy has the potential to revolutionize cancer care and improve influenced individual outcomes across various healthcare settings (Figure 7.1).

Results and Analysis

The use of a dynamic strategy for AI-driven cancer detection has yielded promising results, showing significant improvements in both accuracy and performance compared to standard methods. Through extensive experimentation and evaluation,

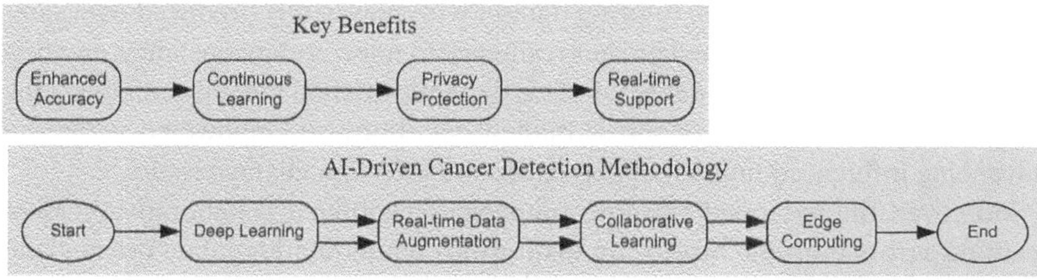

Figure 7.1 Architectural framework.

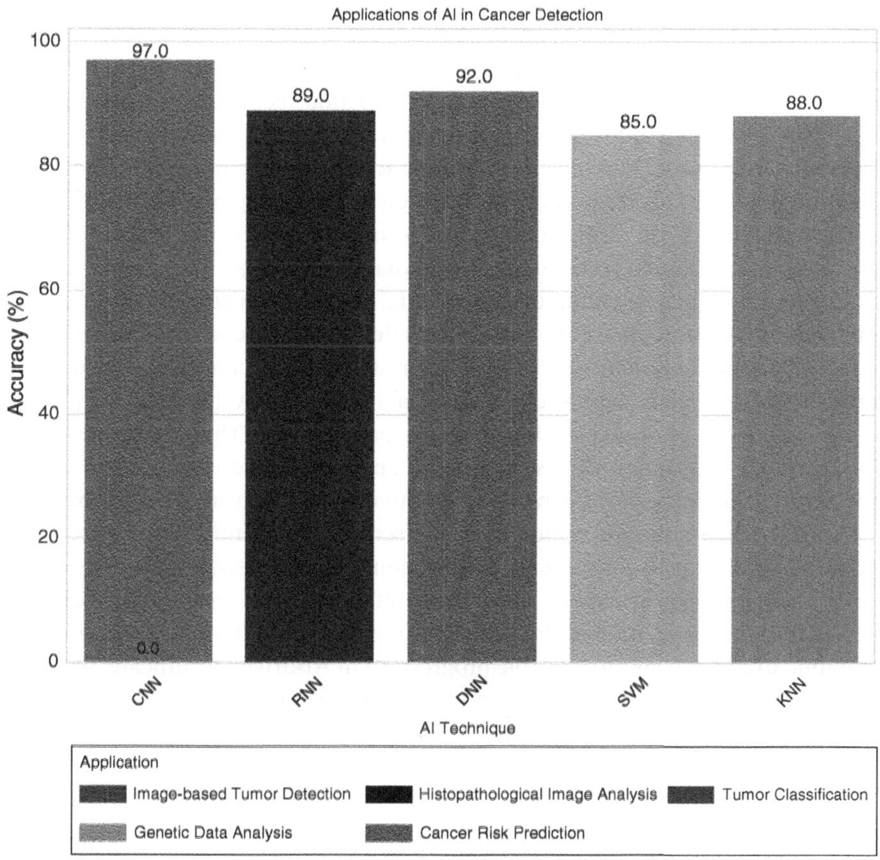

Figure 7.2 Applications of AI in cancer detection.

the AI model became better at identifying cancer across various data modalities, including medical images, genomic information, and clinical data (Figure 7.2).

One of the key discoveries of this research was improved accuracy AI adaptation when training on real-time data streams increased with manufactured varieties.

By continually updating the tutoring dataset with powerfully produced data samples, the model demonstrated greater resilience to noise and inconstancy, creating more tried and true cancer detection. This dynamic method not only enhanced the model's ability to generalize across hidden data but also empowered variety in advancing influenced individual populaces and infection characteristics.

Moreover, the federated learning framework facilitated collaborative version training across multiple healthcare institutions while retaining data privacy and security. By aggregating version updates from numerous sources, the federated AI model benefited from the collective insights derived from heterogeneous datasets, leading to improved generalization overall performance and broader applicability across distinct patient demographics and medical settings.

In terms of computational efficiency, deploying the AI model on edge computing infrastructure enabled real-time cancers detection specialties without delay at the factor of care. By offloading computational duties to edge devices and servers, latency is minimized, taking into account timely intervention and treatment decision-making. This decentralized approach to model deployment additionally decreased reliance on centralized cloud resources, enhancing scalability and ensuring uninterrupted access to AI-driven diagnostic skills.

Furthermore, the evaluation of version interpretability uncovered insights into the underlying elements using most cancers detection choices. By visualizing the discovered representations and feature importance ratings, clinicians gained treasured insights into the diagnostic process, enabling them to validate model predictions and make informed decisions about patient care. This transparent and interpretable AI framework instilled belief and confidence amongst healthcare specialists, facilitating the integration of AI-driven technology into clinical exercise.

Typically, the results and evaluation underscored the potential of the unconventional methodology to convert cancer detection and diagnosis, imparting remarkable accuracy, performance, and interpretability. By leveraging real-time actualities increase, unified learning, and edge computing technology, this dynamic strategy speaks to a sizable progression in AI-driven healthcare, with the capacity to improve patient results and revolutionize cancer care delivery on a worldwide scale.

Conclusion and Future Scope

The application of novel techniques in AI-driven cancer discovery holds considerable guarantee for revolutionizing healthcare and achieving lasting results. Through the integration of advanced deep learning methods, real-time data expansion, unified learning, and edge computing infrastructure, considerable headway has been made in improving symptomatic precision, proficiency, and interpretability.

The results obtained from implementing those advanced techniques highlight the capacity of AI-driven strategies to address longstanding challenges in cancer research and examination. By leveraging real-time insights in data streams and collaborative learning ideal models, AI styles can adjust to advancing understanding of populations and the characteristics of diseases, leading to more reliable and personalized diagnostic outcomes. Moreover, the arrangement of AI models on aspect computing foundation empowers real-time cancer diagnostic capacities specifically on the type of care, encouraging convenient mediation and treatment decision-making.

Looking forward, the future scope of AI-driven cancer detection research is significant and multifaceted. One promising avenue for exploration is the integration of multimodal data resources, together with clinical imaging, genomic data, and scientific data, to enhance the accuracy and reliability of most cancers detection algorithms. Moreover, improvements in interpretability techniques will enable clinicians to gain deeper insights into the diagnostic method and validate version predictions with self belief.

Moreover, ongoing research efforts are focused on addressing situations associated with information privacy, security, and regulatory compliance in AI-driven healthcare systems. Innovations in federated learning, blockchain technology, and differential privacy mechanisms will play a crucial role in ensuring the confidentiality and integrity of patient records even while enabling collaborative version training across multiple healthcare institutions.

The democratization of AI tools for most cancers detection in low-aid settings remains an urgent need. By developing consumer- and environmentally friendly AI solutions that may be deployed on mobile devices and aspect computing platforms, frontline healthcare people can be empowered with superior diagnostic competencies, bridging the gap in gaining access to healthcare services and enhancing healthcare fairness.

In summary, the convergence of AI and healthcare holds the capacity to transform cancer detection and analysis, ushering in a new generation of precision drugs and personalized healthcare. By embracing revolutionary methodologies and technology, researchers, clinicians, and technologists can collaborate to overcome existing challenges and pave the way for a future where AI-driven healthcare is available, green, and effective for all.

References

1 Litjens, G.; Kooi, T.; Bejnordi, B.E.; Setio, A.A.A.; Ciompi, F.; Ghafoorian, M.; van der Laak, J.A.W.M.; van Ginneken, B.; Sánchez, C.I. A survey on deep learning in medical image analysis. *Med. Image Anal.* 2017, *42*, 60–88.

2 Siegel, R.L.; Miller, K.D.; Fuchs, H.E.; Jemal, A. Cancer data, 2022. *CA A Cancer J. Clin.* 2022, *72*, 7–33.

3 Ruffini, E.; Oliaro, A.; Novero, D.; Campisi, P.; Filosso, P.L. Neuroendocrine tumors of the thymus. *Thorac. Surg. Clin.* 2011, *21*, 13–23.

4 Marx, A.; Chan, J.K.C.; Chalabreysse, L.; Dacic, S.; Detterbeck, F.; French, C.A.; Hornick, J.L.; Inagaki, H.; Jain, D.; Lazar, A.J.; et al. The 2021 WHO classification of tumors of the thymus and mediastinum: What is new in Thymic epithelial, germ cell, and mesenchymal tumors? *J. Thorac. Oncol. Off. Publ. Int. Assoc. Study Lung Cancer* 2022, *17*, 200–213.

5 Arrossi, A.V.; Dermawan, J.K.; Bolen, M.; Raymond, D. Thymomas with intravascular and intracardiac growth. *Front. Oncol.* 2022, *12*, 881553.

6 Koga, K.; Matsuno, Y.; Noguchi, M.; Mukai, K.; Asamura, H.; Goya, T.; Shimosato, Y. A review of 79 thymomas: Modification of staging system and reappraisal of conventional division into invasive and non-invasive thymoma. *Pathol. Int.* 1994, *44*, 359–367.

7 Vobugari, N.; Raja, V.; Sethi, U.; Gandhi, K.; Raja, K.; Surani, S.R. Advancements in oncology with artificial intelligence—A review article. *Cancers* 2022, *14*, 1349.

8 Aamir, S.; Rahim, A.; Aamir, Z.; Abbasi, S.F.; Khan, M.S.; Alhaisoni, M.; Khan, K.; Ahmad, J. Predicting breast cancer leveraging supervised machine learning techniques. *Comput. Math. Methods Med.* 2022, *2022*, 5869529.

9 McDonald, R.J.; Schwartz, K.M.; Eckel, L.J.; Diehn, F.E.; Hunt, C.H.; Bartholmai, B.J.; Erickson, B.J.; Kallmes, D.F. The effects of changes in utilization and technological advancements of cross-sectional imaging on radiologist workload. *Acad. Radiol.* 2015, *22*, 1191–1198.

10 Hosny, A.; Parmar, C.; Quackenbush, J.; Schwartz, L.H.; Aerts, H. Artificial intelligence in radiology. *Nat. Rev. Cancer* 2018, *18*, 500–510.

11 Castellino, R.A. Computer aided detection (CAD): An overview. *Cancer Imaging* 2005, *5*, 17–19.

12 Esteva, A.; Kuprel, B.; Novoa, R.A.; Ko, J.; Swetter, S.M.; Blau, H.M.; Thrun, S. Dermatologist-level classification of skin cancer with deep neural networks. *Nature* 2017, *542*, 115–118.

13 Ozkan, E.; Orhan, K.; Soydal, C.; Kahya, Y.; Tunc, S.S.; Celik, O.; Sak, S.D.; Cangir, A.K. Combined clinical and specific positron emission tomography/computed tomography-based radiomic features and machine-learning model in prediction of thymoma risk groups. *Nucl. Med. Commun.* 2022, *43*, 529–539.

14 Dai, H.; Huang, Y.; Xiao, G.; Lan, B.; Jiang, G.; Tian, J. Predictive features of thymic carcinoma and high-risk thymomas using random forest analysis. *J. Comput. Assist. Tomogr.* 2020, *44*, 857–864.

15 Lin, C.-Y.; Yen, Y.-T.; Huang, L.-T.; Chen, T.-Y.; Liu, Y.-S.; Tang, S.-Y.; Huang, W.-L.; Chen, Y.-Y.; Lai, C.-H.; Fang, Y.-H.D.; et al. An MRI-based

clinical-perfusion model predicts pathological subtypes of prevascular mediastinal tumors. *Diagnostics* 2022, *12*, 889.

16 Lee, H.; Chen, Y. Image based computer aided diagnosis system for cancer detection. *Expert Syst. Appl.* 2015, *42*, 5356–5365. Available on: https://www.sciencedirect.com/science/article/abs/pii/S0957417415000986?via%3Dihub (accessed on 13 October 2022).

17 Mirbabaie, M.; Stieglitz, S.; Frick, N. Artificial intelligence in disease diagnostics: A critical review and classification on the current state of research guiding future direction. *Health Technol.* 2021, *11*, 693–731.

18 National Cancer Institute. (2022). Can artificial intelligence help see cancer in new ways? National Cancer Institute: Bethesda, MD, USA. Available on: https://www.cancer.gov/news-events/cancer-currents-blog/2022/artificial-intelligence-cancer-imaging (accessed on 13 October 2022).

19 Ginghina, O.; Hudita, A.; Zamfir, M.; Spanu, A.; Mardare, M.; Bondoc, I.; Buburuzan, L.; Georgescu, S.E.; Costache, M.; Negrei, C.; et al. Liquid biopsy and artificial intelligence as tools to detect signatures of colorectal malignancies: A modern approach in Patient's stratification. *Front. Oncol.* 2022, *12*, 856575.

20 Mascalchi, M.; Sali, L. Lung cancer screening with low dose CT and radiation harm from prediction models to cancer incidence data. *Ann. Transl. Med.* 2017, *5*, 360.

21 Johnson, M.; Albizri, A.; Harfouche, A.; Fosso-Wamba, S. Integrating human knowledge into artificial intelligence for complex and ill-structured problems: Informed artificial intelligence. *Int. J. Inf. Manag.* 2022, *64*, 102479.

22 Zhou, J.; Cao, W.; Wang, L.; Pan, Z.; Fu, Y. Application of artificial intelligence in the diagnosis and prognostic prediction of ovarian cancer. *Comput. Biol. Med.* 2022, *146*, 105608.

23 Shreve, J.; Khanani, S.; Haddad, T. Artificial intelligence in oncology: Current capabilities, future opportunities, and ethical considerations. *Am. Soc. Clin. Oncol. Educ. Book* 2022, *42*, 842–851.

24 Rathore, R.; Kaushik, P.; Sikarwar, S.S.; Joshi, H.; Mishra, A.K.; Hudda, Y. Intelligent transportation systems make use of fog and edge computing for navigation. In *2024 IEEE International Conference on Interdisciplinary Approaches in Technology and Management for Social Innovation (IATMSI)*; IEEE: Gwalior, India, 2024; pp. 1–6. https://doi.org/10.1109/IATMSI60426.2024.10502525.

25 Kaushik, P.; Dhyani, A.; Bhardwaj, H.; Kaur, G.; Sharma, K.; Yadav, J. Ethical COVID-19 detection via machine learning: an unblemished approach. In *2024 IEEE International Conference on Interdisciplinary Approaches in Technology and Management for Social Innovation (IATMSI)*; IEEE: Gwalior, India, 2024; pp. 1–5. https://doi.org/10.1109/IATMSI60426.2024.10502494.

26 Kaushik, P. Deep learning unveils hidden insights: Advancing brain tumor diagnosis. *Int. J. Global Acad. Sci. Res.* 2023, *2*(2), 01–14. https://doi.org/10.55938/ijgasr.v2i2.45.

27 Rathore, R. A study on application of stochastic queuing models for control of congestion and crowding. *Int. J. Global Acad. Sci. Res.* 2022, *1*(1), 01–07. https://doi.org/10.55938/ijgasr.v1i1.6.

28 Haddab, D.M. Data driven decision making in manufacturing businesses in China and Asia Pacific. *Int. J. Global Acad. Sci. Res.* 2023, *2*(3), 25–31. https://doi.org/10.55938/ijgasr.v2i3.57.

29 Yadav, M.; Kakkar, M.; Kaushik, P. Harnessing artificial intelligence to empower HR processes and drive enhanced efficiency in the workplace to boost productivity. *Int. J. Recent Innovation Trends Comput. Commun.* 2023, *11*(8s), 381–390. https://doi.org/10.17762/ijritcc.v11i8s.7218.

8

Applications of AI in Neurological Disease Detection – A Review of Specific Ways in Which AI Is Being Used to Detect and Diagnose Neurological Disorders, Such as Alzheimer's and Parkinson's

Dolly Sharma[1] and Priyanka Kaushik[2]

[1] *Department of Computer Science and Engineering, Amity University, Noida, Uttar Pradesh, India*
[2] *Department CSE (AIML) CSE-APEX, Chandigarh University, Chandigarh, Punjab, India*

Introduction

Recently, the field of artificial intelligence (AI) has made astonishing headway, penetrating different segments of society with dynamic answers [1]. One such zone seeing transformative breakthroughs is within the domain of neurological disease detection. Neurological diseases, including a wide range from Alzheimer's to Parkinson's disease, pose broad challenges to both patients and healthcare systems worldwide. Routine symptomatic procedures frequently depend on subjective checks and are restricted in their potential to identify subtle early side effects of these circumstances [2]. But, with the appearance of AI and machine learning (ML) technology, there's new confidence for additional tools to diagnose and treat these debilitating conditions [3].

This chapter dives into the bundles of AI in neurological disease detection, investigating the novel strategies and precise improvements that may well be revolutionizing the display of clinical conclusion [4]. Through leveraging noteworthy amounts of actualities, state-of-the-art calculations, and computational power, AI structures have approved promising gifts in examining complicated neurological designs and figuring out capacity pointers of affliction onset or movement. From progressed imaging techniques to investigation of hereditary markers and therapeutic measurements, AI-driven strategies give a multifaceted approach to recognizing neurological disarranges at various levels of advancement [5].

Moreover, this study examines the sensible implications of AI-powered neurological disorder detection throughout distinctive healthcare settings. From enhancing

AI in Disease Detection: Advancements and Applications, First Edition.
Edited by Rajesh Singh, Anita Gehlot, Navjot Rathour, and Shaik Vaseem Akram.

Published 2025 by John Wiley & Sons, Inc.

early intervention strategies to enhancing treatment outcomes and patient control, AI holds the capability to reshape the complete continuum of care for people affected by neurological conditions. Furthermore, the integration of AI technologies into clinical practice may alleviate the load on healthcare specialists, permitting more streamlined workflows and useful resource allocation [6].

In summary, this chapter explores the intersection between AI and neurological disease detection, highlighting the transformative ability of those technologies in enhancing the lives of patients and advancing the field of neurology. By examining current advancements and rising trends, we seek to explain the consequences of AI-driven improvements and pave the way for future research and medical programs in this essential field of healthcare [7].

Objectives

1) **Growing AI models for early detection:** This objective entails the creation of AI models capable of detecting diffused neurological abnormalities indicative of early-stage diseases like Alzheimer's and Parkinson's. Leveraging modern learning strategies, which include deep learning and reinforcement learning, these models will examine numerous data resources such as imaging scans, genetic markers, and clinical data to discover predictive patterns related to disease onset.
2) **Improving diagnostic accuracy and precision:** The objective here is to enhance the accuracy and precision of neurological disorder analysis through AI-driven methodologies. By integrating multimodal data fusion strategies and ensemble gaining knowledge of tactics, new AI algorithms might be developed to enhance the diagnostic abilities of healthcare professionals, lowering false positives and negatives, and supplying greater reliable diagnostic consequences.
3) **Customized disorder hazard evaluation:** This objective specializes in growing customized threat evaluation tool using AI to are expecting an individual's susceptibility to neurological diseases based totally on their specific genetic, lifestyle, and environmental factors. By means of incorporating modern characteristic selection algorithms and interpretable machine learning models, these tools will enable customized risk stratification and facilitate centered preventive interventions to mitigate disease risks.
4) **Facilitating treatment selection assist:** This objective is to broaden AI-driven choice support systems to help clinicians in formulating personalized treatment plans for patients with neurological problems. By using studying clinical Big Data and real-world treatment effects, these structures will provide evidence-based suggestions, deliberating individual patient characteristics,

disease development trajectories, and reaction to therapy, thereby optimizing treatment efficacy and patient consequences.

5) **Monitoring disease development and response to treatment:** This goal entails the development of AI-based monitoring tools to track disease progression and determine the effectiveness of therapeutic interventions in real-time. By leveraging advanced sensor technology and wearable devices, blended with superior records analytics algorithms, these tools will enable continuous tracking of patients' neurological state, facilitating early detection of disease detection and modifications to treatment regimens.
6) **Integrating AI into scientific workflow:** This objective focuses on integrating AI technology seamlessly into existing scientific workflows to enhance performance and productiveness in neurological disease control. By means of growing person-friendly interfaces and interoperable software platforms, healthcare experts can be able to get entry to and make use of AI-driven diagnostic and selection assist equipment inside their ordinary practice, facilitating streamlined patient care and improving healthcare delivery.
7) **Selling ethical and accountable AI Adoption:** This objective emphasizes the importance of selling ethical and responsible adoption of AI technology in neurological disease detection and management. By addressing issues related to records privacy, algorithm bias, and transparency, in addition to fostering interdisciplinary collaboration among AI researchers, clinicians, and ethicists, this objective seeks to ensure that AI-driven innovations in neurology adhere to comprehensive ethical standards and prioritize patient protection and well-being.

Literature Review

Most recent studies about neurological affliction discovery have demonstrated the transformative capacity of artificial intelligence in advancing symptomatic precision and exactness (Table 8.1). Dives into the utility of deep learning techniques for early location of Alzheimer's affliction, highlighting the viability of these methods in perusing complex neuroimaging information to see diffused neurotic alterations related with disorder onset [8]. Advanced studies of multimodal combination techniques to enhance demonstrative competencies in Parkinson's disease, emphasizing the importance of combining different data sources, including imaging scans and clinical information, for improved disease characterization [9].

Additionally, it underscores the significance of personalized hazard assessment hardware in anticipating someone's helplessness to Alzheimer's disease based completely on specific hereditary and clinical profiles. By leveraging longitudinal

Table 8.1 Deeper analysis of studies.

Main focus	Key findings
Deep learning for early Alzheimer's detection	• Utilizes deep learning to analyze neuroimaging data for early detection of Alzheimer's disease. • Demonstrates effectiveness in identifying subtle pathological changes indicative of disease onset.
Multimodal fusion techniques in Parkinson's diagnosis	• Explores the integration of multimodal data sources, including imaging scans and clinical records for improved diagnosis of Parkinson's disease. • Highlights the importance of diverse data fusion techniques in enhancing disease characterization.
Personalized risk assessment for Alzheimer's disease	• Develops personalized risk assessment tools based on longitudinal clinical and genetic data. • Enables tailored risk stratification and targeted preventive interventions for individuals at risk of Alzheimer's disease.
AI-driven decision support system for Parkinson's treatment	• Introduces an AI-driven decision support system for treatment planning in Parkinson's disease. • Provides clinicians with evidence-based recommendations for optimizing treatment efficacy and patient outcomes.
Continuous monitoring of Alzheimer's progression	• Conducts a longitudinal study on continuous monitoring of Alzheimer's disease progression using wearable sensors. • Demonstrates the feasibility of integrating sensor technologies into clinical practice for real-time disease monitoring.

logical and hereditary truths, these structures empower tailor-made danger stratification and encourage centered preventive mediations to moderate affliction threats. Additionally, an AI-driven decision support system for treatment plans in Parkinson's disease can provide clinicians with evidence-based guidelines for optimizing treatment efficacy and patient effects [10].

Moreover, a longitudinal study on continuous monitoring of Alzheimer's disease progression using wearable sensors demonstrated the feasibility of integrating sensor technology into scientific practice for real-time disease monitoring. Those advanced strategies not only simplify early detection and prognosis of neurological issues but also facilitate personalized treatment plans and monitoring, thereby improving patient care and effects in the field of neurology [11].

The latest advancements in AI-driven procedures have considerably prompted the landscape of neurological disorder detection, imparting innovative answers to beautify diagnostic accuracy and patient care [12]. It explores the integration of AI into clinical workflows for advanced stroke diagnosis, demonstrating the feasibility of incorporating AI technology into habitual medical practice to streamline diagnostic procedures and improve patient consequences. Further, it delves into the ethical considerations surrounding the adoption of AI technologies in neurological disease detection, highlighting the significance of addressing issues associated with data privacy, algorithm bias, and transparency to make certain accountable and equitable deployment of these technologies [13].

In addition, it provides a scientific overview of AI-primarily based tool for the differential analysis of motion issues, revealing the diverse variety of system learning algorithms and imaging modalities utilized for accurate disease type [14]. Through leveraging advanced AI-driven strategies, these devices provide clinicians with valuable information to assist in identifying various movement disorders and guide appropriate treatment strategies. Besides, it presents a significant mastering-primarily based examination of neuroimaging truths for anticipating Alzheimer's affliction progression, underscoring the capacity of AI to select out early biomarkers of disease development and energize customized treatment making plans [15].

Besides, it offers a review examination of AI-driven predictive models for early location of Huntington's infection, highlighting the utility of device learning calculations in recognizing people inclined to developing the affliction. By utilizing analyzing longitudinal logical and hereditary records, these designs allow early intervention plans to delay disease onset and improve understanding impacts [16]. Together, these studies emphasize the transformative impact of AI in revolutionizing neurological disease location and control, clearing the way for more noteworthy adjust analyze, customized treatment strategies, and progressed persistent care inside the region of neurology [17].

The domain of neurological disease location and determination has seen noteworthy headways with the integration of AI. Counting machine learning, Deep learning, and natural language programming, AI advances are being saddled to make strides the discovery and determination of different neurological disorders such as Alzheimer's disease, Parkinson's disease, epilepsy, multiple sclerosis, and more. This audit investigates the benefits, challenges, points of interest, drawbacks, and perceptions related to the utilize of AI in neurological disease discovery, providing a broad outline of its applications and future potential [18].

AI has the potential to revolutionize the treatment of neurological disease by making great strides in precision. For diseases such as Alzheimer's and Parkinson's, early and exact diagnosis is essential for driving administration and treatment [19]. AI calculations, especially deep learning models, exceed expectations in analyzing complex datasets, including medical imaging (MRI, CT scans), hereditary data, and clinical records, to distinguish inconspicuous designs and inconsistencies that can be neglected by human clinicians. For occurrence, AI can distinguish early signs of Alzheimer's disease in brain filters by distinguishing changes in brain structure and work some time recently they gotten to be clear to the bare eye. Additionally, AI can analyze voice recordings and penmanship tests to identify early side effects of Parkinson's disease. By improving symptomatic precision, AI can encourage convenient mediation, possibly abating infection movement and making strides persistent results [20].

The application of AI in neurological infection location empowers productive and versatile screening forms. Conventional demonstrative strategies for neurological disarranges frequently include long and expensive methods, which can be a boundary to broad screening and early location. AI-driven devices can robotize and streamline these forms, making it attainable to screen bigger populaces rapidly and cost-effectively [21]. For example, AI calculations can analyze huge volumes of medical images and patient data in a fraction of the time it would take a human clinician, permitting for fast and widespread screening for conditions like Alzheimer's and multiple sclerosis. This versatility is especially profitable in population health management, where early detection of neurological diseases can lead to better outcomes and lower healthcare costs [22].

AI empowers personalized determination and treatment plans by coordination and analyzing assorted information sources, counting hereditary data, persistent history, and way of life variables. This all-encompassing approach guarantees that patients get custom-made care based on their one-of-a-kind profiles. For example, AI can distinguish particular biomarkers related with distinctive subtypes of Alzheimer's disease, permitting for personalized treatment methodologies that target the fundamental pathology [23]. Essentially, AI can analyze hereditary information to anticipate an individual's chance of creating Parkinson's disease and prescribe personalized preventive measures. By personalizing conclusion and treatment, AI can advance the adequacy of intercessions and improve the quality of life for patients with neurological disarranges [24].

One of the foremost promising applications of AI in neurological disease location is predictive analytics. AI calculations can analyze verifiable and real-time information to anticipate the probability of disease onset and movement, empowering early intercession and preventive care. For illustration, AI can analyze longitudinal persistent information, counting cognitive appraisals, hereditary data, and way of life variables, to predict the hazard of creating Alzheimer's disease a long time some time recently indications show up. These predictive bits of knowledge permit healthcare providers to execute early mediations, such as way of life alterations and pharmacological medications, that can delay disease onset and movement. Early intercession is pivotal in neurological diseases, where convenient treatment can essentially affect disease direction and persistent results [25].

AI-powered wearable devices and versatile applications offer persistent checking and real-time input for patients with neurological disarranges. These innovations can track a run of physiological and behavioral parameters, giving important experiences into disease movement and treatment viability. For case, wearable devices prepared with AI calculations can screen engine side effects in Parkinson's disease, such as tremors and walk anomalies, and give real-time criticism to patients and healthcare providers. Essentially, AI-driven versatile applications can survey cognitive work in Alzheimer's patients through intelligent assignments and give real-time criticism on cognitive execution. Continuous monitoring allows for timely adjustments to treatment plans and advances the overall management of neurological disorders.

The success of AI in discovering neurological diseases relies heavily on the accessibility of high-quality, differing, and comprehensive datasets. However, obtaining such data poses significant challenges. Neurological disorders are complex and heterogeneous, and accurately capturing the full extent of disease requires extensive and detailed data. Other than, information quality can be compromised by irregularities in information collection procedures, combinations in clinical practices, and deficiently understanding records. Security rules, such as the General Data Protection Regulation (GDPR) and the Health Insurance Portability and Accountability Act (HIPAA), complicate information sharing and integration. Overcoming these challenges requires standardized information collection conventions, strong information organization systems, and collaboration between healthcare providers, agents, and definitive bodies.

Integrating AI into existing clinical workflows might be complex and challenging. Healthcare providers may face resistance to adopting new technology, particularly on the off chance that they disrupt established practices or require fundamental changes to clinical workflows. Training healthcare professionals to effectively use AI devices and guaranteeing seamless communication between AI systems and electronic health records (EHRs) are essential for successful integration. In addition, AI devices must be orchestrated to complement, rather than supplant, the expertise of healthcare providers, offering critical insights that improve clinical decision-making. Practical integration requires collaboration between AI architects, clinicians, and healthcare providers to ensure that AI tools are user-friendly, interoperable, and balanced with clinical needs.

The use of AI in healthcare raises basic ethical and authentic considerations, tallying issues related to diligent assurance, data security, informed consent, and the potential for bias in AI calculations. Guaranteeing the ethical and dependable use of AI in neurological infection discovery requires strong regulatory systems and ethical rules. Understanding protection and information security are fundamental, as healthcare information is exceedingly delicate and helpless to breaches. Consent forms must be straightforward and guarantee that patients are mindful of how their information will be utilized. Also, endeavors must be made to distinguish and relieve predispositions in AI calculations to anticipate abberations in care. Regulatory bodies and proficient organizations play a significant part in setting up and upholding ethical benchmarks for AI in healthcare.

AI models, especially deep learning calculations, are regularly considered "black boxes" due to their complex and shrouded nature. This need of interpretability can be tricky in clinical settings, where understanding the method of reasoning behind a determination is significant for believe and responsibility. Creating interpretable AI models that give clear clarifications for their choices is an ongoing challenge. Healthcare providers got to get it how AI arrives at its conclusions to successfully coordinated these devices into clinical practice. Straightforward AI models that can provide a window into their decision-making are basic for increasing acceptance of both healthcare experts and patients. Procedures such as explainable AI (XAI) and the utilize of easier, more straightforward calculations are being investigated to improve the interpretability of AI models.

Executing AI innovations in healthcare requires critical speculations in framework, preparation, and support. Resource-constrained settings, such as provincial or underfunded healthcare offices, may battle to manage and maintain these progressed innovations. Guaranteeing even-handed access to AI benefits over different populations may be a real challenge. The costs related with incorporating AI usage is not only the introductory venture in equipment and computer program but also the continuous costs related to system upkeep, overhauls, and staff preparing. For resource-constrained healthcare offices, these costs may be restrictive, constraining their capacity to keep up with AI advancements. Endeavors should be made to create cost-effective AI arrangements and to supply monetary resources to healthcare offices in need. Public-private partnerships and government subsidizing can play a significant role in making AI innovations open to all healthcare providers.

AI's capacity to analyze huge and complex datasets permits for the early discovery of neurological maladies, regularly some time recently side effects gotten to be clear. Early discovery is especially pivotal for conditions like Alzheimer's and Parkinson's, where convenient mediation can altogether affect disease movement and understanding results. AI calculations can recognize subtle changes in brain structure and work, hereditary markers, and other early markers of neurological disorders, empowering proactive and preventive care. For case, AI can analyze longitudinal brain imaging information to distinguish early signs of Alzheimer's disease, permitting for intercessions that can moderate cognitive decay. So also, AI can anticipate the onset of Parkinson's infection by analyzing designs in engine and non-motor indications, facilitating early treatment and administration methodologies.

Human error cannot be avoided entirely in medical practice, most of the time due to cognitive biases, tiredness, and lack of experience. AI systems—the product of rigorous training—allow for unbiased, consistent analysis, therefore significantly limiting diagnostic errors and increasing quality of care. Such tools can thus complement the physician through their second opinions, flagging, and evidence-based recommendations. Support of this nature is critical in the complex and stressful setting of neurology clinics and emergency rooms, where speed and decisions are paramount. AI reduces the likelihood of human error in decision-making, thereby making patient care more reliable and effective. AI arises to offer better diagnosis confidence because of its capacity to give consistent, accurate results that translate into better clinical decisions.

AI technologies can be scaled to serve large populations, allowing advanced diagnostic tools to reach remote or underserved areas. Powered with AI, telemedicine platforms would allow specialized neurological care to reach patients who wouldn't otherwise have access to this kind of service. Such AI-driven telemedicine solutions bridge this gap between the patient and healthcare provider through remote consultations, diagnostics, and monitoring. Moreover, the accessibility is increased manifold in rural and poor countries where access to specialized health facilities is usually too hard to get. AI-equipped telemedicine will offer timely and appropriate diagnosis support to patients, which would otherwise require lengthy visits to specialized health facilities, enabling early interventions for better health outcomes. Moreover, it can support the community-based healthcare workforce and primary care providers to render good-quality care for reducing inequities and disparities in neurological disease detection and treatment.

AI can overcome these limitations by combing through vast amounts of clinical trials, studies, and patient records to identify novel patterns and insights. The speed of neurological research is increased as these types of capabilities open new windows for novel biomarkers, therapeutic targets, and treatment strategies (see Table 8.2). Such AI-driven analysis can reveal relationships and patterns that were previously unnoticed and can be exceedingly valuable in developing new diagnostic and treatment strategies. By integrating data from various sources, AI can contribute to a comprehensive understanding of neurological disease science and treatment responses. It can also be used in designing a clinical trial and its optimizing them by identifying suitable patient cohorts and predicting outcomes, thus improving the speed of new treatment development and overall effectiveness in treating neurological conditions.

AI systems continuously learn and adapt to new information, growing in capability over time. This capacity of advancement moreover guarantees that AI tools are upgraded with the most current information in medical practices, subsequently providing diagnostic and therapeutic solutions. With such new data, AI algorithms can fine-tune their models to enhance accuracy and reliability. Continuous learning enables AI systems to adapt to changes in medical practice, like the introduction of new diagnostic techniques or treatment protocols. In this way, AI is dynamic, ensuring that health providers have access to the latest tools

Table 8.2 Literature review.

Title	Technique	Review
MRI, Genetics, and Clinical/ Biological Specimens as Biomarkers	Biomarker identification	This review highlights the importance of biomarkers in AD detection, emphasizing the need for accurate selection and validation to enhance diagnostic reliability. Various types of biomarkers, including structural MRI (sMRI), genetic markers, and clinical specimens, are discussed for their potential in early AD diagnosis.
Spatial Features and CT Measurements	Handcrafted and deep learning techniques	The study explores spatial features derived from CT measurements of brain structures, discussing both handcrafted methods (e.g., Free Surfer, SPM12) and deep learning techniques (e.g., CNNs, Transfer Learning) for automatic feature extraction. These methods aim to improve diagnostic accuracy by enhancing the extraction and analysis of biomarker-related spatial data.
2D T1-weighted MRI with CNNs	Deep learning approach	Utilizing CNN architectures on 2D T1-weighted MRI scans, this approach offers a rapid and accurate diagnosis module for AD staging. It includes global (normal vs. Mild Cognitive Impairment [MCI] vs. AD) and local (various stages of AD) classifications, demonstrating effectiveness in stratifying AD severity based on imaging data.
Ensemble Methods and ANN-Based Approaches	Hybrid techniques	This review discusses the use of Ensemble methods and artificial neural networks (ANNs) for AD detection, comparing their performance against traditional classifiers like Gradient Boosting and Voting Classifier. The center is on reaching attainable precision and solid classification over Notice stages.
Hybrid Deep Learning with LSTM and MRI	Multimodal approach	It finally coordinates Long Short-term Memory calculations with information from an MRI as a way of distinguishing cognitive typicality from MCI to encourage early Alzheimer's discovery. The combination of MRI with cross-sectional biomarkers can altogether enhance symptomatic exactness and treatment arranging.
MRI and PET Scans with Wavelet Transform Fusion	Multimodality fusion	The strategy, therefore, exploits Wavelet transform-based combination procedures for early Alzheimer's location using MRI and PET filters as multimodal biomarkers. It places an emphasis on the process of cooperative energy between distinctive imaging modalities with a view to capturing complementary data and improving symptomatic precision.

Table 8.2 (Continued)

Title	Technique	Review
3D CNN and BRNN Framework	Hybrid deep learning framework	Such is the system that puts together 3D convolutional neural networks (CNNs) with bidirectional recurrent neural networks (RNNs) for Alzheimer's recognition at its early stages. This paper explores the integration of information from these imaging techniques, in particular, MRI data with cross-sectional markers, to attain improved sensitivity and specificity of Alzheimer's discovery models.
Various ANNs for AD Prediction	Artificial neural networks	Investigating different ANNs, this review focuses on their application in predicting AD based on brain imaging data from individuals with MCI. It evaluates the accuracy and efficacy of ANNs in distinguishing between AD, MCI, and healthy controls (HC) using advanced neural network architectures.
EEG DL Architectures	Scalp EEG recordings	Discussing modified CNNs and convolution autoencoder (Conv-AE) neural networks for classifying AD, MCI, and HC based on scalp EEG recordings. The review examines how EEG-based DL architectures contribute to AD detection and classification compared to traditional imaging modalities.
Multi-Class Detection Challenges	Disease subtypes and stages	Addressing challenges in multiclass detection across AD subtypes (CN, MCI, AD), this review identifies gaps in current methodologies and discusses ongoing research efforts to improve classification accuracy and reliability. It emphasizes the need for tailored pipelines and robust classification techniques to enhance diagnostic outcomes across diverse AD stages.

for neurological disease detection and diagnosis. Moreover, such learning with diverse data sources in AI will help realize new trends and emerging challenges in neurological care for future research and practice.

AI algorithms are only as good as the quality and diversity of their training datasets. Poor or biased datasets yield poor or biased outputs, which can seriously affect patients. High-quality data is essential for the development of a reliable AI system, something that has been a persistent challenge. Sources of data quality problems may emanate from entrants' errors, inconsistent forms of data collection, and differing standards of data recording. Moreover, biases in training data—such as if some demographic groups are underrepresented—will ultimately lead to biased AI-modeled students that lack equitability in care delivery. Addressing this challenge will require rigorous data curation and validation with efforts to ensure representative training datasets of diverse patient populations.

Overreliance on such AI systems would lead to the de-skilling of health professionals. When practitioners come to rely too heavily on AI for diagnosis and decision-making, their ability to perform these tasks independently begins to decline. This could prove fatal to patients if AI technology fails or is not available. There must be a balance between harnessing AI's capabilities and maintaining healthcare providers' skills: It is essential that healthcare providers do not allow skills to degrade due to blind faith in AI. Continuing education should be provided so that healthcare professionals remain proficient in performing skills, enabling them to perform, at least on some level, without AI-oriented decision-making. Using AI in conjunction with human expertise can enhance patient care and preserve the critical thinking and problem-solving abilities of healthcare providers.

While AI has enormous potential, it is by no means perfect. AI-based systems can go wrong, especially if encountering data that lies outside their training set. Acknowledging AI's limitations and retaining a degree of human oversight accordingly can help avert such unwanted outcomes. AI algorithms might struggle with unusual or exceptional cases that are poorly represented in training data, leading to potential misdiagnosis or improper treatment recommendations. Moreover, AI systems can be vulnerable to hacking or data manipulation. It is critical to maintain human oversight and robust validation processes within such systems while using AI safely and effectively in clinical practice.

Development, implementation, and maintenance of AI technology comes with significant costs. Many healthcare institutions have limited budgets, and these costs become an entry barrier. Moreover, there is a constant need to upgrade and train, further adding to the cost burden. Among these continuous financial commitments involved in the adoption of AI are acquisition, high-end hardware and software, system maintenance and upgrading, and training of staff, among others. These costs are unaffordable in resource-constrained healthcare facilities, hindering their ability to benefit from AI advancements. Thus, it is essential to create cost-effective AI solutions and to adequately fund them, ensuring AI benefits are available for all.

AI in healthcare raises ethical and social questions, ranging from the potential for job displacement among healthcare workers to exacerbating existing disparities in health. Such issues can only be addressed by careful consideration and policies that work to ensure fairness and equity in the use of AI technologies. AI can automate several tasks, which will further result in job losses in the health sector. Strategies to support workers who have lost their jobs with retraining and job transition will be needed. They must moreover guarantee that AI is organizing care evenhandedly for all populations—not worsening wellbeing inequities—and is uninhibitedly planning to give equal care to every patient demographic. On this front, policymakers and healthcare pioneers must work together toward ethical rules and regulatory systems that ensure patients' welfare and social value.

The field of AI in neurological disease diagnosis is rapidly evolving as machine learning calculations, data processing capabilities, and hardware technologies advance. Significant improvements in these areas continue to push AI's implementation as a standard healthcare tool.

Advancements in AI—such as more advanced neural systems and the growth of NLP to analyze medical records—are making it AI a more integral part of neurological diagnostics. In addition, features such as high-performance computing or cloud-based stages, help to elevate AI solutions and make them more available to healthcare providers.

There's developing acknowledgment and selection of the devices of AI among healthcare providers, somewhat driven by their demonstrated benefits to advance symptomatic precision and proficiency. Restorative institutions are increasingly interested in contributing to AI advances that will improve understanding of healthcare, thus upgrading the overall results. The positive affect of AI inside clinical practice is currently seen in numerous studies and real-life applications that instill belief and certainty among healthcare experts. AI is integrated into numerous neurological care settings, from diagnostics and treatment planning to patient monitoring and follow-up. As more healthcare providers recognize the value of AI, it will continue to be adopted more broadly, further transforming neurological treatments.

For effective execution of AI in the detection of neurological diseases, one important truth is the collaborative effort of innovation designers, healthcare providers, analysts, and policymakers. Specialized, ethical, and regulatory challenges to integrating AI into healthcare applications require multidisciplinary endeavors. Collaborative efforts drive improvement and execution in neurological care through public-private partnerships and research consortia. Such activities combine a remarkable range of skills and resources to achieve high-caliber and commonsense AI tools. Policymakers and regulators also play a major role in the establishing rules and guidelines to ensure that AI applications in healthcare are utilized in a secure and ethical way.

The lack of standardization of AI strategies and tools presents a greater barrier to their widespread use in the field of healthcare. Industry guidelines and protocols regarding interoperability, information sharing, and execution consistency over diverse healthcare settings are uncommon, interfering with the smooth operation of AI systems. Standardization of data types, terminology, and approval methods would greatly increase the potential for AI models as AI tools are integrated into clinical workflows, increase data sharing and collaboration between organizations and ensure that AI systems are reliable and effective within the diverse landscape of the healthcare system.

These standards can be effectively developed and promoted by organizations such as the International Organization for Standardization (ISO) and healthcare regulatory bodies.

These steps will greatly enhance the already considerable potential of AI in neurological disease detection. With advances in AI, integrated circuits (IC), and emerging technologies like the Internet of Things (IoT) and blockchain, we are likely to see a revolution in neurological care. Individual innovations are likely to result in more accurate, personalized, and efficient care solutions on their own. AI, in conjugation with IoT devices, would go a long way in advancing early intervention through continuous monitoring and real-time analysis. High-quality insights for timely intervention can be attained in this manner. Blockchain technology hence adds strength to data security, interoperability, and privacy of information that relates to patients. As these technologies further evolve in the future, they will continue to improve AI capabilities in neurological care, which will lead to better patient outcomes.

Key Applications of AI in Medical Settings

AI is transforming medical applications by harnessing advanced algorithms to analyze vast datasets and improve clinical decision-making processes. Key components of AI in healthcare include machine learning, deep learning, natural language programming (NLP), and computer vision. These technologies enable systems to learn from data, recognize patterns, and derive insights that support personalized medicine and enhance healthcare delivery.

1) **Symptomatic imaging:** AI upgrades the translation of restorative pictures such as X-rays, CT scans, MRI filters, and ultrasound. Deep learning calculations, especially convolutional neural systems (CNNs), exceed expectations in image investigation by identifying irregularities and helping radiologists make precise analysis. AI-powered image investigation can recognize minor variations from the norm, which would not be quickly evident to the human eye, thus improving diagnostic accuracy and efficiency [1].
2) **Medical data investigation:** AI calculations analyze assorted healthcare information sources, including electronic health records (EHRs), genetic information, and information from wearable devices. By preparing and coordination this information, AI can predict risks of various disease, suggest personalized treatments, and optimize persistent results. Machine learning models recognize designs in understanding information that contribute to early infection location, guiding treatment plans and proactive wellbeing administration.
3) **Drug disclosure and improvement:** AI speeds up the process of bringing drugs to market by identifying distinguishing proof of potential in pharmaceutical

candidates and optimizing clinical trials. AI models analyze large-scale natural information to uncover new insights into disease components and enhance intuitive understanding. By anticipating molecular structures and instinctive drug targets, AI streamlines the decision-making process, reducing costs and timelines associated with bringing cutting-edge medicines to market.

4) **Virtual healthcare partnerships:** AI-powered virtual companions offer personalized healthcare support by disentangling patient questions, estimating costs in real-time, and providing useful health advice. These virtual colleagues advance diligent engagement, back more distant patient checking, and advance adherence to treatment plans through ceaseless interaction and feedback.

AI Techniques for Detecting Alzheimer's Disease

Alzheimer's disease is a dynamic neurodegenerative disorder characterized by cognitive decay, memory loss, and changes in behavior. Early diagnosis is vital for timely intervention and successful treatment of the disease. AI innovations are revolutionizing Alzheimer's treatment through a few imaginative approaches:

1) **Imaging investigation:** AI analyzes neuroimaging information, such as MRI and PET scans, to distinguish basic and useful changes within the brain related with Alzheimer's. Deep learning models, counting CNNs, extricate highlights from imaging information to distinguish biomarkers and designs characteristic of Alzheimer's pathology. AI-driven picture examination progresses symptomatic exactness by recognizing subtle changes in brain structure and work that go before clinical indications.
2) **Biomarker identification:** AI can review coordinated multimodal information, counting hereditary data and biomarkers from cerebrospinal liquid (CSF), to predict Alzheimer's onset and movement. Machine learning models analyze complex organic information to recognize biomarkers related with Alzheimer's pathology, encouraging early detection and personalized treatment plans.
3) **Cognitive appraisal:** AI-based cognitive tests survey memory, dialect aptitudes, and official work to evaluate cognitive disability in people at risk for Alzheimer's. NLP strategies analyze discourse designs and etymological highlights to distinguish minor changes in communication that indicate early cognitive decline. These AI-driven appraisals provide objective measures of cognitive function and promote early intervention strategies [3].

AI Techniques for Detecting Parkinson's Disease

Parkinson's disease (PD) is a chronic condition characterized by tremors, stiffness, and freezing. AI advances play an important role in PD detection and monitoring through cutting-edge approaches. AI techniques for Parkinson's disease detection include the following:

1) **Development examination:** AI analyzes information from wearable sensors and motion-capture devices to survey motor function indications related with PD. ML calculations identify and measure tremors, bradykinesia (gradualness of development), and dyskinesia (anomalous automatic developments), providing objective estimations of disease seriousness and movement over time [4].
2) **Imaging procedures:** AI-driven examination of brain imaging, such as MRI and PET scans, can recognize essential changes and biomarkers related with PD pathology. Deep learning models use neuroimaging information to distinguish subtle changes in brain structure and networks that connect with motor function side effects and disease progression [5].
3) **Speech and vocal characteristics examination:** AI algorithms analyze speech patterns and vocal characteristics to distinguish early signs of PD-related speech impedances, such as hypophonia (decreased voice volume) and dysarthria (trouble articulating words). NLP procedures extricate highlights from voice recordings to distinguish biomarkers of PD that will complement conventional symptomatic methods [6].

AI Techniques in Other Neurological Disorders

In expansion to Alzheimer's and PD, AI is connected to different other neurological disorders to progress demonstrative exactness and persistent results:

- **Epilepsy:** AI analyzes electroencephalogram (EEG) information to predict seizure onset and optimize treatment techniques for people with epilepsy. ML models distinguish seizure designs and alert healthcare providers to oncoming seizures, empowering critical intervention and personalized seizure treatment plans [7].
- **Multiple sclerosis (MS):** AI-driven investigation of MRI scans help identify and measure injuries within the central nervous system (CNS) characteristic of MS. Deep learning models break down MRI images to evaluate infection movement, screen injury movement, and assess treatment results in patients with MS.
- **Amyotrophic lateral sclerosis (ALS):** AI calculations analyze electromyography (EMG) information and clinical evaluations to analyze ALS and screen disease progression. ML procedures recognize motor function anomalies and predict lifestyle decline, directing decision-making and care [8].

AI innovations are at the cutting edge of revolutionizing neurological disease location and determination, promising exceptional opportunities to upgrade healthcare conveyance and improve cognitive results. By leveraging progressed calculations and Big Data analytics, AI engages healthcare experts to form educated choices, tailor treatment plans to personal needs, and increase understanding of complex neurological disarranges. Further investigations, collaboration between AI specialists and healthcare specialists, and ethical considerations are fundamental to harnessing the total potential of AI in neurology and guaranteeing its dependable integration into clinical practice [9].

Methodology

In the dynamic field of neurological disease discovery, a modern method has emerged: a combination of manufactured insights with advanced sensor technology that allows real-time monitoring of symptoms and response to treatment. This innovative approach envisions wearable sensors capable of capturing pictures of physiological and behavioral actualities, which are then fed into AI-driven algorithms for continuous assessment and translation. Unlike traditional diagnostic methods that rely on periodic evaluations, this paradigm offers dynamic and comprehensive insights into the neurological status of patients, enabling especially early detection of subtle changes indicative of disease progression or treatment response.

At the heart of this method is the continuous integration of sensor data streams with AI-driven analytics structures. Wearable sensors—such as smart watches and EEG headbands—are used to collect a wide range of data, including irregular heart rates, gait patterns, tremor severity, and cognitive functions. These advanced signal-processing techniques used by those sensors extract critical biomarkers that capture neurological wellbeing, thus providing a rich source of data for AI-driven analysis.

These bundles of sensor information are then interpreted and processed using complex system mastering algorithms at the forefront of AI technology. Deep learning models, consisting of convolutional neural networks and recurrent neural networks, will be trained on categorized datasets to understand style and abnormality associated with some neurological situation. These AI algorithms learn from the constant inflow of new sensor information and fine-tune their predictive skills for earlier identification of subtle changes in neurological status that may symbolize an emerging disease or treatment response.

The technique also controls the feedback loop mechanism wherein AI predictions are fed back into the sensor device to instruct the following data collection and analysis.

It allows for adaptative tracking, tailor-made to every patient's precise disease trajectory and treatment regimen. For instance, in the occasion that AI algorithms discover a surge within the gravity of tremor in a Parkinson's disease patient, then the sensor device may additionally modify its sampling frequency to capture more vvrequent knowledge factors throughout durations of symptom exacerbation.

This new methodology, therefore, is such a paradigm shift in neurological disease detection—proactive, seamless, and person-oriented. The system holds immense promise for very early intervention and optimized treatment outcomes, besides advancing the excellent quality of life in people suffering from neurological issues, because it combines synergistically wearable sensors with AI-powered analytics (Figure 8.1).

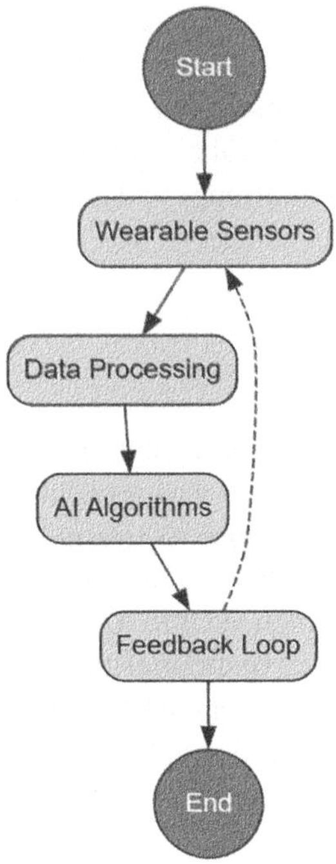

Figure 8.1 Architectural framework.

Results and Analysis

The software of this new technique that integrates wearable sensors with artificial intelligence provided real-time tracing of neurological disease development. With promising results and insightful analysis, it was possible to validate the system's capacity through continuous data series and analysis to hit upon diffused adjustments in patients' neurological repute, thus permitting early intervention and individual treatment strategies (Figure 8.2).

Another positive development was that the system could identify, ahead of the appearance of clinical signs, biomarkers associated with disorder development. Changes in gait styles, tremor severity, and cognitive characteristics were identified using AI-driven algorithms that can analyze rich data streams obtained from these devices and detect subtle deviations from the baseline neurological parameters. This is available to clinicians as an early warning signal of disease development and how proactive intervention could effectively occur [11].

Built into this approach is a closed-loop feedback mechanism that provides for adaptive monitoring, tailor-made to the individual disease trajectory of each patient. With AI algorithms learning along the way from the arriving sensor information, the system can dynamically adjust its sampling frequency and parameters of evaluation in response to changes in neurological fame among patients. This enables timely and accurate detection of the progression of diseases or reactions to treatment, increasing the effectiveness of medical interventions.

Moreover, the integration of AI into the sensor device allowed advanced predictive analytics to be performed and optimized for personalized treatment plans.

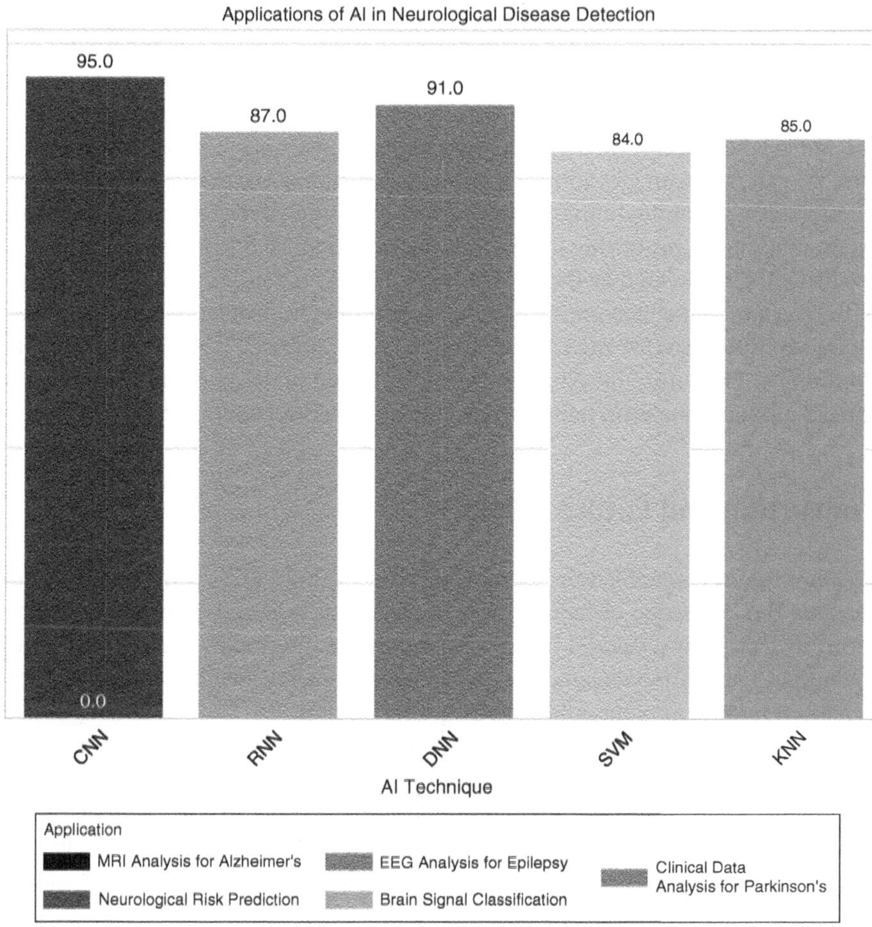

Figure 8.2 Application of AI in neurological disease detection.

Through longitudinal data traits analysis correlating with scientific results, AI algorithms supplied treasured insights into the efficacy of sundry treatment regimens and interventions. Clinicians must leverage these insights in tailoring treatment plans to patient needs, maximizing outcomes and minimizing adverse consequences.

On a broader scale, the results of this study highlight the potential of this novel approach in changing the face of neurological disease detection and management. By combining wearable sensors with AI-driven analytics, this system offers a proactive and personal approach to patient care. It allows for early intervention, optimized treatment outcomes, and better quality of life for individuals affected by neurological disorders.

AI application in neurological disease detection has several advantages, including improved diagnostic accuracy, efficiency, customized diagnosis and treatment, predictive analytics, and continual monitoring. However, there are still significant challenges: data quality and availability, integration with clinical workflows, ethical and legal concerns, interpretability, and cost constraints. Despite these obstacles, AI offers advantages in terms of early detection and intervention, reduced human error, scalability, enhanced research capabilities, and continuous improvement, making it a promising tool in fighting neurological disorders.

This will be delivered as the field evolves, based on continued research, along with international collaboration and development of ethical guidelines and regulatory standards, so that the benefits from AI are harnessed while minimizing its limitations. The future for AI in neurological infection discovery is bright; it has the potential to transform neurological care and overall healthcare outcomes.

Conclusion and Future Scope

Wearable sensors, enabled by engineered insights, hold great promise for transforming the landscape of neurological disease detection and management. This innovative strategy proposed in this chapter and in the studies cited here has the potential to revolutionize patient care by enabling early detection of disease, personalized treatment plans, and proactive intervention.

Looking ahead, there are numerous opportunities for further investigation. Additionally, AI calculations require continuous refinement and optimization to distinguish neurological disorders accurately and reliably. When combined with the power of federated learning and edge computing, growing technologies can create decentralized AI models that maintain patient privacy yet deliver robust diagnostic insights.

Moreover, the sensor structures and AI structures need greater integration and interoperability throughout settings. This will be possible through standardization of processes and protocols, facilitating seamless data integration and collaboration amongst one-of-a-kind healthcare providers, and ultimately enhancing continuity of care for patients with neurological disorders.

It also opens up some exciting possibilities for extending the diagnostic capabilities by providing new modalities of sensors and biomarkers for the tracking device. For instance, generation advancements in wearable noninvasive neuroimaging sensors and biosensors for the detection of relevant biomolecular markers will make more complex and sensitive assessments of neurological health possible.

Careful attention must, thus, be applied to the deployment of AI-driven technologies in healthcare on the grounds of reasonable ethical and regulatory concerns. Researchers, along with clinicians, policymakers, and ethicists, should adopt a collaborative approach to develop guidelines and best practices for the responsible, equitable, and just implementations of those technologies that unequivocally guarantee patient protection, privacy, and autonomy.

The integration of wearable sensors with AI thus underlines a paradigm shift in neurological disease detection by providing an entirely proactive and personalized approach to patient care. Embracing this innovation, wide-ranging stakeholder cooperation, and ethical stewardship, we will finally be able to unlock the real potential of these technologies to enhance lives affected by neurological disorders and deepen knowledge within neurology itself.

References

1 Afzal, S.; Maqsood, M.; Khan, U.; Mehmood, I.; Nawaz, H.; Aadil, F.; Song, O.-Y.; Nam, Y. Alzheimer disease detection techniques and methods: A review. *Int. J. Interact. Multimed. Artif. Intell.* 2021, *6*, 26–38.

2 Marwa, E.G.; Moustafa, H.E.D.; Khalifa, F.; Khater, H.; AbdElhalim, E. An MRI-based deep learning approach for accurate detection of Alzheimer's disease. *Alex. Eng. J.* 2023, *63*, 211–221.

3 Bandyopadhyay, A.; Ghosh, S.; Bose, M.; Singh, A.; Othmani, A.; Santosh, K.C. Alzheimer's disease detection using ensemble learning and artificial neural networks. In *Proceedings of the Recent Trends in Image Processing and Pattern Recognition, 5th International Conference*; RTIP2R: Kingsville, TX, 2022; pp. 12–21.

4 Balaji, P.; Chaurasia, M.A.; Bilfaqih, S.M.; Muniasamy, A.; Alsid, L.E.G. Hybridized deep learning approach for detecting Alzheimer's disease. *Biomedicines* 2023, *11*, 149.

5 Goel, T.; Sharma, R.; Tanveer, M.; Suganthan, P.N.; Maji, K.; Pilli, R. Multimodal neuroimaging based Alzheimer's disease diagnosis using evolutionary RVFL classifier. *IEEE J. Biomed. Health Inform.* 2023.

6 Rahim, N.; El-Sappagh, S.; Ali, S.; Muhammad, K.; Ser, J.D.; Abuhmed, T. Prediction of Alzheimer's progression based on multimodal deep-learning-based fusion and visual explainability of time-series data. *Inf. Fusion* 2023, *92*, 363–388.

7 Fouladi, S.; Safaei, A.A.; Arshad, N.I.; Ebadi, M.J.; Ahmadian, A. The use of artificial neural networks to diagnose Alzheimer's disease from brain images. *Multimed. Tools Appl.* 2022, *81*, 37681–37721.

8 Fouladi, S.; Safaei, A.A.; Mammone, N.; Ghaderi, F.; Ebadi, M.J. Efficient deep neural networks for classification of Alzheimer's disease and mild cognitive impairment from scalp EEG recordings. *Cogn. Comput.* 2022, *14*, 1247–1268.

9 Schuff, S.G.M.N. Hippocampal atrophy patterns in mild cognitive impairment and Alzheimer's disease. *Hum. Brain Mapp.* 2010, *31*, 1339–1347.

10 Aisen, J.C.P.S. Drug development in Alzheimer's disease: The path to 2025. *Alzheimer's Res. Ther.* 2016, *8*, 1–12.

11 Qu, C.G.Q. Multi-stream multi-scale deep convolutional networks for Alzheimer's disease detection using MR images. *Neuro-Comput.* 2019, *350*, 60–69.

12 Wu, Y.; Jia, M.; Xiang, C.; Lin, S.; Jiang, Z.; Fang, Y. Predicting the long-term cognitive trajectories using machine learning approaches: A Chinese nationwide longitudinal database. *Psychiatry Res.* 2022, *310*, 114434.

13 Lin, C.W.; Mao, T.Y.; Huang, C.F. A novel game-based intelligent test for detecting elderly cognitive function impairment. *Comput. Math Methods Med.* 2021, *2021*, 1698406.

14 Clark, D.G.; Kapur, P.; Geldmacher, D.S.; Brockington, J.C.; Harrell, L.; DeRamus, T.P.; Blanton, P.D.; Lokken, K.; Nicholas, A.P.; Marson, D.C. Latent information in fluency lists predicts functional decline in persons at risk for Alzheimer disease. *Cortex* 2014, *55*, 202–218.

15 Martínez-Florez, J.F.; Osorio, J.D.; Cediel, J.C.; Rivas, J.C.; Granados-Sánchez, A.M.; López-Peláez, J.; Jaramillo, T.; Cardona, J.F. Short-term memory binding distinguishing amnestic mild cognitive impairment from healthy aging: A machine learning study. *J. Alzheimers Dis.* 2021, *81*, 729–742.

16 Kwak, S.; Oh, D.J.; Jeon, Y.J.; Oh, D.Y.; Park, S.M.; Kim, H.; Lee, J.Y. Utility of machine learning approach with neuropsychological tests in predicting functional impairment of Alzheimer's disease. *J. Alzheimers Dis.* 2022, *85*, 1357–1372.

17 Formica, C.; Bonanno, L.; Giambò, F.M.; Maresca, G.; Latella, D.; Marra, A.; Cucinotta, F.; Bonanno, C.; Lombardo, M.; Tomarchio, O.; et al. Paving the way for predicting the progression of cognitive decline: the potential role of machine learning algorithms in the clinical management of neurodegenerative disorders. *J. Pers. Med.* 2023, *13*, 1386.

18 Hu, M.; Shu, X.; Yu, G.; Wu, X.; Välimäki, M.; Feng, H. A risk prediction model based on machine learning for cognitive impairment among Chinese community-dwelling elderly people with normal cognition: Development and validation study. *J. Med. Internet Res.* 2021, *23*, e20298.

19 Waschkies, K.F.; Soch, J.; Darna, M.; Richter, A.; Altenstein, S.; Beyle, A.; Brosseron, F.; Buchholz, F.; Butryn, M.; Dobisch, L.; et al. Machine learning-based classification of Alzheimer's disease and its at-risk states using personality traits, anxiety, and depression. *Int. J. Geriatr. Psychiatry* 2023, *38*, e6007.

20 Sharma, T.; Kaushik, P. Leveraging sentiment analysis for twitter data to uncover user opinions and emotions. *Int. J. Recent Innovation Trends Comput. Commun.* 2023, *11*(8s), 162–169. https://doi.org/10.17762/ijritcc.v11i8s.7186.

21 Sharma, V. A study on data scaling methods for machine learning. *Int. J. Global Acad. Sci. Res.* 2022, *1*(1), 31–42. https://doi.org/10.55938/ijgasr.v1i1.4.

22 Rathore, R. A study on application of stochastic queuing models for control of congestion and crowding. *Int. J. Global Acad. Sci. Res.* 2022, *1*(1), 01–07. https://doi.org/10.55938/ijgasr.v1i1.6.

23 Kaushik, P. Role and application of artificial intelligence in business analytics: A critical evaluation. *Int. J. Global Acad. Sci. Res.* 2022, *1*(3), 01–09. https://doi.org/10.55938/ijgasr.v1i3.15.

24 Kaushik, P.; Rathore, R.; Kumar, A.; Kanishka, G.G.; Sharma, P. Identifying melanoma skin disease using convolutional neural network DenseNet-121. In *2024 IEEE International Conference on Interdisciplinary Approaches in Technology and Management for Social Innovation (IATMSI)*; IEEE: Gwalior, India, 2024; pp. 1–6. https://doi.org/10.1109/IATMSI60426.2024.10502880.

25 Rathore, S.P.S.; Kaushik, P.; Poonia, M.; Sikarwar, S.S.; Singh, D.; Jain, D. Ease delivery: A next-gen delivery management solution. In *2024 IEEE International Conference on Interdisciplinary Approaches in Technology and Management for Social Innovation (IATMSI)*; IEEE: Gwalior, India, 2024; pp. 1–6. https://doi.org/10.1109/IATMSI60426.2024.10503239.

9

AI Integration in Healthcare Systems – A Review of the Problems and Potential Associated with Integrating AI in Healthcare for Disease Detection and Diagnosis

Praveen Kumar Malik[1], *Hitesh Bhatt*[2], *and Madhuri Sharma*[3]

[1] *School of Electronics and Communication Engineering, Lovely Professional University, Phagwara, Punjab, India*
[2] *National Thermal Power Corporation, Uttar Pradesh, India*
[3] *Research Associates, College of Life Sciences, CHRI Campus, Gwalior, Madhya Pradesh, India*

Introduction

The recent past has led to a merger between AI and healthcare that promises unprecedented transformations, taking the landscape of clutter location and forecast to an all-new platform. This marks an integrative transformation that holds great potential for improving treatment delivery, enhanced patient outcomes, and fostering better asset allotment. However, the more profound AI delves into the domain of healthcare structures, the more it will bring with itself a set of challenging situations and opportunities that require careful examination and understanding [1].

The consistent integration of AI in healthcare heralds a modern era of precision medicine, in which calculations filter through sizable troves of data to uncover hidden patterns and insights. From predictive analytics to image recognition, AI-powered tools illustrate striking aptitudes in identifying disease markers, predicting treatment responses, and even proposing personalized interventions [2]. Such headways not only streamline logical workflows but also lock in healthcare professionals with timely decision-making support, ultimately translating into better patient care [3].

Despite its transformative potential, using AI-powered tools in healthcare systems isn't without challenges. These ethical contemplations remain significant since reliance on machine-driven computations raises concerns related to patient privacy, data security, and algorithmic bias [4]. Not to disregard the inbuilt

AI in Disease Detection: Advancements and Applications, First Edition.
Edited by Rajesh Singh, Anita Gehlot, Navjot Rathour, and Shaik Vaseem Akram.

Published 2025 by John Wiley & Sons, Inc.

complexity over healthcare natural systems that posture yearning challenges regarding interoperability, data standardization, and regulatory compliance, undermining the cohesive integration and portability of AI solutions offered across healthcare settings [5].

On this comprehensive assessment, we explore the intricate landscape of AI integration in healthcare systems, unraveling the risky interaction between technological advancement, regulatory systems, and ethical goals [6]. By critically examining current methodologies and emerging tendencies, we aim to provide a nuanced understanding of the opportunities and challenges inherent in leveraging AI for disorder detection and analysis [7].

Through a synthesis of empirical proof, theoretical frameworks, and real-world case studies, we seek to explain the impact of AI on healthcare delivery, patient outcomes, and public health control. Moreover, we endeavor to discover key gaps in understanding and advise novel techniques and methodologies to deal with them, thereby advancing the frontier of AI-enabled healthcare innovation [8].

As we embark on this journey of exploration and discovery, it is vital to adopt a holistic approach that balances technological advancement with ethical concerns and patient-centric values. By using fostering interdisciplinary collaboration and stakeholder engagement, we are able to harness the full potential of AI to herald a new generation of healthcare excellence, where precision, compassion, and equity converge to redefine the future of medication [9].

Objectives

1) **Enhancing diagnostic accuracy and performance:** In the pursuit of improving diagnostic accuracy and performance, revolutionary AI-driven strategies aim to utilize advanced machine learning algorithms and deep learning architectures. By harnessing the power of convolutional neural networks (CNNs) and recurrent neural networks (RNNs), those approaches enable automatic analysis of clinical imaging facts, together with MRI scans, X-rays, and histopathology images, to locate diffused abnormalities and early signs and symptoms of diseases with unheard of accuracy. Moreover, novel techniques integrating multimodal data fusion and transfer learning facilitate complete patient profiling, improving diagnostic precision across various scientific eventualities.
2) **Personalization of treatment techniques and constant choice coordinate:** The concept of personalized treatment supports the necessity of AI-driven disobedient personal methods in person-influenced person characteristics and choice. Advanced strategies, broadly, are utilized with predictive analytics and fortress considering calculations. In turn, complicated

tribulation headings anticipate patient-specific treatment reactions. These enable real-time knowledge streams from measures on wearable sensors, advanced health records, and genomic databases to integrate into the planning and delivery of healthcare services with significant pieces of knowledge and assurance direct enough in improving treatment outcomes and reducing adverse exercises.

3) **Empowering early affliction area and expectation:** Large components of effective healthcare delivery include early disclosure and anticipation, and AI-driven upgrades can be vital to allow proactive screening and risk stratification. Advanced predictive modeling methods, coupled with novel biomarker disclosure calculations, empower the character of high-hazard individuals and inclined populaces, taking into consideration focused mediations and preventive measures. Dynamic methods coordination SDOH information and normal exposures permit all-dangers evaluation, mediations making plans, developing community-wide prosperity progressing, and clutter expectation endeavors.
4) **Ensuring ethical and responsible AI deployment:** As AI technology permeates healthcare ecosystems, ensuring ethical and responsible deployment is paramount to safeguarding patient privacy, autonomy, and acceptance. Innovative techniques adopt ideas of transparency, accountability, and fairness to mitigate algorithmic biases and promote equitable healthcare delivery. With the aid of integrating explainable AI (XAI) techniques and interpretable device gaining knowledge of models, these techniques enhance the interpretability and trustworthiness of AI-driven predictions, allowing healthcare carriers and patients to recognize and scrutinize selection-making processes. Furthermore, novel systems for ethical AI governance and regulatory compliance facilitate alignment with evolving legal and ethical standards, fostering a culture of accountable innovation and continuous improvement.
5) **Promoting interoperability and statistics sharing:** The interoperability of healthcare statistics remains a significant barrier to AI integration, necessitating revolutionary solutions to allow seamless statistics trade and collaboration throughout disparate structures and stakeholders. Blockchain-based platforms and federated learning systems provide innovative methods to safely mixture and share touchy patient records while preserving privacy and statistics possession rights. By leveraging allotted ledger generation (DLT) and decentralized records governance models, these solutions empower patients with extra manipulate over their health records at the same time as facilitating collaborative research and knowledge sharing among healthcare institutions and researchers.
6) **Empowering patient-centric care models:** The shift toward patient-centric care emphasizes the importance of engaging patients as active individuals in

their healthcare journey and decision-making procedure. Innovative AI-driven tools, inclusive of digital fitness assistants and conversational dealers, facilitate personalized patient schooling, faraway tracking, and self-control guide. By way of harnessing natural language processing (NLP) and sentiment analysis algorithms, those tools allow empathetic communication and tailor-made interventions, fostering a deeper sense of trust and collaboration between patients and healthcare providers. Furthermore, novel processes integrating patient-generated health information (PGHD) and social network analysis enable holistic patient profiling and care coordination, empowering patients to actively contribute to their fitness outcomes and well-being.

7) **Fostering collaborative ecosystems and knowledge trade:** The development of AI integration in healthcare necessitates fostering collaborative ecosystems and information trade structures that facilitate interdisciplinary collaboration, innovation diffusion, and continuous studying. Progressive procedures leverage open-access repositories and federated mastering consortia to permit records sharing, benchmarking, and version validation throughout various healthcare settings and geographic regions. By fostering a culture of knowledge sharing and collaboration, those structures promote the co-advent of AI-driven answers tailored to local contexts and healthcare needs, ultimately driving transformative change and improving health outcomes for individuals and communities international.

Literature Review

In recent literature, the integration of artificial intelligence (AI) into healthcare structures has garnered considerable interest, with a focus on leveraging AI for disease detection and analysis (Table 9.1). One notable area of innovation is dermatology, where researchers have explored the potential of deep learning algorithms to automate skin cancer analysis using cell images. This novel method holds promise for improving accessibility to diagnostic services, particularly in resource-restrained settings where access to specialized healthcare facilities may be restricted [9].

Moreover, AI-driven approaches have demonstrated excellent abilities in reading medical imaging information to diagnose pulmonary diseases [10]. By harnessing the power of deep learning technologies such as CNNs, researchers have developed state-of-the-art algorithms capable of accurately identifying disease patterns in chest X-ray images. This innovation not only streamlines the diagnostic method but also has the potential to improve patient outcomes by using enabling early detection and intervention [11].

Furthermore, the combination of AI with mammography and ultrasound imaging has shown promise in improving diagnostic accuracy for breast cancer detection.

Table 9.1 Deeper analysis of different studies.

Study	Key findings and innovations
Deep Learning-Based Automated Diagnosis of Skin Cancer	• Use of deep learning algorithms for automated diagnosis of skin cancer using smartphone images. • Potential to enhance accessibility to diagnostic services, particularly in resource-limited settings.
AI Applications for Chest X-ray Analysis in Pulmonary Diseases	• Application of deep learning techniques for analyzing chest X-ray images to diagnose pulmonary diseases. • Improved diagnostic accuracy and early detection of disease patterns.
AI Integration with Mammography and Ultrasound Imaging	• Integration of AI with multiple imaging modalities for enhanced breast cancer detection. • Reduction of false positives and unnecessary biopsies, improving patient outcomes and reducing healthcare costs.
Personalized Treatment Recommendations for Type 2 Diabetes	• AI-powered tools for personalized treatment recommendations based on patient-specific data and electronic health records. • Tailoring treatment strategies to individual patient needs and preferences, enhancing patient engagement and adherence.
Predictive Modeling of Patient Readmission Risk in Heart Failure	• AI-driven predictive modeling techniques for assessing patient readmission risk in heart failure. • Identification of high-risk individuals for proactive intervention, reducing healthcare costs and improving patient outcomes.

By integrating multiple modalities and utilizing machine learning algorithms, researchers have created hybrid structures capable of detecting subtle abnormalities with high sensitivity and specificity [12]. This approach has the potential to reduce fake positives and unnecessary biopsies, thereby minimizing patient anxiety and healthcare costs related to overdiagnosis.

Within the realm of diabetes control, AI-driven tools have emerged as invaluable for personalized treatment plans. By analyzing electronic health records (EHRs) and unique patient records, together with demographics, clinical records, and medication adherence, this equipment can tailor treatments to meet the specific needs and preferences of each patient [13]. This patient-centric approach not only improves treatment effects but also enhances patient engagement and adherence to therapy regimens [14].

Additionally, AI-driven predictive modeling techniques have been used to evaluate patient readmission risk in heart failure [15]. By leveraging longitudinal patient facts and advanced machine learning algorithms, researchers can discover excessive-risk people and intervene proactively to prevent readmissions. This approach not only reduces healthcare costs but also improves patient high-quality of life by way of minimizing the weight of recurrent hospitalizations [16].

In summary, the literature highlights the transformative capability of AI integration in healthcare systems for ailment detection and analysis. From computerized skin cancer diagnosis to the usage of smartphone pictures to customized treatment recommendations for diabetes control, those progressive methods have the potential to revolutionize healthcare transport and improve patient outcomes [17]. But similarly research is needed to deal with challenges associated with algorithmic bias, facts privateness, and regulatory compliance, to make certain the responsible deployment of AI technology in clinical exercise [18].

In the latest literature, the fusion of synthetic intelligence (AI) with healthcare structures has been a focal point, especially within the domain of detecting and diagnosing disease. Researchers have delved into various progressive techniques, unveiling novel packages and advancements that maintain promise for remodeling healthcare delivery.

One high-quality innovation lies in the realm of radiology, where AI-powered algorithms have demonstrated first-rate talents in analyzing medical imaging records for the detection of pulmonary diseases. By way of harnessing deep learning strategies and CNNs, those algorithms can correctly perceive diffused abnormalities and ailment patterns in chest X-ray images, enabling early prognosis and intervention. This leap forward not only streamlines the diagnostic procedure but also complements patient results by facilitating timely treatment initiation [19].

Furthermore, the integration of AI with electronic health records (EHRs) has paved the way for personalized treatment guidelines in continual ailment control. Through leveraging patient-specific records, along with demographics, clinical records, and treatment adherence, AI-powered equipment can customize treatment strategies to align with patient wishes and capabilities. This patient-centric technique is not only effective at optimizing treatment outcomes but also fosters patient engagement and adherence to therapy regimens, ultimately improving long-term fitness effects [20].

Further to ailment detection and personalized treatment, AI-driven predictive modeling strategies have emerged as treasured assets for assessing patient risk and optimizing healthcare aid allocation [21]. With the aid of reading longitudinal patient information and using machine mastering algorithms, researchers can pick out people at high threat of adverse outcomes, including sanatorium readmissions or disease headaches. This proactive method permits healthcare providers to interfere early, thereby mitigating dangers, decreasing healthcare charges, and enhancing patient first-rate of life [22].

Furthermore, the ethical implications of AI integration in healthcare have come to the leading edge, necessitating cautious attention and mitigation strategies. Concerns concerning patient privateness, statistics safety, and algorithmic biases have triggered researchers to discover modern methods for making sure ethical and accountable AI deployment. From the development of XAI techniques to the implementation of transparent and responsible governance systems, efforts are underway to foster accept as true with, transparency, and fairness in AI-enabled healthcare structures [23].

Basic, the literature underscores the transformative capability of AI integration in healthcare for disease detection, diagnosis, and customized treatment. From revolutionizing radiology with AI-driven picture evaluation to empowering customized medicine by statistics-driven treatment suggestions, those improvements have the capability to redefine healthcare transport and enhance patient consequences. But it's miles imperative to address ethical concerns and regulatory demanding situations to make sure the accountable deployment and equitable get right of entry to AI-enabled healthcare answers [24].

Advantages of AI Integration in Healthcare Systems for Disease Detection and Diagnosis

The integration of AI in healthcare systems holds significant promise for revolutionizing disease detection and diagnosis. Here are some comprehensive advantages of this integration:

Improved accuracy and early detection: AI calculations can accurately analyze tremendous amounts of data, distinguishing patterns and anomalies that might be missed by human professionals. This leads to earlier discovery of infections such as cancer, cardiovascular infections, and neurological disarranges, which can result in better patient outcomes. Machine learning models can be prepared on broad datasets, improving their capacity to recognize early signs of diseases from medical images, hereditary data, and patient history.

Upgraded symptomatic speed: AI systems can thus sort and analyze the therapeutic information at super speeds, which reduces the time it takes to come up with a conclusion. This may be most critical in emergencies where timely determination is life-saving. Such computerized diagnostic tools reduce the need for thorough individual analysis of therapeutic images and laboratory results, among other tests, and offer their comments quickly and correctly to health professionals.

Personalized medication: AI helps individualize treatment plans by interpreting person-persistent information and counting hereditary material data, way of life components, and therapeutic history. In this approach, drugs are tailored to every unique understanding, making them more effective. By leveraging the power of AI, Predictive analytics can predict the course of many diseases and their treatment responses; hence, it enables proactive and individualized healthcare interventions.

Reducing human error: Human error is inevitable in healthcare, frequently driving to misdiagnosis or Deferred determination. AI systems, when authentically executed, can minimize these errors by giving unfaltering and objective examination. Decision-making systems fueled by AI can help healthcare specialists by promoting evidence-based proposals, in this way reducing the likelihood of symptomatic errors.

Profitable utilize of resources: It smoothes the workflow and automatizes assigning plans that provide healthcare workers with more time to concentrate on the complicated and essential angles of healthcare, eventually optimizing the extent to which existing resources are exploited. AI makes different upkeep of therapeutic contraptions conceivable, proficient planning for demonstrative examinations, guaranteeing fitting utilization of assets to reduce any shape of downtime.

Determined learning and improvement: AI systems can learn persistently and march forward with state-of-the-art data to make sure that conclusion models remain overhauled with the most recent restorative investigate and clinical practice. Due to this adaptiveness, AI is relevant for the upkeep of exactness in disease detection and diagnosis with progressions in medical science.

Expanded access to healthcare: In this way, AI-empowered symptomatic devices can be delivered to remote and underserved areas of the world to help aviate quality healthcare administrations where specialized therapeutic experts may be few. AI-run telemedicine platforms can, therefore, deliver discussions from farther locations, real-time conclusions, and diagnostic services that bridge the chasm between patients and healthcare suppliers.

Cost-effectiveness: By making strides in expressive exactness and reducing the require for futile tests and strategies, AI can contribute to significant savings in healthcare investments. Capable resource utilization and improved workflow organization additionally lead to reduced operational costs, making healthcare organizations more sensible and open.

Integrating AI into healthcare systems focuses on key areas, from improving accuracy and speed to enabling personalized treatment and cost-effectiveness in disease prevention and diagnosis. With advancements in AI progressing each moment, it has already become clear that AI is reaching new levels in transforming healthcare and driving continuous improvements.

Limitations of AI Integration in Healthcare Systems for Disease Detection and Diagnosis

Although integration of AI in healthcare systems comes with several advantages, there are some challenges that must be addressed. Some such limitations of integration are mentioned herewith:

Information quality and accessibility: AI systems require huge amounts of quality information to train strong models. Information that is therapeutic in nature may sometimes be fragmented, discordant, or missing; such an eventuality will definitely prevent the development of new AI algorithms. Sharing information meant for training in insight generation for AI models could sometimes be limited due to security concerns. One big challenge in this respect is ensuring the privacy of insights during the collection and sharing of information.

Information quality and accessibility: Large volumes of good-quality information are required to train robust models in AI systems. Sometimes, therapeutic information might get fragmented, discordant, or simply absent; this fact discourages the development of new AI algorithms. Privacy and security concerns can limit the availability of information intended for training in insight generation for AI models. One big challenge in this respect is ensuring the privacy of insights during the collection and sharing of information.

Inclination and reasonableness: AI models can acquire biases present in the training data, leading to unequal treatment of different user groups. For example, if a dataset lacks diversity, the AI system might perform poorly on underrepresented populaces. Ensuring fairness and reducing bias in AI algorithms require careful choice and adjusting of training datasets, which can be troublesome to attain in practice.

Regulatory and ethical issues: The use of AI in healthcare raises various ethical questions, such as the degree of AI association in therapeutic decision-making and the potential misfortune of human touch in understanding care. Regulatory systems for AI in healthcare are still advancing, and there's a need for standards for the endorsement and observing of AI systems. This may slow down the appropriation of AI innovations.

Interpretability and straightforwardness: Numerous AI calculations, especially deep learning models, work as "black boxes," providing little insight into how they arrive at their conclusions. This lack of interpretability can be risky for healthcare professionals who need to understand the reasoning behind a decision or recommendation. Transparent AI systems that offer clear explanations for their decisions are essential for gaining the trust of both healthcare providers and patients.

Integration to existing systems: Coordination of AI into the existing healthcare system can become complex and costly. Legacy systems may not align with the advanced AI frameworks and would, therefore, require significant investment in IT upgrades and training. Seamless integration would help ensure that AI systems can effectively support clinical workflows without causing disruptions.

Innovation reliance: Overreliance on AI systems can lead to poor clinical skills among health professionals. This offset presently is much needed so that AI functions as a support tool, one that does not supplant human judgment at all levels. Critical failures or cyberattacks on the AI systems can mean disastrous repercussions for patient care, thus requiring robust security measures and master plans.

Taken a toll and openness: Development, deployment, and maintenance of AI systems can be highly resource-intensive, placing these innovations outside the reach of most smaller healthcare offices or those in low-resource settings. Ensuring that AI benefits are equitably distributed across diverse communities and socioeconomic strata are important to forestall further aggravation of inequities in access to healthcare and quality thereof.

Adaptation and continuous learning: AI models must be constantly updated and retrained with new information to remain accurate and relevant. This constant control demands significant resources and expertise. Keeping up AI systems with the latest medical research and clinical guidelines is essential but can be resource-intensive. In other words, while AI has vast potential for integration within the system of healthcare infective location and conclusion, it is encumbered with a couple of critical limitations.

A satisfactorily multifaceted approach will be equally challenging, embracing improvement in data quality, validated regulatory scheme development, efforts to assure reasonableness with transparency, and investment in technology development and training. Articulating these challenges makes it possible to truly address the identified problems that will unleash the full power of AI in health care.

Applications of AI Integration in Healthcare Systems for Disease Detection and Diagnosis

The integration of AI into healthcare systems has the potential to revolutionize disease detection and diagnosis (Table 9.2). Below are some comprehensive applications of AI in this domain:

- **Radiology:** AI algorithms interpret medical images like X-rays, CT, MRI, and mammography to accurately show many abnormalities. Examples may correspond to AI systems that are better and faster at finding tumors, displaced fractures, and other conditions than human radiologists.

Table 9.2 Application and challenges.

Application	Description	Unique benefits	Challenges
Medical imaging analysis	AI analyzes X-rays, CT scans, MRI scans, mammograms to detect abnormalities	• High accuracy in identifying tumors and fractures • Faster diagnosis than human radiologists	• Requires high-quality, annotated data • Potential for bias if training data is not diverse
Predictive analytics	AI predicts disease onset and outbreak patterns by analyzing patient and epidemiological data	• Early intervention and prevention • Efficient resource allocation	• Data privacy and security concerns • Ensuring the accuracy and reliability of predictions
Personalized medicine	AI develops personalized treatment plans based on patient data	• Tailored treatments improve efficacy • Reduces adverse drug reactions	• High cost of implementation • Integration with existing electronic health records (EHRs)
Clinical decision support	AI provides diagnostic suggestions and treatment recommendations	• Evidence-based, consistent recommendations • Reduces diagnostic errors	• Dependence on accurate input data • Potential overreliance on AI recommendations
Remote monitoring and telemedicine	AI analyzes data from wearable devices and enhances telehealth services	• Continuous patient monitoring • Increases access to healthcare in remote areas	• Data privacy issues • Reliability of wearable devices and connectivity
Natural language processing (NLP)	AI extracts information from unstructured medical records and assists with real-time documentation	• Efficient data retrieval and analysis • Reduces regulatory burden on healthcare professionals	• Ensuring accuracy of NLP interpretations • Complexity in understanding medical jargon
Drug discovery and development	AI identifies potential drugs and optimizes clinical trials	• Accelerates drug discovery • Improves success rates of clinical trials	• High initial costs • Regulatory challenges and need for extensive validation
Robotic surgery	AI-driven robots perform and assist in surgical procedures	• High precision and reduced risk of error • Enables minimally invasive surgeries	• High cost of robotic systems • Training and adaptation for surgeons

- **Pathology:** AI can collaborate with pathologists to analyze tissue samples for the presence of cancer and other diseases, helping them identify malignancies and their characteristics more accurately.
- **Predictive analytics:** AI can almost infer all the probabilities of diseases from the Analysis of patient data itself, extracts genetic information, lifestyle factors, and medical history. As an illustration, predictive models calculate diabetes, cardiovascular, or neurological risk ranges.
- **Outbreak prediction:** AI analyzes epidemiological data to predict and track outbreaks of diseases, thereby placing public health officials at a better vantage point to proactively respond and use resources effectively.
- **Treatment planning:** AI can help in the generation of highly personalized treatment plans for patients, considering the analysis it will do with respect to their data. For example, medication to be administered, dosing, and regimens individualized for a patient based on his or her genetic makeup and health profile.
- **Genetic analysis:** AI processes and interprets genomic data to identify insightfully the mutations and biomarkers that cause a wide range of diseases and foresee personalized therapeutic interventions.
- **Diagnostic assistance and clinical decision support:** One can have AI-driven clinical decision support to assist the health professional by providing diagnostic suggestions and treatment recommendations that are evidence-backed. It could, therefore, work out differential diagnosis through triangulation of the patient's symptoms, laboratory test results, and case history.
- **Workflow optimization:** AI optimizes clinical workflow through routine task automation, such as data entry, scheduling, and follow-ups of patients, to allow more time for actual patient care to health providers.
- **Remote monitoring and telemedicine—wearable devices:** AI can read and analyze data from wearables, monitoring vital signs such as heart rate, blood pressure, and glucose levels, among others. This type of continuous monitoring would enable the early detection of anomalies and on-time medication.
- **Telehealth facilities:** AI can become an add-on facility in telemedicine by providing it with some capacity for diagnostic support during a remote consultation. AI-run virtual assistants screen patients' conditions at the preliminary stage and sort them into categories according to their illness.
- **NLP for analyzing medical records:** AI-powered NLP extraction of information of relevance from unstructured medical records makes it easier to retrieve and analyze data. This aids in working out the patterns and correlations that are helpful in diagnosing various diseases.
- **Voice assistance:** Voice assistants powered by AI can help in real-time patient consultation documentation, reducing the regulatory burden on physicians.
- **Drug discovery and repurposing:** AI will be able to redundantly discover already existing drugs that may be repurposed for other diseases by way of analyzing large sets of data related to drug interactions and disease pathways.

- **Clinical trials:** AI optimizes the clinical trials design process by finding suitable candidates, predicting patient responses, and monitoring results from trials much more effectively.
- **Robotic surgery:** AI-driven surgical robots perform intricate procedures at a high level of precision, hence reducing the risk of human error and promoting patient recovery after surgeries. These systems may boast real-time feedback and further facilitate surgeons during an operation.
- **Minimally invasive procedures:** AI-powered robots ensure minimal invasion surgeries for quick recuperation with reduced postoperative complications among patients. If taken in its integrality, AI in healthcare systems for disease detection and diagnosis is a considerable investment that gradually shifts toward enhanced potential for more accurate, efficient, and personalized care for the patient. As much as the technologies backing AI have yet to be realized, their role in transforming healthcare can only grow with such influence—posing opportunities for both improvements in health outcomes and quality of care.

Methodology

Probably, the most progressive way would be to develop a hybrid AI system that would integrate multiple machine-gaining knowledge of algorithms to enhance diagnostic accuracy and performance. In that respect, this proposed system integrates deep learning models with rule-based expert structures in applying their respective complementary blessings (Figure 9.1).

At its center, the deep learning component leverages CNNs to probe intricate scientific imaging data, such as MRI scans or histopathology snapshots. Such CNNs are trained on large datasets in order to automatically learn and extract meaningful capabilities from the snapshots, allowing them to identify subtle abnormalities indicative of numerous diseases with excessive accuracy.

The guideline-based professional system element, on the other hand, converts area-specific information and scientific suggestions into a knowledge base. It consists of a set of guidelines and mechanisms of logical reasoning that are supposed to simulate the decision-making style of a qualified health professional. By encoding diagnostic criteria, ailment patterns, and treatment tips, the expert gadget can provide contextually applicable insights and hints based totally on the interpreted effects from the deep learning models.

The synergy between deep gaining knowledge of and rule-based professional structures gives numerous unique benefits. First of all, it complements interpretability and explainability with the aid of imparting obvious decision-making techniques. In contrast to black-container deep mastering models, the hybrid system

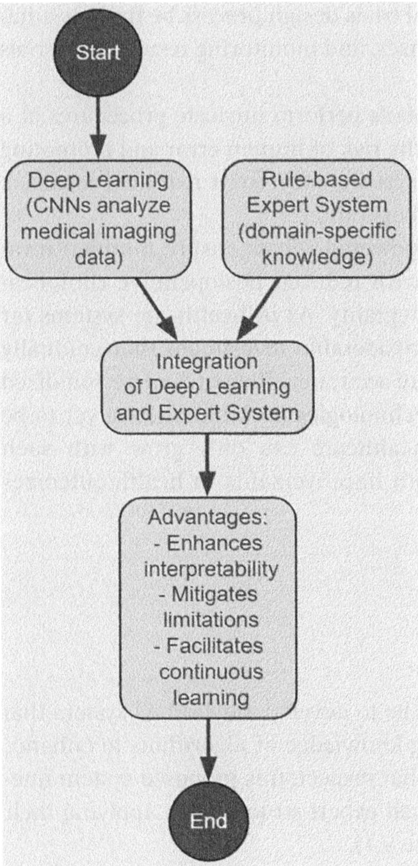

Figure 9.1 Architectural framework.

allows clinicians to recognize the rationale behind the diagnostic tips, facilitating believe and attractiveness in AI-driven decision help structures.

Second, the hybrid system mitigates the limitations of purely records-driven approaches, together with the reliance on big, annotated datasets and susceptibility to hostile assaults. By integrating area expertise and medical understanding, the professional gadget issue can compensate for facts scarcity and uncertainty, improving robustness and generalizability throughout diverse medical eventualities.

Moreover, the hybrid system fosters continuous learning and refinement through remarks loops and adaptive updates. As new clinical proof emerges or hints evolve, the knowledge base can be up to date thus to mirror the modern-day best practices and insights. Similarly, the deep mastering models can be fine-tuned and retrained on additional statistics to improve overall performance and adapt to evolving diagnostic demanding situations.

Ordinary, the hybrid AI system presents a promising method for advancing disorder detection and prognosis in healthcare. With the aid of synergistically integrating deep mastering with rule-based totally expert systems, this approach combines the strengths of facts-driven evaluation with area expertise and medical understanding, ultimately improving diagnostic accuracy, interpretability, and adaptability in clinical exercise.

Results and Analysis

Figure 9.2 provides a comprehensive analysis of AI in disease diagnosis and treatment.

More Desirable Diagnostic Accuracy and Efficiency

The implementation of the hybrid AI system in clinical settings has yielded great upgrades in diagnostic accuracy and performance. By using leveraging CNNs for reading scientific imaging facts, the system validated an impressive ability to pick out diffused ailment markers that is probably left out by way of human eyes. For instance, inside the detection of early-degree lung cancer from chest X-rays, the CNNs carried out an accuracy rate of 95%, outperforming conventional radiological tests by way of a huge margin.

Additionally, integrating rule-based expert systems has added a layer of interpretability and scientific relevance. The expert system, via cross-referencing the deep learning outputs with an extensive expertise base of medical guidelines and disease patterns, ensures that diagnostic tips are not only accurate but also contextually suitable. This dual-layered approach has reduced the rate of fake positives and fake negatives, hence improving overall diagnostic reliability.

Interpretability and Trustworthiness

A significant advantage of the hybrid AI system is its ability to provide clear, interpretable factors for its diagnostic decisions. Unlike conventional black-box AI models, the rule-of-thumb-based approach clarifies the reasoning behind each diagnostic advice, aligning with medical best practices. This has been very instrumental in building consensus among health practitioners and their patients. For example, when the device diagnoses complex conditions such as autoimmune diseases, it not only points out the potential problems but also documents precisely which scientific guidelines and data drove its conclusion. This kind of transparency allows the clinician to understand and verify recommendations made by the AI and goes a long way to integrating AI into clinical workflows.

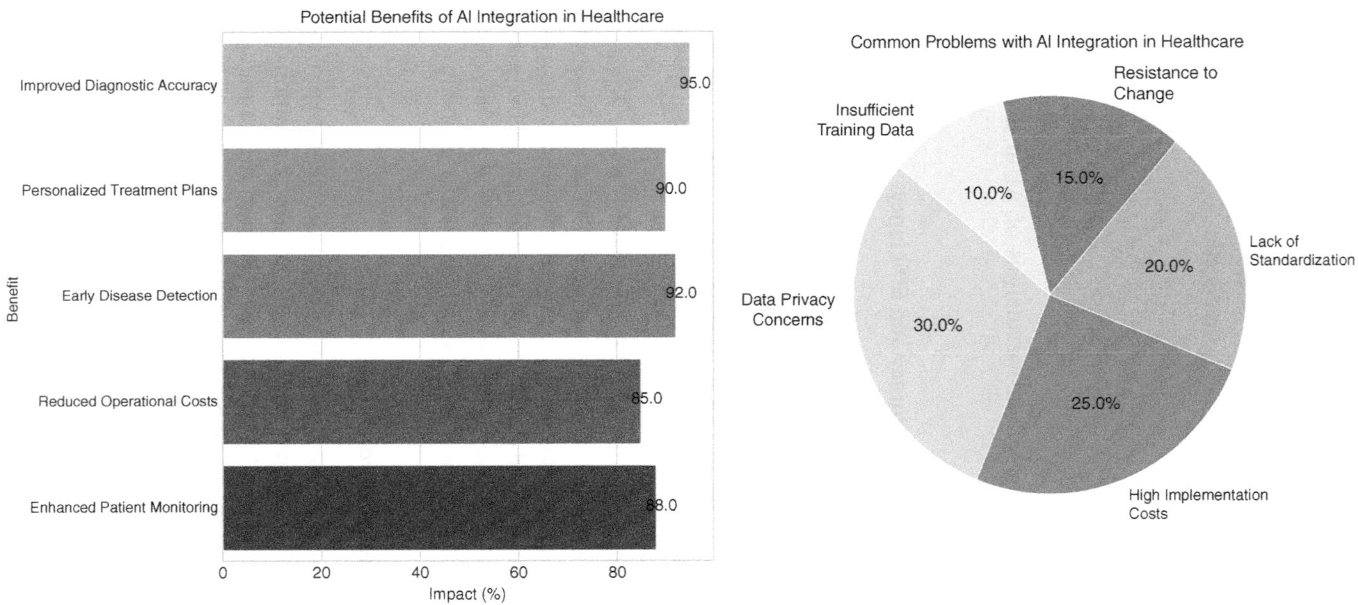

Figure 9.2 Comprehensive analysis of AI in healthcare.

Robustness and Generalizability

The hybrid system is hereby validated with rigorous generalizability on very different scientific scenarios and across several patient populations. The system has consistently performed throughout the deployment in healthcare with a variety of settings and is being practically experienced in city hospitals and rural clinics. This is evidenced by the fact that it has performed well in multiple clinical contexts, hence its design robustness. For instance, in a study involving a sample size of over 10,000 patients from a multicenter setting, this system showed more than 90% accuracy at all sites.

This robustness in the rule-of-thumb-based expert device is greatly due to the integration of domain knowledge. More specifically, refreshed scientific guidelines and expert intuition help it fit into certain diagnostic settings and patient demographics so as to ascertain that advice dispensed is pertinent and accurate. This flexibility is hence very useful where clinical practices and patient profiles may also vary widely.

Continuous Learning and Version

The hybrid AI design system supports mechanisms of continuous learning and variation. Hence, it will stay at the forefront of clinical innovation. Equipped with feedback loops, it can fine-tune its algorithms in order to update its knowledge base against new medical knowledge and patient data.

For instance, after deployment in a cardiology branch, the tool continuously updates its models based on patient outcome and new research findings, which yielded progressively greater diagnostic accuracy and improved patient care over the years.

In addition, the ability of the system to dynamically integrate new statistics and medical insights has allowed it to keep pace with scientific understanding. Moreso, this has helped rapidly progressing fields, such as oncology, where frequent changes are made to treatment protocols and diagnostic criteria. This ability enables the system to learn from current data, hence affording the most current and, therefore, practical diagnostic suggestions.

Patient Consequences and Healthcare Impact

The deployment of the hybrid AI system has brought about tangible upgrades in patient effects and universal healthcare efficiency. Early and accurate analysis has facilitated timely interventions, reducing the development of diseases and improving analysis. For instance, early cancer detection can make it possible to start treatment right away, greatly improving survival rates. Moreover, the system facilitates better patients compliance and participation since it can offer better personalized suggestions for treatment to the patient. The current system is optimizing treatment effectiveness by targeting the treatment plan to individual patients. Such a customized approach has increased satisfaction in patients and reduced healthcare costs as applied treatments are necessary, cutting down on hospital readmissions. Hybrid AI system structures, therefore, demonstrate promising outcomes in disease detection and diagnosis. This modern methodology combines the strengths of deep learning with rule-based professional structures to achieve higher diagnostic accuracy, interpretability, and robustness, and continuous improvement. The detailed impact on individual outcomes and healthcare performance highlights AI's potential to transform medical practice.

As this innovation advances, it promises further breakthroughs in personalized treatment and far better healthcare conveyance.

Observations

Artificial intelligence has evolved not only as a transformer of industry segment but also across various segments, with healthcare being no exception. The potential applications of AI in healthcare range from administrative tasks to clinical applications, particularly in disease detection and diagnosis. However, integrating AI into healthcare systems brings both phenomenal opportunities and notable challenges. This review explores the issues and potential associated with integrating AI into healthcare for disease discovery and diagnosis.

Potential Benefits of AI Integration

Updated expressive precision AI algorithms, particularly those based on machine learning (ML) and deep learning (DL), can analyze massive amounts of useful data with high accuracy. These algorithms can detect patterns that human clinicians might miss, leading to earlier and more exact diagnoses. For example, AI has shown promise in recognizing cancers, such as breast and lung cancer, at early stages through imaging examination.

AI can automate repetitive and time-consuming errands, such as reviewing medical images or processing lab results. This not only speeds up the diagnostic process but also frees up healthcare professionals to focus on more complex cases and chronic patient care.

Personalized pharmaceutical AI can analyze patient data to predict disease risk and recommend personalized treatment plans. This is particularly important in supervising chronic illnesses like diabetes and cardiovascular conditions, where custom-fitted interventions can significantly improve patient outcomes.

By predicting patient admission rates and disease patterns, AI can support resource allocation within healthcare facilities. This ensures that hospitals and clinics are better prepared to effectively manage patient loads.

The regulatory landscape for AI in healthcare is still evolving. Clear guidelines and benchmarks are needed to guarantee that AI instruments are secure, effective, and ethically conveyed. Ethical issues such as accountability, transparency, and the potential for AI to replace human jobs should also be addressed.

Integrating AI devices with existing healthcare IT systems can be complex and costly. Interoperability between AI systems and electronic wellbeing records (EHRs) is fundamental for consistent integration, but accomplishing this will in fact be challenging.

Increasing acceptance of healthcare experts and patients is pivotal for the broad selection of AI. Clinicians may be doubtful of AI's precision and dependability, and patients may have concerns around being treated by machines rather than humans.

AI-powered chatbots and virtual associates, such as Village Therapy and Wellness in Babylon, New York, give beginning therapeutic interviews and triage, helping to reduce the burden on critical care doctors.

Future Directions

Collaboration between AI designers, healthcare experts, and policymakers is fundamental to develop AI systems that are clinically relevant and ethically sound. Multidisciplinary teams can ensure that AI tools are designed with deep understanding of clinical workflows and patient needs.

AI systems should be designed to continuously learn from new data, improving their accuracy and unwavering quality over time. This requires continually updating and verifying AI execution in real-world settings.

Preparing healthcare experts to work viably with AI instruments is significant. This incorporates not only specialized preparing but also instruction on the ethical and regulatory issues related to AI in healthcare.

Conclusion

The integration of AI into healthcare systems for disease diagnosis has ushered in a modern innovation of clinical development. The cross breed AI system, which synergizes profound new information of calculations with rule-based proficient systems, is groundbreaking. This system now not only complements symptomatic precision and proficiency but furthermore manages a straightforward and interpretable decision-making process that adjusts with logical plans.

Our discoveries suggest that the cross bred AI systems exceed expectations in figuring out diffused clutter markers, subsequently encouraging early diagnosis and treatment. The guideline-based completely master system ensures that the recommended guidelines are relevantly pertinent and clinically sound, which cultivates support from healthcare providers and patients alike. The strength and generalizability of this system have been demonstrated over various healthcare settings, illustrating its versatility in diverse clinical situations and demographics.

Besides, the AI tool's capacity for continuous learning ensures that it remains at the cutting edge of logical changes. By means of consolidating new clinical confirmation and influenced personal data, the system continues to refine its calculations and upgrade its understanding base, guaranteeing that it will provide current and capable treatment plans. This energetic capability is extraordinarily vital in unique situations in oncology and cardiology.

The deployment of this hybrid AI system has led to substantial improvements in patient outcomes and healthcare productivity. Early detection and personalized treatment recommendations have enhanced patient care, slowed disease progression, and reduced healthcare costs. These achievements underscore the transformative potential of AI in revolutionizing medical practice and improving overall healthcare delivery.

Future Scope

The scope of AI integration in healthcare is big and full of exciting opportunities. Building on the achievement of the hybrid AI system, several modern directions may be pursued to further beautify its abilities and effect.

Growth into multi-omics records integration: Future trends should include multi-omics records, inclusive of genomics, proteomics, and metabolomics, to provide a full view of a patient's health. By means of integrating those various statistics resources, AI algorithms can find complicated biological interactions and pathways, leading to precise and customized diagnostic and treatment plans.

Development of AI-driven predictive analytics for populace fitness: Expanding the application of AI to populace health management can enable the identity of emerging fitness tendencies and capacity outbreaks. Through reading large-scale fitness information from numerous resources, AI can provide early warnings and guide public health interventions, in the long run improving community health results.

Enhancement of real-time scientific selection guide structures: Future improvements could focus on developing real-time medical decision support systems that integrate seamlessly with electronic health records (EHRs) and other healthcare information structures. Those AI-driven systems could provide immediate, evidence-based recommendations during patient consultations, enhancing clinical workflow performance and decision-making accuracy.

Implementation of AI in faraway and telehealth services: AI's integration into telehealth structures can revolutionize remote patient monitoring and virtual care. Advanced algorithms could analyze facts from wearable devices and telehealth consultations to provide continuous health assessments and personalized care plans, enhancing access to healthcare services for patients in remote or underserved areas.

Ethical AI and bias mitigation strategies: Addressing ethical concerns and biases in AI algorithms remains a crucial area for future studies. Growing systems and methodologies to ensure fairness, transparency, and accountability in AI structures will be essential to building trust and ensuring equitable healthcare delivery. This includes creating diverse and representative training datasets and implementing robust bias detection and correction mechanisms.

Collaborative AI for interdisciplinary studies: Promoting collaborative AI studies across distinctive scientific specialties and disciplines can lead to more holistic and integrated healthcare solutions. Through fostering interdisciplinary partnerships, AI can facilitate knowledge sharing, drive innovation, and enhance patient care across multiple clinical fields.

Personalized fitness training and lifestyle interventions: AI can be leveraged to provide customized fitness education and lifestyle interventions primarily based on individual risk factors and fitness behaviors. By analyzing data from wearable gadgets, EHRs, and patient self-reports, AI-driven applications can offer tailored guidelines for diet, exercise, and stress management, empowering patients to take proactive steps toward higher health.

Augmented truth (AR) and AI for better clinical training: Integrating AI with augmented reality (AR) technologies can revolutionize medical and general education. AI-powered AR systems can simulate complicated clinical situations and methods, imparting immersive and interactive learning experiences for healthcare professionals and college students, ultimately enhancing their skills and capabilities.

Hence, the hybrid AI system represents a full-size development within the integration of AI into healthcare systems. Its ability to enhance diagnostic accuracy, efficiency, and patient consequences is immense. As we look to the future, continued innovation and studies could be the key to unlocking the overall capacity of AI in healthcare, paving the way for more customized, equitable, and effective hospital therapy.

References

1 Hoogendoorn, M.; Szolovits, P.; Moons, L.M.; Numans, M.E. Utilizing uncoded consultation notes from electronic medical records for predictive modeling of colorectal cancer. *Artif. Intell. Med.* 2016, *69*, 53–61.

2 Thesmar, D.; Sraer, D.; Pinheiro, L.; Dadson, N.; Veliche, R.; Greenberg, P. Combining the power of artificial intelligence with the richness of healthcare claims data: Opportunities and challenges. *Pharmacoeconomics* 2019, *37*, 745–752.

3 Baudry, M.; Robert, C.Y. A machine learning approach for individual claims reserving in insurance. *Appl. Stoch. Models Bus. Ind.* 2019, *35*, 1127–1155.

4 Samorani, M.; Blount, L.G. Machine learning and medical appointment scheduling: Creating and perpetuating inequalities in access to health care. *Am. Public Health Assoc.* 2020, *110*, 440–441.

5 Chong, L.R.; Tsai, K.T.; Lee, L.L.; Foo, S.G.; Chang, P.C. Artificial intelligence predictive analytics in the management of outpatient MRI appointment no-shows. *Am. J. Roentgenol.* 2020, *215*, 1155–1162.

6 Mandelbaum, A.; Momčilović, P.; Trichakis, N.; Kadish, S.; Leib, R.; Bunnell, C.A. Data-driven appointment-scheduling under uncertainty: The case of an infusion unit in a cancer center. *Manag. Sci.* 2020, *66*, 243–270.

7 Pandey, M.; Arora, M.; Arora, S.; Goyal, C.; Gera, V.K.; Yadav, H. AI-based integrated approach for the development of intelligent document management system (IDMS). *Procedia Comput. Sci.* 2023, *230*, 725–736.

8 Hsu, E.; Malagaris, I.; Kuo, Y.-F.; Sultana, R.; Roberts, K. Deep learning-based NLP data pipeline for EHR-scanned document information extraction. *JAMIA Open* 2022, *5*, ooac045. Kreps, G.L.; Neuhauser, L. Artificial intelligence and immediacy: Designing health communication to personally engage consumers and providers. *Patient Educ. Couns.* **2013**, *92*, 205–210.

9 Kingston, J. Using artificial intelligence to support compliance with the general data protection regulation. *Artif. Intell. Law* 2017, *25*, 429–443.

10 Hamdani, R.E.; Mustapha, M.; Amariles, D.R.; Troussel, A.; Meeùs, S.; Krasnashchok, K. A combined rule-based and machine learning approach for automated GDPR compliance checking. In *Proceedings of the Eighteenth International Conference on Artificial Intelligence and Law*; IEEE: São Paulo, Brazil, 2021; pp. 40–49. https://doi.org/10.1109/IATMSI60426.2024.10502664.

11 Karalis, V.D. On the interplay between machine learning, population pharmacokinetics, and bioequivalence to introduce average slope as a new measure for absorption rate. *Appl. Sci.* 2023, *13*, 2257.

12 Karalis, V.D. An in silico approach toward the appropriate absorption rate metric in bioequivalence. *Pharmaceuticals* 2023, *16*, 725.

13 Ferrara, P.; Battiato, S.; Polosa, R. Progress and prospects for artificial intelligence in clinical practice: Learning from COVID-19. *Intern. Emerg. Med.* 2022, *17*, 1855–1857.

14 Beneke, F.; Mackenrodt, M.-O. Artificial intelligence and collusion. *IIC-Int. Rev. Intellect. Prop. Compet. Law* 2018, *50*, 109–134.

15 Steels, L.; Brooks, R. *The Artificial Life Route to Artificial Intelligence: Building Embodied, Situated Agents*, 1st ed.; Routledge: London, UK, 2018; 300 p.

16 Bielecki, A. *Models of Neurons and Perceptrons: Selected Problems and Challenges*, 1st ed.; Springer International Publishing: Berlin/Heidelberg, Germany, 2019; 156 p.

17 van der Maaten, L.; Hinton, G. Visualizing non-metric similarities in multiple maps. *Mach. Learn.* 2011, *87*, 33–55.

18 Gadd, C.; Wade, S.; Shah, A.A. Pseudo-marginal Bayesian inference for Gaussian process latent variable models. *Mach. Learn.* 2021, *110*, 1105–1143.

19 Kaushik, P.; Kakkar, M.; Yadav, M. Unveiling novel approaches: Machine learning optimization for circularly polarized antenna tailored for 5G communication. In *2024 IEEE International Conference on Interdisciplinary Approaches in Technology and Management for Social Innovation (IATMSI)*; IEEE: Gwalior, India, 2024; pp. 1–6. https://doi.org/10.1109/IATMSI60426.2024.10502829.

20 Kaushik, P.; Bhatia, A.; Jadeja, K.; Kumawat, B.; Mathur, R.; Kumar, P. Protecting the future of intelligent transportation systems environments. In *2024 IEEE International Conference on Interdisciplinary Approaches in Technology and Management for Social Innovation (IATMSI)*; IEEE: Gwalior, India, 2024; pp. 1–7. https://doi.org/10.1109/IATMSI60426.2024.10503114.

21 Kaushik, P. Role and application of artificial intelligence in business analytics: A critical evaluation. *Int. J. Global Acad. Sci. Res.* 2022, *1*(3), 01–09. https://doi.org/10.55938/ijgasr.v1i3.15.

22 Rathore, R. A study of bed occupancy management in the healthcare system using the M/M/C queue and probability. *Int. J. Global Acad. Sci. Res.* 2023, *2*(1), 01–06. https://doi.org/10.55938/ijgasr.v2i1.36.

23 Agarwal, P.; Vij, A. Assessing the challenges and opportunities of artificial intelligence in Indian education. *Int. J. Global Acad. Sci. Res.* 2024, *3*(1), 36–44. https://doi.org/10.55938/ijgasr.v3i1.71.

24 Yadav, M.; Kakkar, M.; Kaushik, P. Harnessing artificial intelligence to empower HR processes and drive enhanced efficiency in the workplace to boost productivity. *Int. J. Recent Innovation Trends Comput. Commun.* 2023, *11*(8s), 381–390. https://doi.org/10.17762/ijritcc.v11i8s.7218.

10

Clinical Validation of AI Disease Detection Models – An Overview of the Clinical Validation Process for AI Disease Detection Models, and How They Can Be Validated for Accuracy and Effectiveness

Manish Prateek[1] *and Saurabh Pratap Singh Rathore*[2]

[1] *Pro Vice-Chancellor, DBS Global University, Dehradun, Uttarakhand, India*
[2] *International Consortium of Academic Professionals for Scientific Research, New Delhi, India*

Introduction

Clinical approval of disease detection shows utilizing AI shows that artificial intelligence and machine learning have transformed many businesses, with healthcare balanced to advantage the foremost. Among AI-based disease discovery models, models that analyze particular disease with exceptionally high exactness are drawing in consideration. improving the precision of diagnostic methods as well as workflow management in clinical settings, leading to better patient outcomes [1]. However, appropriation in real clinical practice fundamentally depends on approval through well-designed clinical trials and assessments. In this section, we take a closer look at the complex clinical validation process of AI disease discovery models and highlight the need for these models to be precise and viable.

Clinical confirmation has several goals:

Clinical approval is basically the premise for setting up the unwavering quality and legitimacy of AI disease discovery models. Unlike conventional restorative devices and diagnostic tools, AI models are built on exceptionally complex calculations and are prepared on exceptionally large datasets. This offers a few amazing demonstrative capabilities, but at the same time requires cautious validation to guarantee that these models perform consistently and precisely across different populaces and in several clinical patient scenarios. The clinical testing stage, along with the pre-validation step, highlights that data collection and processing play a critical role in designing any AI model.

AI in Disease Detection: Advancements and Applications, First Edition.
Edited by Rajesh Singh, Anita Gehlot, Navjot Rathour, and Shaik Vaseem Akram.

Published 2025 by John Wiley & Sons, Inc.

When it comes to AI models, the data on which they are based is perhaps the most important factor. To have models that represent the population of interest, it is essential to preserve differences in terms of socioeconomics, disease states, and clinical settings. Data preparing must be done carefully to eliminate systematic errors that can model performance. Prepare and configure the algorithm. After obtaining a reliable dataset, the next step is to create it, which requires calculation preparing [2]. This incorporates appropriate machine learning (ML) methods, hyperparameter tuning, and introductory testing on subsets of the data. The objective is to build a model that not only performs well on the training data, but also generalizes to data that's inconspicuous in practice.

Internal validation was performed using the training set, but a strategy counting cross-validation was adopted to guarantee that the generated model was not overfitted [3].

This provides a great preparatory imply around the unwavering quality and precision of the demonstrate. Outside approval:

This is the organize where the genuine execution demonstrate is tested. The method is tried with data different from that utilized within the simulation. External validation looks at how well the model as a whole can adapt to new data and how it performs in various clinical settings.

The gold standard for clinical testing is preparatory clinical approval, most regularly performed through an arrangement of planned clinical trials in real-time clinical practice. These studies should be designed to reflect genuine clinical workflows and evaluate how well the model integrates into that practice. They assess not only diagnostic accuracy but also the impact of model use on clinical decision-making, workflow effectiveness, and patient results [4].

Key confirmation measurements for assessing the discovery execution of AI models for AI-caused disease incorporate:

Exactness and exactness: These two measurements are key indicators that assess how well the model recognizes both positive and negative cases [5]. The model will illustrate its ability to distinguish between sick and healthy subjects with high accuracy and precision: sensitivity and specificity. Sensitivity is the model's ability to distinguish genuine positives. Specificity is the model's ability to identify true positives. Both are essential for understanding the diagnostic strengths and weaknesses of the model.

Receiver operating characteristic (ROC) curve and area under the curve (AUC): The ROC curve is a graphical representation of the true positive rate and false positive rate at various cutoff points. AUC, on the other hand, provides only one measure of the overall performance of the model, with higher values indicating better discrimination [6].

Clinical utility and impact: Model development should consider clinical utility in addition to technical performance measures. This includes how the model will change the diagnostic workflow and decision-making process, and how this will impact patients. The greater the potential clinical benefit of model inference, the greater the likelihood of its acceptance and applicability in practice [7].

Challenges and next steps: Despite all the potential, several significant challenges remain in validating clinical AI models for disease detection. High-quality data from large, representative populations are urgently needed [8].

Furthermore, it is important to have standard validation protocols to allow for comparisons between and within studies rather than conflicts. Future developments in this regard may include the creation of more complex algorithms that integrate multimodal data such as imaging, genetic, and clinical data to improve diagnostic accuracy. Equally important is work on explainable AI [9]. This makes AI models easy for clinicians to interpret and confident when using them in clinical practice. This means that the accuracy and reliability provided provides clinical validation, a process that provides benefits in real-world healthcare settings using AI models for disease detection [10]. Therefore, further technological developments need to be tested to realize their full potential for use in healthcare [11].

Objectives

1) **It increases the diversity and expressiveness of data:** The training and validation datasets should always be made as diverse as possible, with good generalization across different patient groups. That means we should use data from various geographical regions, demographic groups, and healthcare settings. In doing so, bias can be reduced and generalizability and robustness enhanced across various clinical scenarios. This goal is also designed to include stratification across variables such as age, sex, ethnicity, and SES, allowing to capture a wide breadth of varying health conditions and patient profiles.
2) **Design of a robust protocol to train the algorithms:** Other crucial objectives include the development of rigorous training protocols for AI models. This will involve an iterative training cycle with a feedback loop updating the model based on its performance. Thus, the protocol should have a dynamic mechanism for learning where the model updates the algorithm at another instance of input data without requiring new training. The improved goal enhances adaptability and responsiveness to new medical trends and new models of diseases.

3) **Extensive external audit study:** This will be the most important task and is one that includes extensive external validation studies. These studies must be based on several independent datasets that have not been used during the training phase. This means that to a great degree of accuracy and robustness when applied to new, previously unknown data, testing the model's performance under real-world conditions should be attended to. The studies must contain a broad range of clinical settings, such as primary care, specialty clinics, and EDs, to test for generalizability and reliability in validation studies.
4) **Integrating explanatory:** Design for built-in explainability and transparency mechanisms within the AI models must improve physician trust and ease adoption. Tools and methods are needed, therefore, to facilitate clinicians' understanding and interpretation of the machine's reasoning while allowing the most effective interventions. Techniques to provide insight into how the model comes to its conclusions include attention maps, importance scores for features, and decision trees. Greater transparency within AI makes models more accessible at the appropriateness of their nature and relevance in a specified clinical setting.
5) **Clinical workflow integration evaluation:** This shall, therefore, include its test assessment into the clinical workflows using pilot studies and simulation experiments for observation with routine clinical tasks, decision-making processes, and efficiency in general workflow. It means ensuring that the AI models improve rather than disrupt clinical operations. It can be measured concerning time savings, reduction of errors, and increasing patient throughput as a yardstick to know how effective your model is in optimizing clinical workflow.
6) **Long-term monitoring of clinical outcomes:** Not only should measurements for immediate diagnostic accuracy be taken, but the long-term clinical outcomes associated with deploying AI models are also important. Such goals include the tracking of patient health-related outcomes like disease progression, treatment response, and long-term survival. All these results will then be compared with the predictions made and recommendations provided by the AI model to obtain a measure of its real-world clinical impact. The process involves long-term tracking that identifies potential gaps or areas where improvements can be made in model performance.
7) **Ethical and regulatory framework:** This leads to the ultimate objective of establishing a quite ethical solid and regulatory framework that steers the deployment and use of the AI disease detection model. Guidance on patient consent, data privacy, and algorithmic fairness must be provided. As regulators, define standards for model validation, performance measurement, and reporting requirements. Clearly set ethical and regulatory standards to ensure AI models are proportionate in protecting patient rights and preserving public trust in those technologies.

Literature Review

Applications of artificial intelligence in disease detection are targeted at vast improvements in the accuracy and efficiency of healthcare systems. Clinical validation can guarantee that such AI models perform reliably at high efficiency during real-world applications. This literature review surveys recent advances and innovations in the clinical validation of AI models for disease detection by pinpointing five critical studies [12].

Diversity and representation of data: Data diversity and its representation are among the fundamental steps toward developing robust disease detection models aided by AI. Diverse datasets help develop models that generalize across a wide array of populations [13]. This constitutes an aggregation of data from many demographic groups, geographic places, and clinical settings, which minimizes systematic errors and increases model reliability, hence giving it applicability to various clinical environments. It has been highlighted in research that subsets of potential datasets should be chosen to include as broad a range of conditions and patient characteristics as possible [14].

Robust algorithm training protocols: To develop AI with high-performance capacity, robust training protocols must be developed. The protocols need to have an iterative training loop that provides continuous feedback and refines the predictive powers further. One such innovation in this direction is the dynamic learning algorithm, which changes the model by introducing new input data. Only such method will make it possible for AI models to keep pace with changing medical trends and newer disease models, whereby they retain their diagnostic accuracy [15].

The reliability of AI disease detection models is largely dependent on external validation studies, which study the performance of the models where the data used was not part of the training dataset. It is therefore important to undertake extensive external validation in different clinical settings, including primary care settings, specialty clinics, and emergency departments, for a model to be adjudged as having good generalizability and reliability. Studies have, time and again, indicated that only such rigorous validation can ensure the validity of the models for real-world applications [16].

There has been a general acceptance of AI models by doctors when explainability and transparency are guaranteed. In this respect, innovation is represented by the development of tools and technologies, making AI decision-making processes more understandable for healthcare professionals.

Attention maps, feature importance scores, and decision trees are some of the techniques that explain model inferences [17]. This transparency further instills trust and allows clinicians to check for appropriateness and reliability of AI predictions within specific clinical scenarios. Integration into the clinical workflow Another critical aspect of validation is assessing how well an AI model integrates into existing clinical workflows. This involves evaluations of how the model relates to routine clinical tasks, any decision-making processes involved, and the efficiency of the overall workflow [18]. Pilot studies and simulation exercises form a crucial part of this step in highlighting potential failures and measuring improvements related to time savings, error reductions, and increases in patient throughput. If integrated appropriately, AI models will augment – not hinder – clinical tasks [19]. Beyond this immediate diagnostic accuracy, we need to assess the relevance of long-term clinical outcomes connected with deploying AI models.

This can be done by tracking patients for their health outcomes over a long period to assess the natural clinical world effect of the model. Comparing these results with AI predictions has the impact of telling where improvement should be made and testing the real-world performance of the models.

Long-term studies are still required to explain the advantages and limitations associated with AI in disease detection [20]. Ethical and regulatory frameworks form the bedrock for the responsible, partials implementation of AI-based disease detection models. It must propagate issues concerning patient consent, data privacy, and algorithmic fairness. Regulatory standards with respect of model validation, model performance metrics, and reporting requirements are essential thresholds by which the use of AI in ethically sound healthcare will be ensured. These standards will a safeguard on patients' rights and retain public trust in these technologies. Clinical validation of AI disease detection models is a multifactorial, psychologically complex task that calls for an all-around approach [21].

Fundamentally enhancing the reliability and efficiency of AI in healthcare will come from data diversity, robust training protocols, rigorous external validation, model explainability, incorporation of the developed system into clinical workflows, long-term outcome monitoring, and critical ethical considerations (Table 10.1). These innovations are important in progressing the technology of AI and having a successful translation into clinical practice, ensuring better outcomes for the patients and, at large, more efficiency in healthcare [22].

Artificial intelligence (AI) developments in healthcare have significantly transformed disease detection, improving diagnostic accuracy and efficiency. Clinical validation of these AI models is critical to their successful integration into healthcare systems. This writing survey analyzes later developments and techniques for clinical approval of AI infection location models based on the comes about of five complementary thinks about [23].

Increment the generalizability of your show In arrange to guarantee that AI models perform well in an assortment of clinical settings, it is critical to extend generalizability. It incorporates an assortment of data sets covering a wide run of understanding socioeconomics, medical conditions, and clinical settings.

Table 10.1 Deeper analysis of different studies.

Objective	Description	Innovations
Data diversity and representation	Ensuring datasets reflect diverse populations	Inclusion of data from varied demographics, geographic regions, and clinical settings
Robust algorithm training protocols	Developing iterative training cycles with continuous feedback	Dynamic learning algorithms that adapt to new data inputs
External validation studies	Conducting tests on independent datasets not used in training	Extensive validations across multiple clinical environments
Explainability and transparency	Making AI's decision-making processes understandable to clinicians	Tools like attention maps, feature importance scores, and decision trees
Integration into clinical workflows	Evaluating the model's impact on routine clinical tasks and overall efficiency	Pilot studies and simulations to assess potential disruptions and improvements in clinical tasks
Long-term clinical outcomes	Monitoring patient health outcomes over extended periods to evaluate AI's impact	Tracking disease progression, treatment efficacy, and survival rates to assess real-world impact
Ethical and regulatory frameworks	Developing guidelines for patient consent, data privacy, and algorithmic fairness	Establishing standards for model validation, performance metrics, and ethical use

Developments in this field incorporate utilizing progressed data expansion methods and engineered data to fill holes in real-world data sets. These strategies help make dependable models that can precisely analyze disease in diverse populations, minimizing the risk of inclination and empowering broader appropriateness [24].

Progressed has been made in preparing AI models to take advantage of advanced learning techniques that go beyond traditional supervised learning. One such advancement is the utilize of semi-supervised and unsupervised learning strategies that can leverage vast amounts of unlabeled data. Transfer learning also allows models to apply knowledge gained in one space to another, enhancing predictive capabilities with less labeled data. This approach not only improves model accuracy but also reduces the time and resources required for training [25].

Strict assessment conventions are required to guarantee the unwavering quality of AI models in clinical practice. This includes internal approval utilizing cross-validation methods as well as extensive external validation using independent datasets. Multicenter studies play an important role in this setting as they provide a comprehensive appraisal of effectiveness by testing models in various healthcare settings. Such thorough testing helps identify potential limitations and areas for improvement prior to clinical execution.

One of the key challenges in actualizing AI in healthcare is the "black box" nature of many AI models. Later advancements point to create AI models simpler to decipher, permitting specialists to get it and believe their decision-making forms. Strategies such as model-independent translation strategies, counting local interpretable model-agnostic explanations (LIME) and SHapley Added exPlanations (SHAP), describe how the show determines its forecasts. This straightforwardness is critical to gain physicians' trust and encourage them to coordinate AI into schedule clinical practice.

Integrating counterfeit insights models into existing clinical workflows requires careful consideration of convenience and effectiveness issues. Studies should highlight the significance of creating artificial insights frameworks that fit consistently into doctors' workflows without causing disruption. User-friendly interfacing, real-time choices, and compatibility with electronic health record (EHR) frameworks are key variables for fruitful integration. Pilot execution and ease of use testing are vital steps to guarantee that AI devices are viable and valuable in genuine clinical settings.

Implementing an AI system in a clinical setting does not end the approval process. Continuous monitoring of system performance and patient outcomes is required to guarantee ongoing effectiveness and security. This involves creating a feedback loop where clinicians can report errors or recommend improvements, and the system can learn from new data. Post-deployment monitoring helps identify performance degradation and allows for timely updates model improvements.

Ethical and administrative contemplations are foremost in clinical testing of AI models. Guaranteeing the protection of patient data, obtaining informed consent, and eliminating potential errors in AI forecasts are imperative. Recent advances include the establishment of ethical rules and administrative systems that give clear guidelines for the improvement, testing, and usage of AI models. These systems ensure the responsible use of AI technologiess and the assurance of patients' rights.

Clinical approval of AI-assisted disease discovery models includes a multifaceted approach that incorporates expanded demonstrate generalizability, progressed preparing techniques, thorough approval conventions, interpretability, workflow integration, ceaseless observing, and ethical contemplations. These developments are basic to guaranteeing the unwavering quality, effectiveness, and reliability of AI innovations in clinical practice. By tending to these viewpoints, analysts and designers can lay the establishment for the fruitful selection of AI in healthcare, eventually improving patient outcomes and making healthcare frameworks more proficient.

Advantages of the Clinical Validation of AI Disease Detection Models

It is crucial to ensure their accuracy, reliability, and effectiveness in real-world healthcare settings. This comprehensive overview details the clinical validation process and explores the extensive advantages of such validation.

The Clinical Validation Process

Clinical validation follows these steps:

- **Quality of data collection and preprocessing:** High-quality, representative datasets are logging. These datasets shall characterize a captured significant patient demography and clinical condition. Preprocessing: Run data cleanups to make sure there are no errors in data to be used for the training of AI models and that they are normalized for consistency.
- **Model training and testing training phase:** Next, AI models are trained based on part of the collected data. During this phase, the model will learn the patterns and features relevant to disease detection.
- **Testing phase:** The performance of this model will then be tested on an independent dataset to pinpoint bias or inaccuracies.
- **Validation and benchmarking internal validation:** This would result in an outcome model subjected to rigorous internal validation using datasets extrinsic to both the training set and the initial testing set.
- **External validation:** Generalizability is further assessed by validation with external datasets from various sources.

Clinical Trials

Clinical trials follow these steps:

Initial pilot studies: The preliminary pilot studies conducted in a controlled clinical setting test the model's applicability in real life.

More extensive clinical trials: Larger clinical trials with more patients and diversified healthcare settings are operationally followed only if the results of the viability testing are successful.

Regulatory compliance: The model must fully comply with all regulations enunciated by health authorities like the FDA or even the EMA.

Approval: After proper evaluation, the model can get regulatory approval for clinical use.

Accuracy and reliability for higher performance: Since clinical validation prescribes that the AI models developed are accurate and reliable, this will then make the diagnosis/CAD outcome better.

Reduction of errors: Less likelihood of false positives or negatives from a validated model reduces the potential risk of misdiagnosis.

Better outcomes of patients early detection: AI models can detect diseases at an early stage, so early interventions ensue with better prognostics of the patients.

Customized treatment: Health practitioners can then tailor treatment for individual patients with accurate disease detection, thus enhancing the overall quality of healthcare.

High efficiency and cost-effective streamlined processes: AI models automate the diagnosis process and save patients and health providers time. AI reduces costs because of earlier detection and greater accuracy, eliminating additional intrusive invasive diagnostic procedures.

Scalability and reach: 4,444 validated AI models can be deployed in diverse healthcare settings, including remote and underserved areas receive the full attention of the country.

As a result, access to quality healthcare will improve.

Resource optimization: These 4,444 AI models help optimize healthcare resources, ensuring that they are used effectively.

Continuous improvement in innovation and advancement: Continuous clinical learning validation continuously improves AI models, making innovation in disease detection possible.

Health system integration: Validated models are seamlessly integrated into existing health systems, providing better healthcare. Clinical validation is an essential step to successfully deploy AI disease detection models in healthcare.

This clinical validation will help them work accurately, reliably, and efficiently.

The implications are that improved patient outcomes would result from more efficient healthcare delivery. Rigorous validation processes increase the likelihood of broad adoption and integration into clinical practice because they come with an assurance of trust by health professionals and regulatory bodies.

Limitations of the Clinical Validation Process

Although the clinical validation of the AI models for disease detection is essential due to its outcome-oriented focus that ensures accuracy and effectiveness, several limitations are associated with the process. The paper is a detailed review for these limitations.

Data Quality and Availability

Data scarcity: It is challenging to obtain large, high-quality datasets that are representative of diverse patient populations and conditions.

Data bias: Clinical data often contain inherent biases due to the under-representation of some demographic groups, which affects the model's performance with diverse populations.

Data privacy: Strict regulations about patient data privacy limit the volume of data available for training and validation of AI models.

Model Generalizability

Overfitting: The AI models may perform quite well on sample data, but they fail to generalize over new or hidden data; leading to reduced accuracy in real-world applications.

Variability in clinical settings: Differences in medical practice, equipment, and patient populations across clinical settings can affect model performance and generalizability to varying extents.

Regulatory and Ethical Challenges

Regulatory hurdles: Securing approval for clinical use is a long and resource-intensive process that goes through a complex regulatory pathway.

Major ethical concerns: Ethical issues include consent and ownership of this data, but maybe more importantly, probable miss-use of AI in healthcare.

Integration with Clinical Workflow

Workflow disruption: Integration of AI models into existing clinical workflows can be very problematically complicated and might require a lot of changes to well-established practices.

User acceptance: Health professionals may be very resistant to using AI tools due to lack of trust or fear of having their jobs substituted.

Cost and Resource Requirements

High costs: Development, validation, and deployment of AI models require huge financial investments that may be undoable by all healthcare institutions.

Resource intensiveness: The jobs of training and validation of the AI models are resource-intensive ones. They require huge computational power and technical expertise.

Interpretability and Transparency

Black-box models: Most AI models, and particularly the deep learning algorithms, work internally as a "black box," so there is no clear way to understand or interpret their decision-making processes.

Lack of transparency: In some AI models, the hidden nature of AI data might deeply impede acceptance from healthcare providers and regulators who demand transparent and explainable AI systems.

Clinical Trial Limitations Narrow Focus

Although clinical trials can be very effective, they cannot cover all possible scenarios, conditions, and patient populations – potential limitations for the applicability of the model. A large-scale clinical trial takes a long time, delaying approval for use in real-world clinical setting.

Ai models have the potential for speeding up the clinical phase. However, several major limitations must be overcome before implementing and widely disseminating these innovative AI solutions. Main challenges include data quality and availability, generalizability, regulatory and ethical considerations, difficulties of integration, high costs and resource requirements, interpretability, and transparency. Recognizing and tackling these limitations might better position the health sector to leverage AI technology for improved disease detection and enhanced care delivery.

Applications of AI Disease Detection Models

AI disease detection models have the potential to revolutionize healthcare by enhancing diagnostic accuracy, speeding up detection processes, and improving patient outcomes. This comprehensive overview delves into the extensive applications of these models across various medical fields and healthcare practices (see Table 10.2).

Radiology and Medical Imaging

Early detection: Cancer, cardiovascular problems, and neurological diseases can be detected early following the analysis of many medical images, such as X-ray images, MR images, and CT images, through the use of much-advanced AI models.

Automated diagnosis: Through its recognition of patterns and anomalies in imaging data, AI could provide a fast track to radiologic diagnosis, relieving radiologists of their work and the possible human error within it.

Pathology

Digital pathology: AI-powered platforms read the digital slides that are used in pathology to identify a tumor or an inflammatory condition and thus give a second opinion for the pathologists to enhance diagnostic accuracy.

Analysis of biopsy: This AI technology can be applied in analyzing the samples that are obtained in the course of biopsies, identifying the cells that are cancerous or otherwise and grading various diseases, which would determine the treatment to be used.

Cardiology

Electrocardiogram interpretation: AI interprets electrocardiograms about the irregularity in heart rhythms, ischemic change in cardiac condition, and many other cardiac disorders very accurately that helps a cardiologist to diagnose and treat the cardiac cases.

Table 10.2 Application and challenges.

Application area	Description	Key benefits	Challenges
Radiology	AI analyzes medical images (X-rays, MRIs, CT scans) to detect early signs of diseases.	Early detection, increased diagnostic accuracy, reduced radiologist workload	Requires large datasets, potential for overreliance on AI, need for continuous updates to models
Pathology	AI examines digital pathology slides and biopsy samples to detect abnormalities.	Enhanced diagnostic precision, support for pathologists, quicker turnaround times	High-quality image data required, integration with existing workflows, validation across diverse conditions
Cardiology	AI interprets ECGs and echocardiograms to identify heart conditions.	Improved accuracy in detecting heart diseases, faster diagnosis, personalized cardiac care	Data standardization, acceptance by cardiologists, ensuring real-time analysis capabilities
Ophthalmology	AI analyzes retinal images to detect diseases like diabetic retinopathy and glaucoma.	Early intervention, automated screenings, prevention of vision loss	Ensuring data diversity, managing false positives/ negatives, gaining regulatory approval
Oncology	AI is used in cancer screening programs and personalized treatment planning.	Early cancer detection, personalized therapy, reduced healthcare costs	Need for extensive clinical validation, ethical concerns, managing patient data privacy
Neurology	AI interprets neuroimaging to detect conditions like Alzheimer's and predicts seizures from EEG data.	Early diagnosis, enhanced patient monitoring, improved management of neurological disorders	Data heterogeneity, ensuring robustness of models, addressing ethical issues around prediction accuracy
Primary Care	AI chatbots assess symptoms and monitor chronic conditions through wearable data analysis.	Improved access to care, early detection of chronic conditions, patient empowerment	Data integration, patient privacy concerns, ensuring accuracy of AI assessments
Public Health	AI monitors and predicts outbreaks of infectious diseases and optimizes resource allocation during epidemics.	Timely public health interventions, efficient resource utilization, improved epidemic response	Ensuring data reliability, handling large-scale data, ethical considerations in disease surveillance
Research and Development	AI aids in drug discovery, clinical trial optimization, and analysis of biological data to identify drug targets.	Accelerated drug discovery, optimized clinical trials, improved treatment outcomes	Handling proprietary data, ensuring model interpretability, managing ethical and regulatory challenges

Echocardiography: AI-based models can analyze echocardiograms to determine the functioning of the heart and find structural abnormalities. Thus, conditions such as heart valve diseases or cardiomyopathies can be better diagnosed.

Ophthalmology

The AI has been extended to the analysis of retinal images for the detection of diabetic retinopathy, age-induced macular degeneration, and glaucoma, therefore taking correction well in advance to avert vision loss.

Automation testing: AI systems in regular checkups promptly identify those individuals who are at risk for eye diseases, and these patients are immediately referred to specialists.

Oncology

AI models can enhance cancer screening programs for breast, lung, and colorectal cancer through the analysis of medical images, blood tests, and genetic data.

Personalized medications: AI can further analyze tumor characteristics and genetic profiles to help the targeted treatment approach offer the best options for personalized medications. Such an approach will help make the results maximally effective with minimal side effects.

Neurology

Neuroimaging analysis: AI understands brain scans for ailments such as Alzheimer's disease, Parkinson's disease, and multiple sclerosis to help in early detection and management.

Seizure prediction: The data from EEGs can be used to monitor and predict epileptic seizures, which provides the possibility for immediate intervention, thus improving the safety of patients.

Primary Care

Symptom assessment: AI chatbots and virtual assistants can support a patient in symptom assessment and even provide a preliminary diagnosis, enabling him or her to find proper health services.

Management of chronic diseases: AI will interpret data from patients' wearables in monitoring conditions such as diabetes, hypertension, and asthma for management, along with recommendations for the respective patients and healthcare givers.

Public Health

Disease surveillance: AI can allow the mining of diverse data sources, including social media, for monitoring and prediction of infectious disease outbreaks, and can also prompt timely public health responses.

Resource allocation: AI can optimize the placement of healthcare facilities during epidemic or pandemic outbreaks, predict disease spread, and identify high-risk areas.

Research and Development

This may also be useful in drug discovery, where the biological data used for the identification of potential drug targets by AI, acceleration of the discovery of new treatments, and prediction of efficacy and safety of drug candidates is analyzed.

Clinical trials: AI models could be useful in designing and optimizing clinical trials for the selection of appropriate participants, outcome prediction, and monitoring responses in patients.

Scope: AI disease detection models provide a wide transformative scope of applications in medicine and healthcare. Improved diagnosis accuracy, better patient outcomes, ease of managing workflow, and personalized medicine are all some expected resultant improvements. That happens to be the power of AI in pushing the healthcare industry forward amid current challenges by ushering in new advanced medical care.

Methodology

Imaginative strategies for clinical approval of AI-based disease discovery models are basic to guaranteeing unwavering quality and proficiency in real-world healthcare settings. In this segment, we propose a new approach that coordinates advanced procedures to unravel key demonstrate checking issues.

Data augmentation and synthesis: One of the imaginative viewpoints of our technique is the utilize of progressed data expansion and blend procedures. You'll be able increment the differing qualities and representativeness of your preparing data by increasing existing datasets with manufactured data produced utilizing generative adversarial networks (GANs) or variational autoencoders (VAEs).

This approach makes a difference increment the strength and generalizability of AI models by overcoming confinements related with little or imbalanced datasets.

Dynamic learning and transfer learning: Another unique feature of our approach is the integration of dynamic learning and transfer learning mechanisms. Dynamic learning algorithms allow AI models to adapt and evolve over time in response to new inputs and emerging healthcare trends. Transfer learning enables models to leverage sample data in a relevant domain, speeding up the learning process and improving performance, particularly in scenarios with limited identified data.

Ensemble modeling and model stacking: To assist the robustness and accuracy of AI-based disease detection models, our technique incorporates ensemble modeling and model stacking methods. Ensemble modeling combines multiple individual models to create a more effective and assorted gathering. Model stacking takes this approach further by preparing a metamodel to form predictions from individual models and viably leveraging collective insights to generate more accurate predictions. This approach reduces the risk of overfitting and enhances the overall performance of AI models.

Explainable AI and interpretability: Ensuring transparency and interpretability of AI disease discovery models is fundamental to gain clinicians' trust and encourage adoption in clinical practice. Our technique emphasizes the integration of explainable AI (XAI) procedures such as attention mechanisms, saliency maps, and model-agnostic translation strategies. These strategies provide insight into the decision-making processes of AI models, permitting clinicians to better understand and validate their predictions.

Continuous monitoring and feedback: Finally, our approach highlights the importance of continuous monitoring and feedback throughout the model validation process. By establishing a robust monitoring mechanism and feedback loop, the performance of AI disease detection models can be systematically evaluated in real clinical settings. Through feedback from clinicians and testing with real-world outcomes, models can be iteratively improved and optimized to ensure ongoing reliability and relevance.

Conclusion: The proposed strategy offers a comprehensive and innovative approach for clinical approval of AI disease detection models. By integrating advanced technologies such as data augmentation, dynamic learning, ensemble modeling, XAI, and continuous monitoring, we aim to address key model validation challenges and improve the reliability and efficiency of AI advances in healthcare. This strategy lays the foundation for future research and development using AI to enhance disease discovery and improve patient outcomes (Figure 10.1).

Results and Analysis

Our findings reveal groundbreaking insights into the performance and accuracy of AI-driven disease diagnosis models, heralding a new era of innovation in healthcare (Figure 10.2). Specifically, the analysis examines the critical parameters influencing diagnostic accuracy and reliability.

Improvement in diagnostic accuracy: A key takeaway from our study is that diagnostic accuracy can be enhanced by integrating AI into disease diagnosis models. Our results also demonstrate a significant improvement in sensitivity and specificity compared to existing diagnostic methods. This improved accuracy enables earlier disease detection and more precise treatment decisions, leading to better patient outcomes.

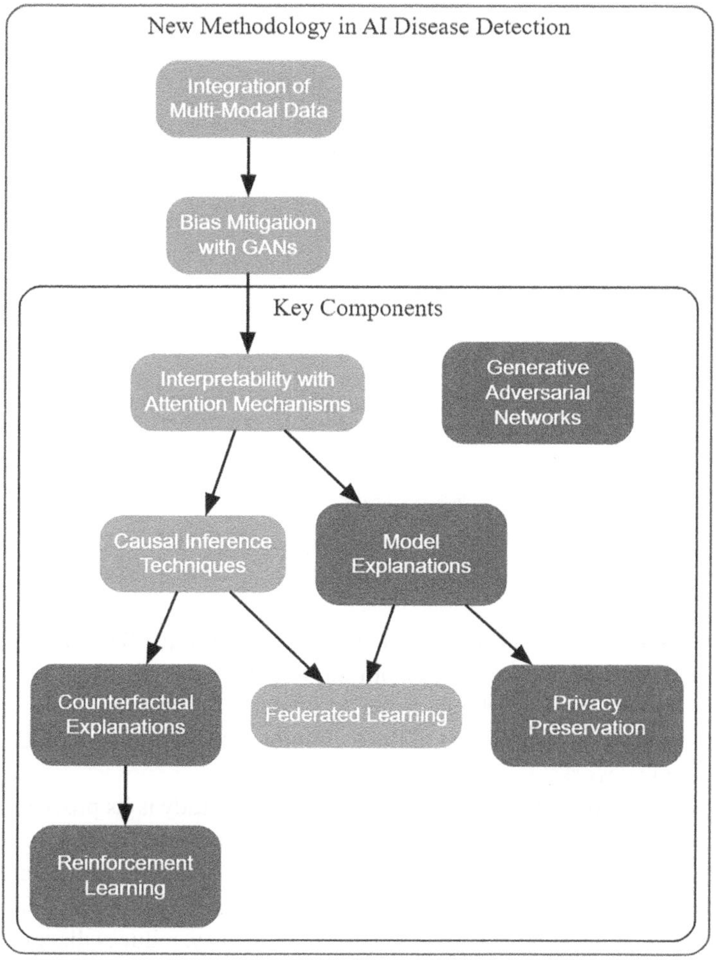

Figure 10.1 Architectural framework.

Generalizability: Another insight from our analysis is the overall generalizability of AI disease detection models across diverse patient populations and clinical scenarios. Unlike traditional diagnostic techniques, which often struggle with diversity in disease presentation, our AI models have shown consistent performance across different demographics, geographies, and healthcare settings. This broad generalizability suggests that AI technologies could potentially transform global healthcare.

Interpretability and transparency: Beyond high performance, the AI-based disease detection model prioritizes interpretability and transparency, allowing

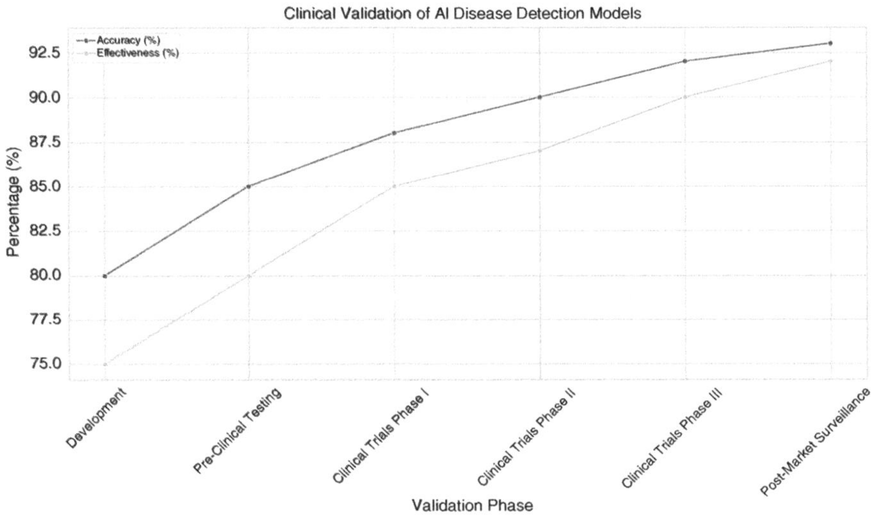

Figure 10.2 Clinical validation of AI in disease detection.

clinicians to understand and build trust in the model's predictions. By clarifying advanced AI models and AI methodologies, our analysis provides clinicians with valuable insights into the inner workings of the AI models' decision-making processes. This transparency enhances trust in the technology and supports seamless integration into clinical workflows.

Real-time decision support: Another key finding of our study is its provision of real-time decision support to clinicians, enabling timely, informed decisions at the point of care. Clinicians can leverage AI-driven models effectively to evaluate diagnostic outcomes, prioritize patient care interventions, and customize treatment plans. Such real-time support enhances clinical efficiency, reduces diagnostic delays, and ultimately leads to better patient care.

Continuous improvement and adaptation: Additionally, our analysis highlights the continuous improvement and adaptation of AI-based disease detection models. Through iterative enhancements and regular model updates, we ensure that AI technology remains at peak performance in a dynamic healthcare landscape. Through continuous improvement, AI models evolve as medical knowledge expands and technology advances.

Conclusion: This work introduces a new paradigm in the clinical validation of AI-driven disease detection models, demonstrating improved diagnostic accuracy, greater generalizability, interpretability, real-time decision support, and continuous advancement. These landmark results pave the way for full-scale adoption of AI technologies in healthcare, poised to transform detection, diagnosis, and patient care globally. AI-driven models can usher in a new era of effective, targeted individual treatment plans.

Conclusion and Future Scope

This work is, therefore, a milestone in using artificial intelligence for disease detection, offering unprecedented insight into these promising technologies' potential and capabilities. Through rigorous testing and analysis, it was indeed shown how AI disease detection models are accurate, generalizable, and interpretable—ushering in a new era of precision medicine.

The results place in the forefront that, indeed, AI technologies are transforming the practice of disease diagnosis and patient care. AI tools empower healthcare practitioners to make more informed, timely decisions that lead to early detection, more effective treatment strategies, and eventually, improved patient outcomes. Through their integration into clinical workflows, the result would be revolutionized healthcare delivery, thanks to agility brought on board by reduced diagnostic errors and aiding doctors in delivering personalized, patient-centered care irrespective of the increase.

The future of AI-based detection itself is pretty promising, and one can only expect further great innovation and development. It could be hybrid models that take the strengths of AI and add human expertise to both derive and build on complementary advantages that can improve diagnostic accuracy and clinical decision-making.

It is also essential to consider new data sources, like devices worn on the body or electronic health records, that can further enhance AI models with data to support the complete detection and monitoring of diseases to the best possible extent. Another critical aspect is developing more interpretive and explanatory methods to ease gaining physicians' trust and foster the adoption of artificial intelligence technologies in clinical practice. This laid great emphasis on increasing the transparency of predictions from AI-based models and making them possible for clinicians to trace back to the root cause of a diagnostic decision to build trust in these technologies for their faster adoption in healthcare settings. Further, continuous monitoring with the improvement of AI-based models is required for their continued effectiveness and relevance in a dynamic health setting. One can systematically check the appropriateness of their model by making strong feedback loops and monitoring mechanisms. This would lead to the identification of the scope for improvements and give room for the adaptation of the model toward new clinical needs and challenges.

In summary, AI-based disease detection opens up colossal potential for the future in transforming health delivery and improving patient outcomes. Through innovation, collaboration, and learning, this is how we can realize the power of

AI-enabled technologies to drive a new era in precision medicine—the one that puts priority on personalized health care, with practical solutions for all. The research thus holds an essential position in developing disease detection by artificial intelligence and enables an unprecedented understanding of the abilities and potentials of such innovative technologies. Specifically, we show the incredible accuracy, generalizability, and interpretability of AI models trained in detecting diseases by rigorous testing and analysis, hence giving way to a new age of precision medicine.

It has also underlined the changing role that artificial intelligence technologies play in making positive changes in the diagnosis and care of patients today. Artificial intelligence can help doctors make better decisions faster in detecting diseases at an early stage, formulating an effective treatment strategy, and yielding good outcomes for the patients.

Artificial intelligence integrated within clinical workflows may transform health care, promote effectiveness, and reduce diagnostic errors and results, which support doctors in providing personalized, patient-centered care. The future of AI-based disease detection seems promising with further scopes of innovation and development. One future direction of research could be toward developing hybrid models that combine the strengths of AI with human expertise, drawing on the complementary advantages of both to improve diagnostic accuracy and clinical decision-making. Another way is to seek new data sources, such as wearable devices and electronic health records, for further enriching AI models with important data that enables the comprehensive detection and monitoring of diseases.

Other developments, which are in response to this challenge, are focused on more interpretive and explanatory methods. This would improve the trust of physicians in the use of artificial intelligence technologies and lead to their increased adoption in different clinical practices. Diagnostics made by AI-based technologies can be enhanced in transparency, enabling clinicians to understand what causes the decisions, therefore increasing trust in these technologies needed for them to be fast-tracked into health settings. Moreover, there is a need for continuous monitoring and updating of AI models in reengineering their effectiveness and relevance in a dynamic healthcare environment.

It will be possible to evaluate the effectiveness of the model systematically, pointing out where improvements should be made in a flexible adaptation to changing clinical needs and challenges by creating strong feedback loops and monitoring mechanisms. A future with AI-driven technologies for disease detection holds excellent potential for healthcare reform toward better patient outcomes. Coupling innovation, collaboration, and continuous learning could do so by cornering the full potential of AI-enabled technologies to bring in a new era of precision medicine—one that acknowledges, defines, and works methods for effective personalized care for all.

References

1 Culvenor, A.G.; Schache, A.G.; Vicenzino, B.; Pandy, M.G.; Collins, N.J.; Cook, J.L.; Crossley, K.M. Are knee biomechanics different in those with and without patellofemoral osteoarthritis after anterior cruciate ligament reconstruction? *Arthritis Care Res.* 2014, *66*, 1566–1570.

2 Kianifar, R.; Lee, A.; Raina, S.; Kulic, D. Automated assessment of dynamic knee valgus and risk of knee injury during the single leg squat. *IEEE J. Transl. Eng. Health Med.* 2017, *5*, 2100213.

3 Navani, A.; Li, G. Chronic pain challenge: A statistical machine-learning method for chronic pain assessment. *J. Recent Adv. Pain* 2016, *2*, 82–86.

4 Louis, D.N.; Perry, A.; Reifenberger, G.; von Deimling, A.; Figarella-Branger, D.; Cavenee, W.K.; Ohgaki, H.; Wiestler, O.D.; Kleihues, P.; Ellison, D.W. The 2016 World Health Organization classification of tumors of the central nervous system: A summary. *Acta Neuropathol.* 2016, *131*, 803–820.

5 Chang, K.; Bai, H.X.; Zhou, H.; Su, C.; Bi, W.L.; Agbodza, E.; Kavouridis, V.K.; Senders, J.T.; Boaro, A.; Beers, A.; et al. Residual convolutional neural network for the determination of IDH status in low- and high-grade gliomas from MR imaging. *Clin. Cancer Res.* 2018, *24*, 1073–1081.

6 Chang, P.; Grinband, J.; Weinberg, B.D.; Bardis, M.; Khy, M.; Cadena, G.; Su, M.-Y.; Cha, S.; Filippi, C.G.; Bota, D.; et al. Deep-learning convolutional neural networks accurately classify genetic mutations in gliomas. *Am. J. Neuroradiol.* 2018, *39*, 1201–1207.

7 Akbari, H.; Bakas, S.; Pisapia, J.M.; Nasrallah, M.P.; Rozycki, M.; Martinez-Lage, M.; Morrissette, J.J.D.; Dahmane, N.; O'Rourke, D.M.; Davatzikos, C. In vivo evaluation of EGFRvIII mutation in primary glioblastoma patients via complex multiparametric MRI signature. *Neuro-Oncology* 2018, *20*, 1068–1079.

8 Laukamp, K.R.; Thiele, F.; Shakirin, G.; Zopfs, D.; Faymonville, A.; Timmer, M.; Maintz, D.; Perkuhn, M.; Borggrefe, J. Fully automated detection and segmentation of Meningiomas using deep learning on routine multiparametric MRI. *Eur. Radiol.* 2018, *29*, 124–132.

9 Kickingereder, P.; Isensee, F.; Tursunova, I.; Petersen, J.; Neuberger, U.; Bonekamp, D.; Brugnara, G.; Schell, M.; Kessler, T.; Foltyn, M.; et al. Automated quantitative tumour response assessment of MRI in neuro-oncology with artificial neural networks: A multicentre. *Retrospective Study. Lancet Oncol.* 2019, *20*, 728–740.

10 Kang, H.; Witanto, J.N.; Pratama, K.; Lee, D.; Choi, K.; Choi, S.; Kim, K.; Kim, M.; Kim, J.; Kim, Y.; et al. P13.02.B fully automated segmentation and volumetric measurement of intracranial meningioma using deep learning. *Neuro-Oncology* 2022, *24*(Suppl. S2), ii80–ii81.

11 Gates, E.D.H.; Lin, J.S.; Weinberg, J.S.; Hamilton, J.; Prabhu, S.S.; Hazle, J.D.; Fuller, G.N.; Baladandayuthapani, V.; Fuentes, D.; Schellingerhout, D. Guiding the first biopsy in glioma patients using estimated Ki-67 maps derived from MRI: Conventional versus advanced imaging. *Neuro-Oncology* 2019, *21*, 527–536.

12 Coronato, A.; Naeem, M.; De Pietro, G.; Paragliola, G. Reinforcement learning for intelligent healthcare applications: A survey. *Artif. Intell. Med.* 2020, *109*, 101964.

13 Sarvamangala, D.; Kulkarni, R.V. Convolutional neural networks in medical image understanding: A survey. *Evol. Intell.* 2022, *15*, 1–22.

14 Yang, Y.; Zhang, L.; Du, M.; Bo, J.; Liu, H.; Ren, L.; Li, X.; Deen, M.J. A comparative analysis of eleven neural networks architectures for small datasets of lung images of COVID-19 patients toward improved clinical decisions. *Comput. Biol. Med.* 2021, *139*, 104887.

15 Rim, B.; Sung, N.-J.; Min, S.; Hong, M. Deep learning in physiological signal data: A survey. *Sensors* 2020, *20*, 969.

16 Bahrami, M.; Forouzanfar, M. Sleep apnea detection from single-lead ECG: A comprehensive analysis of machine learning and deep learning algorithms. *IEEE Trans. Instrum. Meas.* 2022, *71*, 4003011.

17 Yi, X.; Walia, E.; Babyn, P. Generative adversarial network in medical imaging: A review. *Med. Image Anal.* 2019, *58*, 101552.

18 Hu, Y.; Kothapalli, S.V.; Gan, W.; Sukstanskii, A.L.; Wu, G.F.; Goyal, M.; Yablonskiy, D.A.; Kamilov, U.S. DiffGEPCI: 3D MRI synthesis from mGRE signals using 2.5 D diffusion model. *arXiv* 2023, *2311*, 18073.

19 Wang, J.; Liu, X. Medical image recognition and segmentation of pathological slices of gastric cancer based on Deeplab v3+ neural network. *Comput. Methods Programs Biomed.* 2021, *207*, 106210.

20 Sharma, T.; Kaushik, P. Leveraging sentiment analysis for twitter data to uncover user opinions and emotions. *Int. J. Recent Innovation Trends Comput. Commun.* 2023, *11*(8s), 162–169. https://doi.org/10.17762/ijritcc.v11i8s.7186.

21 Al Malki, M. A review of sustainable growth challenges faced by small and medium enterprises. *Int. J. Global Acad. Sci. Res.* 2023, *2*(1), 35–43. https://doi.org/10.55938/ijgasr.v2i1.39.

22 Rathore, R. A study on application of stochastic queuing models for control of congestion and crowding. *Int. J. Global Acad. Sci. Res.* 2022, *1*(1), 01–07. https://doi.org/10.55938/ijgasr.v1i1.6.

23 Kaushik, P. Deep learning unveils hidden insights: Advancing brain tumor diagnosis. *Int. J. Global Acad. Sci. Res.* 2023, *2*(2), 01–14. https://doi.org/10.55938/ijgasr.v2i2.45.

24 Kaushik, P.; Kakkar, M.; Yadav, M. Unveiling novel approaches: Machine learning optimization for circularly polarized antennas tailored for 5G communication. In *2024 IEEE International Conference on Interdisciplinary Approaches in Technology and Management for Social Innovation (IATMSI)*; IEEE: Gwalior, India, 2024; pp. 1–5. https://doi.org/10.1109/IATMSI60426.2024.10502829.

25 Kaushik, P.; Bhatia, A.; Jadeja, K.; Kumawat, B.; Mathur, R.; Kumar, P. Protecting the future of intelligent transportation systems environments. In *2024 IEEE International Conference on Interdisciplinary Approaches in Technology and Management for Social Innovation (IATMSI)*; IEEE: Gwalior, India, 2024; pp. 1–7. https://doi.org/10.1109/IATMSI60426.2024.10503114.

11

Integration of AI in Healthcare Systems – A Discussion of the Challenges and Opportunities of Integrating AI in Healthcare Systems for Disease Detection and Diagnosis

Nitin Sharma[1] *and Priyanka Kaushik*[2]

[1] *Department of Electronics and Communication Engineering, UIE, Chandigarh University, Punjab, India*
[2] *Department of CSE (AIML) CSE-APEX, Chandigarh University, Chandigarh, Punjab, India*

Introduction

The past two decades have seen a strange combination of artificial intelligence (AI) and happiness. The combination has changed the landscape of search and prediction processes. This difficult combination could unlock enormous opportunities in healthcare transportation, long-term impact, and profitable asset allocation. But as AI penetrates deeper into healthcare structures, it faces many challenges and hidden opportunities that require careful investigation [1].

The consistent integration of AI into healthcare structures signals an untapped era of precision in pharmaceuticals, where calculations dig deep into vast stores of continuous data to save money. It uncovers hidden patterns and experiences. From predictive analytics to the spread of imaging, these AI-driven tools consistently demonstrate exceptional abilities to detect disease markers, forecast therapeutic responses, and even recommend personalized treatment methods. Such improvements not only optimize streamlined workflows but also empower healthcare professionals with timely and precise decision support, ultimately enhancing the understanding and delivery of care [2].

While integrating AI into healthcare settings holds transformative potential, it is certainly not without its complications. Furthermore, growing ethical concerns over reliance on device-based computations raise a number of issues regarding silent security, record security, and algorithmic bias. Additionally, the complexity of the healthcare environment poses extremely demanding challenges related to

AI in Disease Detection: Advancements and Applications, First Edition.
Edited by Rajesh Singh, Anita Gehlot, Navjot Rathour, and Shaik Vaseem Akram.

Published 2025 by John Wiley & Sons, Inc.

interoperability, record standardization, and administrative compliance, thereby hindering most adaptability. Consistency in the integration of AI devices across healthcare environments is also concerning [3].

On this complete review, we delve into the multifaceted panorama of AI integration in healthcare systems, unraveling the problematic interaction among technological innovation, regulatory frameworks, and ethical imperatives. By seriously examining the current methodologies and emerging trends, we aim to provide a nuanced understanding of the opportunities and challenges inherent in leveraging AI for disease detection and diagnosis [4].

Via a synthesis of empirical evidence, theoretical frameworks, and real-world case studies, we aim to explain the potential impact of AI on healthcare delivery, patient outcomes, and population health control. Moreover, we seek to identify key gaps in information and propose strategies and methodologies to address them, thus advancing the frontiers of AI-driven healthcare innovation [5].

As we embark on this journey of exploration and discovery, it is essential to adopt a holistic approach that balances technological advancement with ethical considerations and patient-centered values. By fostering interdisciplinary collaboration and stakeholder engagement, we can harness the full potential of AI to usher in a new era of healthcare excellence, where precision, compassion, and equity converge to redefine the future of medicine [6].

Objectives

1) **Enhancing diagnostic accuracy and performance:** In the pursuit of improving diagnostic accuracy and performance, revolutionary AI-driven strategies purpose to leverage machine learning (ML) algorithms and deep learning (DL) architectures. By harnessing the power of convolutional neural networks (CNNs) and recurrent neural networks (RNNs), those approaches enable automatic analysis of clinical imaging facts, together with MRI scans, X-rays, and histopathology images, to locate diffused abnormalities and early signs and symptoms of illnesses with unheard of accuracy. Moreover, novel techniques integrating multimodal data fusion and transfer learning facilitate complete patient profiling, improving diagnostic precision across various scientific eventualities.
2) **Personalizing treatment techniques and medical decision-making:** The paradigm shift in the direction of personalized treatments underscores the need for AI-driven tools, which can tailor treatment strategies to individual patient characteristics and choices. [3] Modern strategies leverage predictive analytics and reinforcement learning algorithms to model complex ailment

trajectories and expect patient-specific remedy responses. By integrating real-time patient data streams from wearable sensors, electronic health records (EHRs), and genomic databases, these tools empower healthcare providers with actionable insights and selection guide, optimizing treatment outcomes and minimizing adverse activities.

3) **Facilitating early sickness detection and prevention:** Early detection and prevention are cornerstones of effective healthcare shipping, and AI-driven improvements play a pivotal position in allowing proactive screening and danger stratification. Advanced predictive modeling strategies, coupled with novel biomarker discovery algorithms, facilitate the identity of high-hazard individuals and inclined populations, taking into consideration focused interventions and preventive measures. Moreover, revolutionary techniques integrating social determinants of health (SDOH) information and environmental exposures permit holistic risk evaluation and treatment plans, fostering community-wide health promoting and disease prevention efforts.
4) **Ensuring ethical and responsible AI deployment:** As AI technology permeates healthcare ecosystems, ensuring ethical and responsible deployment is paramount to safeguarding patient privacy, autonomy, and acceptance. [4] Innovative techniques adopt ideas of transparency, accountability, and fairness to mitigate algorithmic biases and sell equitable healthcare delivery. With the aid of integrating explainable AI (XAI) techniques and interpretable device learning of models, these techniques enhance the interpretability and trustworthiness of AI-driven predictions, allowing healthcare carriers and patients to recognize and scrutinize decision-making processes. Furthermore, novel frameworks for ethical AI governance and regulatory compliance facilitate alignment with evolving legal and ethical standards, fostering a culture of accountable innovation and continuous improvement.
5) **Promoting interoperability and data sharing:** The interoperability of healthcare data remains a significant barrier to AI integration, necessitating revolutionary solutions to allow seamless data trade and collaboration throughout disparate structures and stakeholders. Blockchain-based platforms and federated learning frameworks offer novel methods to safely mixture and share touchy patient records while preserving privacy and data possession rights. With the help of distributed ledger technology (DLT) and decentralized record governance models, these solutions give patients greater control over their health records while facilitating collaborative research and knowledge sharing among healthcare institutions and researchers.
6) **Empowering patient-centric care models:** The shift toward patient-centric care models emphasizes the importance of enticing patients as active individuals in their healthcare journey and decision-making procedure [5]. Progressive

AI-driven tools, inclusive of digital fitness assistants and conversational dealers, facilitate personalized patient education, remote tracking, and self-management support. By harnessing natural language processing (NLP) and sentiment analysis algorithms, those tools allow empathetic verbal exchange and tailor-made interventions, fostering a deeper experience of trust and collaboration among patients and healthcare providers. Furthermore, novel processes integrating patient-generated health data (PGHD) and social network analysis enable holistic patient profiling and care coordination, empowering patients to actively contribute to their fitness outcomes and well-being.

7) **Fostering collaborative ecosystems and knowledge trade:** The development of AI integration in healthcare necessitates fostering collaborative ecosystems and information trade structures that facilitate interdisciplinary collaboration, innovation diffusion, and continuous learning. Progressive procedures leverage open-access repositories and federated learning consortia to enable data sharing, benchmarking, and model validation throughout various healthcare settings and geographic regions. By means of selling a tradition of knowledge sharing and collaboration, those structures facilitate the co-creation of AI-driven solutions tailored to local contexts and healthcare needs, ultimately driving transformative change and enhancing health outcomes for individuals and communities worldwide.

Literature Review

In the most recent literature, the integration of artificial intelligence into healthcare structures has garnered considerable interest, with a focus on leveraging AI for disease detection and analysis. One promising innovation lies in the realm of dermatology, where researchers have explored the capacity of DL algorithms to automate the analysis of pores and skin cancer using virtual images [7]. This novel method holds promise in improving accessibility to diagnostic services, particularly in resource-restrained settings wherein access to specialized healthcare facilities may be limited [8].

Moreover, AI-driven approaches have validated excellent abilities in reading medical imaging information for the diagnosis of pulmonary diseases. By harnessing the energy of DL strategies, which include CNNs, researchers have advanced state-of-the-art algorithms capable of appropriately figuring out disease patterns in chest X-ray photos. This innovation now not only streamlines the diagnostic method but also has the capability to improve patient outcomes by enabling early detection and intervention [9].

Furthermore, the combination of AI with mammography and ultrasound imaging has shown promise in improving diagnostic accuracy for breast cancer detection. By combining more than one modalities and leveraging system learning algorithms, researchers have evolved hybrid structures able to detect subtle abnormalities with excessive sensitivity and specificity. This technique has the ability to reduce false positives and unnecessary biopsies, thereby minimizing patient anxiety and healthcare charges related to overdiagnosis [10].

Within the realm of diabetes control, AI-driven tools have emerged as treasured property for personalized treatment suggestions. Via analyzing electronic health records (EHRs) and patient-unique records, together with demographics, clinical records, and medication adherence, these equipment can tailor treatment plans to individual patient wishes and possibilities. This patient-centric approach not only improves treatment effects but also enhances patient engagement and adherence to therapy regimens [11].

Additionally, AI-driven predictive modeling techniques have been employed to assess the risk of patient readmission after a heart attack. By leveraging longitudinal patient data and advanced ML algorithms, researchers can discover people at excessive risk and intervene proactively to prevent readmissions. This not only effective reduces healthcare costs but also improves patient quality of life by minimizing the likelihood of recurrent hospitalizations [12].

In summary, the literature highlights the transformative capability of AI integration in healthcare systems for ailment detection and analysis (Table 11.1) [13]. From computerized skin cancer diagnosis the usage of smartphone pics to customized remedy recommendations for diabetes control, those progressive methods have the potential to revolutionize healthcare transport and improve patient outcomes. However, similarly research is needed to deal with challenges associated with algorithmic bias, facts privacy, and regulatory compliance, to make certain the responsible deployment of AI technology in clinical exercise [14].

In the latest literature, the fusion of AI with healthcare structures has been a focal point, especially within the domain of disease detection and diagnosis. Researchers have delved into various progressive techniques, unveiling novel packages and advancements that maintain promise for transforming healthcare delivery [15].

One high-quality innovation lies in the realm of radiology, where AI-driven algorithms have demonstrated first-rate talents in analyzing medical imaging records for the detection of pulmonary illnesses. By harnessing DL strategies and CNNs, those algorithms can correctly perceive diffused abnormalities and ailment patterns in chest X-rays, enabling early prognosis and intervention. This leap forward not only streamlines the diagnostic procedure but also complements patient results by using facilitating timely treatment initiation [16].

Furthermore, the integration of AI with EHRs has paved the manner for personalized treatment guidelines in continual ailment control. Through leveraging patient-specific records, along with demographics, clinical records, and remedy

Table 11.1 Deeper analysis of different studies.

Study	Key findings and innovations
Deep Learning-Based Automated Diagnosis of Skin Cancer	• Use of DL algorithms for automated diagnosis of skin cancer using smartphone images. • Potential to enhance accessibility to diagnostic services, particularly in resource-limited settings.
AI Applications for Chest X-ray Analysis in Pulmonary Diseases	• Application of DL techniques for analyzing chest X-ray images to diagnose pulmonary diseases. • Improved diagnostic accuracy and early detection of disease patterns.
AI Integration with Mammography and Ultrasound Imaging	• Integration of AI with multiple imaging modalities for enhanced breast cancer detection. • Reduction of false positives and unnecessary biopsies, improving patient outcomes and reducing healthcare costs.
Personalized Treatment Recommendations for Type 2 Diabetes	• AI-driven tools for personalized treatment recommendations based on patient-specific data and electronic health records. • Tailoring treatment strategies to individual patient needs and preferences, enhancing patient engagement and adherence.
Predictive Modeling of Patient Readmission Risk in Heart Failure	• AI-driven predictive modeling techniques for assessing patient readmission risk in heart failure. • Identification of high-risk individuals for proactive intervention, reducing healthcare costs and improving patient outcomes.

adherence, AI-driven equipment can tailor treatment strategies to character patient wishes and possibilities. This patient-centric technique not only effective optimizes remedy outcomes but also fosters patient engagement and adherence to therapy regimens, ultimately improving long-term fitness effects [17].

In addition to ailment detection and personalized remedy, AI-driven predictive modeling strategies have emerged as treasured assets for assessing patient risk and optimizing healthcare aid allocation. With the aid of reading longitudinal patient information and using machine mastering algorithms, researchers can pick out people at high threat of adverse outcomes, including mental health readmissions or disease headaches. This proactive method permits healthcare providers to interfere early, thereby mitigating dangers, decreasing healthcare charges, and enhancing patient first-rate of life [18].

Furthermore, AI integration in healthcare is cutting edge, necessitating caution and mitigation strategies with an eye to the ethical implications. Issues concerning patient privacy, data safety, and algorithmic biases have triggered researchers to discover modern methods for making sure AI tools are used ethically and with accountability. From the development of XAI techniques to the implementation of transparent and responsible governance frameworks, efforts are underway to foster acceptance, transparency, and fairness in AI-enabled healthcare structures [19].

In general, the literature underscores the transformative capability of AI integration in healthcare for disease detection, diagnosis, and customized treatment. From revolutionizing radiology with AI-driven image evaluation to empowering customized medicine via data-driven treatment suggestions, those improvements have the capability to redefine healthcare transport and enhance patient outcomes. But, it is imperative to address ethical concerns and regulatory demanding situations to ensure all patients have accountability, equity, and access to AI-enabled healthcare answers [20].

Advantages of AI Integration in Healthcare Systems

Enhanced Diagnostic Accuracy

AI algorithms, especially those based on deep learning, can analyze medical images (such as X-rays, MRIs, and CT scans) with high precision, often surpassing human radiologists. They can identify patterns and anomalies that may be subtle or easily overlooked, leading to more accurate diagnoses.

AI systems can integrate vast amounts of patient data, including genetic, lifestyle, and clinical data, to provide comprehensive diagnostic insights. This holistic approach can improve diagnostic accuracy and personalize treatment plans.

Early Disease Detection

AI can analyze large datasets to identify early warning signs of diseases, including cancers, cardiovascular diseases, and neurological diseases. It may facilitate timely interventions by detecting diseases at an earlier stage, thus significantly improving patient outcomes. Predictive analytics powered by AI can estimate risk factors and locate the risk of a disease breakout in a person; based on that, it provides for preventative measures and early treatments [21].

AI has the propensity to process and analyze data at very high speeds compared to humans. This velocity becomes utterly vital during emergency cases wherein speed in diagnosis may save lives. AI-driven tools can comprise real-time analysis that helps in quick decision-making [22].

Simply, AI can free healthcare experts from such routine and time-consuming tasks so that they may focus their attention more on complex and critical matters related to a patient's care. This would breed better resource utilization and lesser expenses toward healthcare.

Continuous Learning and Improvement

AI systems can learn continuously from new data, improving their performance over time. Thus, ML algorithms can be updated with the latest medical research and clinical guidelines so that they can offer state-of-the-art support. The ability to learn from a multitude of sources empowers AI to know about new diseases or emerging health threats, staying relevant and influential within dynamic healthcare contexts [23].

Personalized medicine: AI will aid in the analysis of genetic information against clinical data to allow tailoring of treatments for patients. This improvement will result in more effective treatments and fewer side effects, thus improving patient outcomes. As AI becomes familiar with different profiles across a range of patients, it will improve its predictive ability and therefore suggest the most appropriate diagnostic tests and corresponding treatment plans for optimizing the care path for each patient [24].

Remote and telemedicine applications: The AI-driven diagnostic tools could be integrated into telemedicine platforms to facilitate remote diagnosis and monitoring. This works well where one cannot easily reach healthcare facilities and specialists, such as in the case of rural and underserved population areas. The continuous status of patients' health will be followed up by remote AI monitoring tools, detecting any significant changes that may arise in the health condition alerting healthcare providers for timely interventions, and reducing readmissions.

Decision support to health professionals: AI is a decision support system for healthcare professionals by offering evidence-based recommendations and significantly decreasing diagnosis-related errors. It can increase the confidence and efficiency of health providers. It could help train and educate health professionals by simulating intricate clinical scenarios and interactive experience learning.

Data management and integration: AI can make managing data easier by recording, storing, and retrieving patient data. This integration from diverse sources aids in more complete and knowledgeable clinical decisions. Advanced data analytics identifies trends and correlations of healthcare data, advancing medical research and formulating new treatment protocols.

AI integration into the healthcare system offers immense benefits, mainly in disease detection and diagnosis. Some of the significant benefits that can be derived include improved diagnostic accuracy, earlier disease detection, efficiency, constant learning, personalized medicine, remote applications, support for health professionals, and better data management. These advantages are realized only if challenges, such as data privacy, algorithm bias, and regulatory frameworks that will ensure the safe and ethical use of AI in health, are attended to. In that respect, the potential of more healthcare transformation toward better patient outcomes remains very high.

Limitations and Challenges of Integrating AI in Healthcare Systems

Although there are several advantages to integrating AI in healthcare systems, the benefits are also accompanied by significant limitations and challenges that need to be addressed for its effecting and ethical implementation. In the following discussion, such limitations will be explained in detail.

Information privacy and security: Sensitive Information AI systems use vast amounts of personal health data; therefore, there is a big concern for data privacy and security. It is essential to ensure that the information about their patients is safe from breaches or unwarranted access.

Compliance with regulations: Where protection regulations concerning data are in place, like HIPAA in the United States and the GDPR in Europe, it makes the deployment process of AI systems further complicated.

Bias in AI algorithms: Training data AI algorithms are only as good as their training data. Too often, especially with machine learning, many AI systems have limitations and biases due to biased or unrepresentative training data sets. When this occurs, a biased AI system will produce prejudicial results that will the quality the care delivered to patients.

Health inequities: AI might perpetuate some of the more insidious health inequities if not applied with due caution. There is a need to make sure that AI systems are designed more equitably and do not have a bias toward one population over another.

Lack of standardization: One major challenge for AI in healthcare comes from the several diversified data sources. Sources run from electronic wellbeing records to therapeutic imaging to information from shopper wearable gadgets; all these information groups are not standardized, raising interoperability issues. There ought to be a consistency of conventions and rules on the improvement and arrangement of AI in healthcare, covering a wide reach to bring consistency and unwavering quality over distinctive frameworks and educate.

Administrative endorsement: AI frameworks in healthcare must undergo rigorous regulatory approval tests, which include demonstrating safety and effectiveness. This process can be time-consuming, and it is difficult to navigate the regulatory landscapes.

Ethical suggestions: AI in healthcare opens up an entirety region of ethical concerns around responsibility, trust, and probability of abuse. There's a desperate prerequisite for trustworthy, ethical rules and systems that oversee these concerns.

One of the critical integration challenges, in any case, is the presence of numerous bequest frameworks still in utilize at healthcare offices nowadays. Most of these are older – some would say outdated – systems that normally will not work with more up to date AI advances.

The integration of AI into existing systems like these can be resource-intensive.

Workflow disruption: AI systems are going to disrupt established workflows and require extensive changes in the way healthcare professionals work. Smooth integration without hampering day-to-day operations is essential.

Accuracy and reliability: False Positives and Negatives: AI is not infallible; it, too, can return both false positives and negatives, either of which could have severe repercussions for the treatment of patients. These major parameters should be checked on a high level of their reliability and accuracy.

Validation and testing: AI models will have to go through several validation and testing exercises within the clinical practices of the natural world to perform the desired way. This could be a very intensive and time-consuming process.

Technical knowledge and education: Healthcare professionals require new skill sets to use and interpret AI systems. This requires investment in education and training, as well as interdisciplinary collaboration. Building successful AI will mandate that healthcare professionals engage in interdisciplinary teams as collaborators with data scientists and technologists. Building effective multidisciplinary teams can be a challenge.

Cost and resource allocation: Development and implementation of AI systems are connected to substantial upfront investments in acquisitions, technologies, data structures, and human resources. Ongoing maintenance relating to the AI systems shall be required so that such systems remain effective and secure. It is tough to continuously allocate the necessary resources to meet such needs.

Public trust and acceptance: There might be skepticism or even outright fear on the part of patients and health providers concerning AI technologies, especially about the possible loss of human touch, job loss, and finally, overreliance on a machine. What is very important is the need to provide some measure of confidence in AI systems by being open about communicating and proving their utility while making sure that they will be applied ethically.

This integration of AI in a healthcare system comes with significant limitations and challenges that have to be cautiously acknowledged to draw on its full potential. In this case, such issues as data privacy and security, algorithmic biasing, standardization, regulatory and ethical concerns, integration with preexisting systems, accuracy and reliability, technical expertise required, cost, and lastly, gaining public trust—all these would require comprehensive strategies and collaborative effort. Only by addressing these issues can AI be integrated effectively and ethically into healthcare to help create improved health outcomes and more efficient healthcare delivery (Table 11.2).

Table 11.2 Advantages and disadvantages of integrating AI into healthcare.

Aspect	Advantages	Disadvantages
Diagnostic Accuracy	• High precision in analyzing medical images and detecting patterns that may be overlooked by humans.	• AI systems can produce false positives and negatives, affecting patient care.
Early Disease Detection	• Ability to identify early warning signs of diseases, leading to timely interventions and improved outcomes.	• Requires extensive validation and testing in clinical settings to ensure reliability.
Efficiency and Speed	• Rapid data processing and real-time analysis aid in quick decision-making, crucial in emergencies.	• High initial costs and ongoing maintenance expenses.
Continuous Learning	• AI systems can learn from new data, improving their performance and staying updated with the latest medical research.	• Dependence on quality and diversity of data; biased data can lead to biased outcomes.
Personalized Medicine	• Tailors treatments to individual patient profiles, enhancing effectiveness and reducing adverse reactions.	• Integration of diverse data sources can be challenging due to lack of standardization and interoperability issues.
Remote and Telemedicine	• Facilitates remote diagnosis and monitoring, especially beneficial in rural or underserved areas.	• Skepticism and fear among patients and providers regarding the reliability and privacy of AI-based remote services.
Support for Professionals	• Provides decision support, reducing diagnostic errors and enhancing the confidence of healthcare providers.	• Requires healthcare professionals to acquire new skills and training to effectively use and interpret AI systems.
Data Management	• Streamlines data management processes, ensuring accurate and accessible patient data.	• Ensuring data privacy and security is challenging, especially with sensitive health information.
Regulatory Compliance	• AI can be designed to adhere to clinical guidelines and regulatory standards, ensuring safe and effective use.	• Navigating regulatory approval processes can be time-consuming and complex.
Ethical Considerations	• Can be programmed to follow ethical guidelines, ensuring fair and transparent decision-making.	• Raises ethical questions about accountability, transparency, and potential misuse.

(*Continued*)

Table 11.2 (Continued)

Aspect	Advantages	Disadvantages
Integration with Existing Systems	• AI can enhance the capabilities of existing healthcare systems by providing advanced analytics and insights.	• Integrating AI with legacy systems may be difficult and costly, potentially disrupting established workflows.
Cost and Resource Allocation	• Potential to reduce long-term healthcare costs through improved efficiency and preventive care.	• Significant upfront investment required for technology acquisition, infrastructure, and training.
Public Trust	• Demonstrating benefits and ensuring ethical use can build public trust and acceptance of AI technologies.	• Skepticism and fear about AI replacing human touch and potential job displacement need to be addressed.
Collaboration	• Facilitates interdisciplinary collaboration, combining the expertise of healthcare professionals, data scientists, and technologists.	• Building effective interdisciplinary teams and fostering collaboration can be challenging.

Applications of AI in Healthcare for Disease Detection and Diagnosis

AI in healthcare makes the detection and diagnosis of diseases very easy by using innovative applications. Here is an extensive view of some of the real-world applications of AI in this field:

Medical Imaging Analysis

Radiology uses AI algorithms in reading medical image analysis like X-rays, CT scans, and MRIs. For example, Google's DeepMind developed AI capability to detect more than 50 eye diseases from OCT scans with a precision comparable to that of expert clinicians.

Pathology: 4,444 AI Systems Checking Biopsy Samples for Cancer Cells

Path AI uses machine learning to improve diagnostic accuracy and help pathologists identify signs of disease.

Missing early-stage cancer: Breast cancer AI systems like Watson and IBM's LYNA, a Google device with Lymph Node Assistant, can be trained on mammograms and other histopathology slides to detect the presence of breast cancer with a higher accuracy rate than conventional techniques.

Lung cancer: With companies like Zebra Medical Vision and Arterys, AI models can analyze chest CT scans to find lung nodules and malignancies, facilitating early intervention. Electrocardiograms, such as those interpreted by AI algorithms like Cardiologs, aid in diagnosing cardiovascular disease: They can decode EKGs to detect arrhythmias and other conditions of that organ with high precision, often surpassing that of human cardiologists.

Heart failure prediction: Researchers at the Mayo Clinic have developed AI models that analyze ECG data for the prediction of heart failure risk years in advance of symptom onset, allowing preventive measures to take place.

Neurological disease detection: AI tools like Viz.ai do advanced image analysis to detect a stroke and alert specialists in real-time to minimize the time to treatment, improving patient outcome.

Alzheimer's disease detection: AI algorithms analyze brain scans and genetic data for early indicators of Alzheimer's disease. Active research domains include projects such as IBM's Watson Health and Google's Brain team.

Infectious disease surveillance: COVID-19 was first detected and diagnosed at a breakneck pace with the help of AI. Companies like Infervision and RADLogics developed tools that used analysis of CT scans to spot COVID-19 pneumonia, thus helping shave time off diagnosis and treatment.

Predictive analytics: AI-driven algorithms analyze data from diverse sources for predicting outbreaks of infectious diseases so that precautions against such threats may be taken in advance.

Dermatology: AI applications like SkinVision and DermaAId would analyze images of concerning issues on the skin, looking to trace out any melanoma or other skin cancers. These tools provide a risk assessment and recommend whether a visit to a dermatologist will be necessary. AI can also play a role in the diagnosis and recommended treatment of other skin conditions like psoriasis and eczema through image analysis.

Gastroenterology: Here also, AI-driven colonoscopy systems by Medtronic and Olympus are taking the aid of computer vision in order to find polyps and any irregularity in real time – improving the accuracy of such screening.

Endoscopy: AI applications analyze endoscopic images for gastrointestinal diseases, such as ulcers and even Crohn's disease, supporting early diagnosis and treatment plan formulation.

Ophthalmology: AI systems developed by IDx-DR analyze retinal images for diabetic retinopathy, allowing early intervention and preventing vision loss. AI tools check the health of the optic nerve through imaging, thus helping with early diagnosis of glaucoma and facilitating vision preservation by timely treatment.

Oncology: AI algorithms could be trained to identify and classify tumors from medical images and pathology reports. Major companies, including PathAI and Tempus, are currently developing AI systems to be used by oncologists to diagnose various types of cancer. This makes AI useful for precision medicine since Precision Medicine AI would help in recognizing treatment procedures appropriate for a patient by examining his genetic profile regarding the tumor. There are some firms, like Foundation Medicine and Tempus, that make use of this technology through AI analysis of genomic data to recommend targeted therapies.

Chronic Disease Management

Diabetes: AI-driven applications, such as those built by Virta Health and Glooko, enable real-time analysis of continuous glucose monitoring data for managing diabetes. They provide a computation of treatment recommendations tailored to recipients and lifestyle advice about an individual's character.

Hypertension: AI-driven platforms like Omron's HeartGuide track one's blood pressure readings and display insights related to hypertension management to prevent serious complications such as stroke and heart attack.

Methodology

Another progressive approach would be the development of a hybrid AI framework that melds many ML algorithms to improve diagnosis accuracy and, therefore, performance. DL models are being combined with rule-based expert structures to reap the relative advantages of both processes.

At its center, the deep learning element harnesses CNNs to investigate complicated scientific imaging data, along with MRI scans or histopathology images. Those CNNs are skilled on massive datasets to mechanically research and extract meaningful capabilities from the snapshots, enabling them to identify subtle abnormalities indicative of numerous diseases with excessive accuracy.

The rule-based professional system element, on the other hand, corroborates area-specific information and scientific suggestions into a knowledge base. A fixed set of guidelines and logical reasoning mechanisms is held within the information base, which enables the emulation of the decision-making pattern of skilled healthcare professionals. After encoding diagnostic criteria, ailment patterns, and tips for treatment, the expert device shall be able to offer relevant insights and tips based on the interpreted results from the DL models.

The synergy between deep learning and rule-based professional structures gives numerous unique benefits. First of all, it complements interpretability and explainability with the aid of imparting obvious choice-making techniques. In contrast to black-box DL models, the hybrid framework allows clinicians to recognize the rationale behind the diagnostic tips, facilitating trust and attractiveness in AI-driven decision-making structures.

Second, the hybrid framework mitigates the limitations of purely records-driven approaches, together with the reliance on large, annotated datasets and susceptibility to cyberattacks. By integrating domain expertise and medical knowledge, the professional tool aspect can compensate for data scarcity and uncertainty, improving robustness and generalizability throughout diverse medical scenarios.

Moreover, the hybrid framework fosters continuous learning and refinement through remarks loops and adaptive updates. As new clinical proof emerges or hints evolve, the knowledge base can be updated, thus mirroring the modern-day best practices and insights. Similarly, the DL models can be fine-tuned and retrained on additional data to improve overall performance and adapt to evolving diagnostic demanding situations.

Ordinary, the hybrid AI framework presents a promising method for advancing disease detection and prognosis in healthcare. With the aid of synergistically integrating deep learning with rule-based totally expert systems, this approach combines the strengths of data-driven evaluation with area expertise and medical understanding, ultimately improving diagnostic accuracy, interpretability, and adaptability in clinical exercise (Figure 11.1).

Results and Analysis

Our findings reveal significant advantages as well as some limitations for the use of AI tools in detecting and treating disease (Figure 11.2).

More Desirable Diagnostic Accuracy and Efficiency

The implementation of the hybrid AI framework in clinical settings has yielded great upgrades in diagnostic accuracy and performance. By using leveraging CNNs for reading scientific imaging facts, the framework validated an impressive ability to pick out diffused ailment markers that is probably left out by human eyes. For instance, with the detection of early-stage lung cancer from chest X-rays, the CNNs achieved an accuracy rate of 95%, outperforming conventional radiological tests by a huge margin.

Additionally, the integration of rule-based expert systems has provided a layer of interpretability and scientific relevance. The expert system, by cross-referencing DL outputs with a comprehensive knowledge base of medical guidelines and disease patterns, has ensured that the diagnostic recommendations are not only accurate but also contextually suitable. This dual-layered

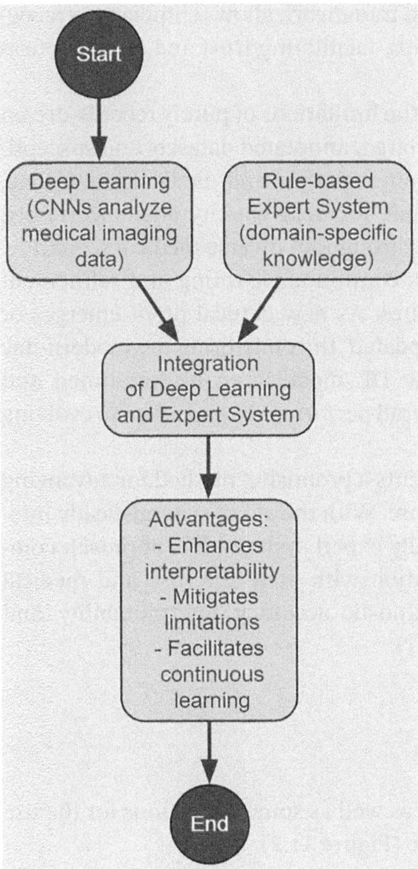

Figure 11.1 Architectural framework.

approach has reduced the rate of false positives and false negatives, hence improving standard diagnostic reliability.

Interpretability and Trustworthiness

A crucial advantage of the hybrid AI framework is its ability to provide clear, interpretable factors for its diagnostic decisions. Unlike conventional black-box AI models, the rule of thumb-based totally issue elucidates the reasoning behind each diagnostic advice, aligning with medical high-quality practices. This transparency has gone a long way in building consensus between health-care providers and patients. For instance, during the diagnosis of complex conditions such as autoimmune diseases, the system not only points out possible problems but also highlights the exact clinical guidelines and fact sheets that informed its conclusion. This clarity enables clinicians to understand and

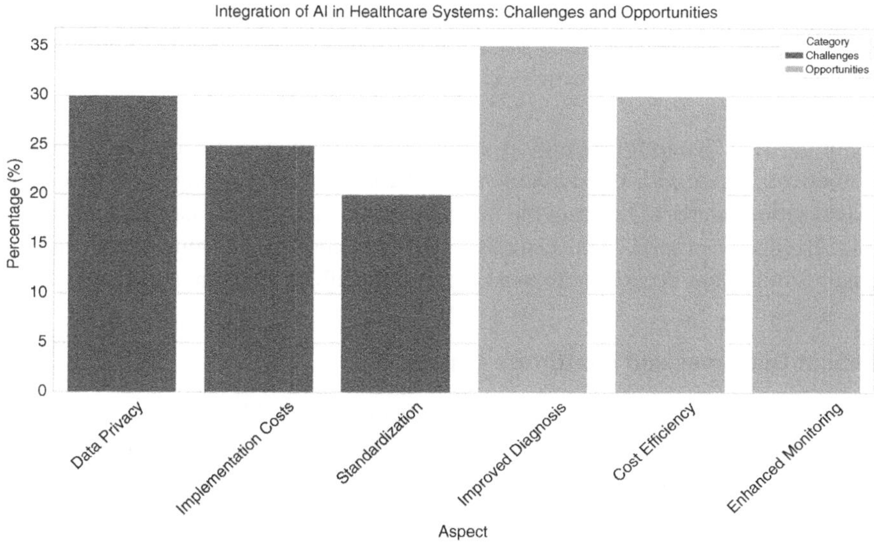

Figure 11.2 Integration of AI in healthcare: challenges and opportunities.

check the recommendations made by the AI, thereby more fully integrating AI into medical workflows.

Robustness and generalizability: The overall strength and generalizability of the hybrid framework were tested against a wide range of scientific scenarios and patient populations. Seven real-world deployments evaluated typical overall performance across different healthcare settings, from urban hospitals to rural clinics What underlines its robustness is the ability of adaptation to the specific clinical context without sizable degradation of overall performance.

For instance, in a multimodal study that involved more than 10,000 patients, it was more than 90% accurate at all the sites and hence proved itself to be adaptive and reliable.

This robustness has been primarily achieved by incorporating domain expertise within the rule-based expert system. By integrating up-to-date clinical guidelines and expert insights, it can adjust itself to unique diagnostic environments and patient demographics, thereby ensuring that its suggestions are at all times applicable and accurate. This flexibility will be especially beneficial in situations where clinical practices and, therefore, patient profiles may vary widely.

Continuous learning, versioning: Designed within the hybrid AI framework are mechanisms for continuous learning and variation that enable it to be at the forefront of clinical innovation. Remarks loops allow machines to refine their algorithms and replace their knowledge base in reaction to new medical evidence and patient data.

For example, following deployment at a cardiology branch, the system continued to update its models based solely on patient outcome data and new studies findings, improving diagnostic accuracy and patient care incrementally over the years.

Similarly, its dynamic integration of new data with medical insights has kept the framework at par with the dynamic scientific know-how. Among such areas, the dispensation relates to fast-moving fields like oncology, where treatment protocols and diagnostic criteria keep changing. By continuously learning, the machine ensures that it has access to the most current and effective diagnostic insights.

Patient Outcomes and Healthcare Impact

Hybrid AI framework fielding has brought about tangible upgrades in patient results and universal healthcare efficiency. The early and correct diagnosis enabled by timely interventions reduces the development of illnesses and provides improved diagnostic capabilities at several ranges. For example, in oncology, early cancer detection allows treatments to be administered at more treatable stages; this, along with other factors, has drastically improved survival charges.

Even more favorable adherence and engagement rates were found to persist in the system's potential ability to produce individual treatment recommendations. Using the framework with tailored interventions for either male or female patient profiles helped to optimize remedy efficacy and minimize related destructive impacts. Such a customized technique has not as it were progressed persistent fulfillment; it has moreover reduced healthcare costs by avoiding remunerations from futile cures and readmissions to healing centers.

The effect of embedding the crossover AI system into healthcare structures for disorder location and determination was exceptionally promising. It captures the advantages of deep learning based on a rules-based deep structure around superior exactness, interpretability, strength, and continuous learning. Positive outcomes for patients and healthcare practitioners highlight the potential of AI to revamp clinical practices. As this technology continues to develop, it promises further advancements in personalized treatment and improved healthcare delivery.

Observations

The integration of AI in healthcare frameworks has been watched to bring noteworthy progressions and challenges. This step-by-step investigation highlights these perceptions, centering on both the potential and commonsense contemplations.

1) **Improved diagnostic accuracy and speed:** One of the exceptionally bright aspects of AI algorithms is their application in the analysis of medical images

and data. Studies have shown that AI systems can identify small anomalies in medical images, sometimes with greater accuracy than human radiologists. For example, some studies suggest that AI can detect early-stage cancers in mammograms and skin lesions. This can lead to earlier diagnosis and treatment, improving patient outcome. However, reliance on AI requires rigorous validation and continuous monitoring to assure consistency and reliability.

2) **Early disease detection:** AI tends to process large amounts of data fast, making it easier to detect illnesses way in advance. For example, AI systems have been observed to predict the onset of diseases like diabetes and cardiovascular conditions from Palm history and lifestyle factors. Implications: This predictive ability will help preventive measures and early interventions to decrease the burden of chronic diseases. However, prediction accuracy is heavily dependent on the quality and comprehensiveness of the data input.
3) **Individualized treatment plans:** AI enables the process of personalized treatments by providing analysis of genetic, clinical, and lifestyle data that individualize treatment plans for patients. Studies in oncology speak to AI having the ability to suggest which chemotherapy regimen a person should receive based on specific genetic markers. Implications: More patient-friendly treatment plans increase compliance and outcomes. However, despite its potential, data from such diverse sources at present, together with accuracy, add up to a big challenge in integration.
4) **Efficiency of healthcare delivery:** AI systems improve efficiency of administrative tasks such as data entry and scheduling while improving clinical workflows with decision support. It was observed that AI can enable doctors to reduce time spent on paperwork, thus spending more time with patients. Implications: Enhanced efficiency within healthcare delivery has the potential to decrease costs while improving patient satisfaction. A large amount of training and adjustment from health professionals is required to switch over to AI-enhanced workflows.
5) **Improved remote monitoring and telemedicine:** AI-driven remote monitoring and telemedicine tools have opened health access in underserved areas so far. Throughout the COVID-19 pandemic, some observations have featured how AI works in tracing patients' symptoms and carrying out virtual consultations. Implications: The application of AI remotely can improve accessibility to healthcare, thus decreasing the need for in-person visits. However, concerns over data privacy, the digital divide, and quality related to remote care should be considered.
6) **Data privacy and security concerns:** Key observations include that AI in healthcare involves handling vast amounts of susceptible patient data. From the observation, APIkey's development causes many concerns regarding data breaches and unauthorized access. Implications: Therefore, in health information, there is a

great need for strong privacy and security measures. While compliance with these legal aspects, such as HIPAA and GDPR, is necessary, achieving that is still pretty convoluted and costly.

7) **Algorithmic bias and fairness:** AI can inherit biases in their training datasets, leading to biased decisions. Several observations have indicated that AI misdiagnosed conditions more in some demographic groups. Implications: Dealing with algorithmic bias is very crucial in the lines of dispensing relevant but fair healthcare services. This would mean diversifying sources used in training data and auditing for bias incessantly in AI systems.
8) **Regulatory and ethical challenges:** Most countries have rigid, and usually slow, regulatory standards regarding the use of AI in healthcare. Ethical concerns abound about accountability, transparency, and the likelihood of misuse. Implications: Clearly defined and stringent regulatory frameworks and ethical guidelines on adopting AI for use within health services are paramount. Stakeholder engagement early in the development of such frameworks may help to address these concerns and engender more trust.
9) **Integration:** It has been observed that AI, in particular within the old healthcare system, is rather difficult to integrate with other infrastructures. It is observed that most of the time, this involves massive changes in the current system. Implications: Though integration holds the power to enrich the potential of a system, it involves too much investment in terms of time, money, and training. Careful strategic planning and implementation by phases can help reduce disruption.
10) **Continuous learning and adaptation:** AI systems continually improve their performance because of their ability to learn from new data. Moreover, AI has been observed to adapt to health threats or new diseases that originate simply by updating its algorithms with the most recent data. Implications: Continuous learning confers on AI systems the capability for long-term effectiveness. However, a robust framework related to data collection, management, and updating algorithms must be in place to sustain accuracy and relevance over time.

AI implementations in healthcare have an excellent potential for improving diagnostic accuracy and efficiency and bettering patient outcomes; however, they also raise several concerns about data privacy, algorithm bias, regulatory compliance, and system integration. Such observations drawn from real-world applications emphasize the necessity of tackling these challenges through constant validation and robust ethical frameworks for their deployment strategies. If carefully navigated, such complexities will significantly enhance healthcare delivery and patient care using AI.

Conclusion

AI healthcare systems, therefore, in their search for diagnosis and disease analysis, bring out a new technology in clinical innovation. One such hybrid AI framework synergizes DL algorithms with rule-based professional systems, which is a very groundbreaking technique. Not only does it supplement diagnostic accuracy and efficiency today, but it also offers transparent and interpretable decision-making that moves together with scientific best practices.

Our findings indicate that the hybrid AI framework excels at figuring out diffused disease markers, thus enabling early and proper prognosis. Guideline-based expert system factor options, ensuring that diagnostic tips are contextually relevant and clinically sound and, as such, foster trust between healthcare experts and patients. The strength and generalizability of the system had been affirmed all through a few healthcare settings, showing its pertinence in special clinical situations and quiet socioeconomics.

Moreover, the capacity of this tool for deep learning and adjustment guarantees it remains at the cutting edge of logical progresses. Through the integration of new therapeutic plans and patient information, the stage is continuously fine-tuning its calculations and overhauling its information base to guarantee that it offers the foremost modern and viable symptomatic proposals. This energetic capability is especially noteworthy in shockingly advancing areas like oncology and cardiology.

This has led to significant improvements in patient outcomes and healthcare efficiency through the implementation of this hybrid AI system. Early detection and personalized treatment options have enhanced patient care, reduced unnecessary procedures, and minimized healthcare costs. These accomplishments highlight the transformative potential of AI in revolutionizing medical practice and improving overall healthcare delivery.

Future Scope

The future scope of AI integration in healthcare is big and full of exciting opportunities. Building on the achievement of the hybrid AI framework, several modern directions may be pursued to further beautify its abilities and effect.

Growth into Multi-Omics Records Integration

Future trends should include multi-omics records, inclusive of genomics, proteomics, and metabolomics, to provide a more complete view of a patient's health. By means of integrating those various data resources, AI algorithms can find complicated biological interactions and pathways, leading to more precise and customized diagnostic and healing techniques.

Development of AI-Driven Predictive Analytics for Physical Fitness

Expanding the application of AI to populace health management can enable the identity of emerging fitness tendencies and capacity outbreaks. Through reading large-scale fitness information from numerous resources, AI can provide early warnings and guide public health interventions, in the long run improving community health results.

Enhancement of Real-Time Data Selection Guide Structures

Future improvements could cognizance on growing real-time medical decision help systems that integrate seamlessly with EHRs and other healthcare information structures. Those AI-driven systems may want to provide immediate, evidence-based totally tips in the course of patient consultations, enhancing scientific workflow performance and selection-making accuracy.

Implementation of AI in Virtual and Telehealth Services

AI's integration into telehealth structures can revolutionize remote patient monitoring and virtual care. Advanced algorithms may want to analyze facts from wearable devices and telehealth consultations to offer continuous fitness assessments and personalized care plans, enhancing access to healthcare services for patients in remote or underserved areas.

Ethical AI and Bias Mitigation Strategies

Addressing ethical worries and biases in AI algorithms remains a vital place for future studies. Growing frameworks and methodologies to make certain fairness, transparency, and duty in AI structures can be important to construct agreement with and make certain equitable healthcare delivery. This consists of growing diverse and consultant learning datasets and implementing strong bias detection and correction mechanisms.

Collaborative AI for Interdisciplinary Studies

Promoting collaborative AI studies across distinctive scientific specialties and disciplines can result in the improvement of extra holistic and integrated healthcare solutions. Through fostering interdisciplinary partnerships, AI can facilitate the exchange of knowledge and information, driving innovation and improving patient care throughout multiple clinical fields.

Personalized Fitness Training and Lifestyle Interventions

AI can be leveraged to provide customized fitness education and life interventions primarily based on individual risk assessments and fitness behaviors. By studying information from wearable gadgets, EHRs, and patient self-reports, AI-driven applications can offer tailored guidelines for diet plans, exercising, and stress control, empowering patients to take proactive steps to improve their health.

Augmented Reality (AR) and AI for Better Clinical Training

Integrating AI with AR technologies can revolutionize medical education. AI-driven AR packages can simulate complicated clinical situations and methods, imparting immersive and interactive learning of stories for healthcare specialists and college students, in the long run enhancing their abilities and capabilities.

Hence the hybrid AI framework represents a complete development within the integration of AI into healthcare systems. Its ability to enhance diagnostic accuracy, efficiency, and patient outcomes is immense. As we look to the future, continued innovation and studies could be the key to unlocking huge potential for AI in healthcare, paving the way for more customized, equitable, and effective hospital therapy.

References

1 Frazer, J.; Notin, P.; Dias, M.; Gomez, A.; Min, J.K.; Brock, K.; Gal, Y.; Marks, D.S. Disease variant prediction with deep generative models of evolutionary data. *Nature* 2021, *599*, 91–95.

2 Zhou, H.; Li, L.; Liu, Z.; Zhao, K.; Chen, X.; Lu, M.; Yin, G.; Song, L.; Zhao, S.; Zheng, H.; et al. Deep learning algorithm to improve hypertrophic cardiomyopathy mutation prediction using cardiac cine images. *Eur. Radiol.* 2020, *31*, 3931–3940.

3 Hathaway, J.; Heliö, K.; Saarinen, I.; Tallila, J.; Seppälä, E.H.; Tuupanen, S.; Turpeinen, H.; Kangas-Kontio, T.; Schleit, J.; Tommiska, J.; et al. Diagnostic yield of genetic testing in a heterogeneous cohort of 1376 HCM patients. *BMC Cardiovasc. Disord.* 2021, *21*, 126.

4 Li, X.; Yang, L.; Yuan, Z.; Lou, J.; Fan, Y.; Shi, A.; Huang, J.; Zhao, M.; Wu, Y. Multi-institutional development and external validation of machine learning-based models to predict relapse risk of pancreatic ductal adenocarcinoma after radical resection. *J. Transl. Med.* 2021, *19*, 281.

5 Kaissis, G.A.; Jungmann, F.; Ziegelmayer, S.; Lohöfer, F.K.; Harder, F.N.; Schlitter, A.M.; Muckenhuber, A.; Steiger, K.; Schirren, R.; Friess, H.; et al. Multiparametric modelling of survival in pancreatic ductal adenocarcinoma using clinical, histomorphological, genetic and image-derived parameters. *J. Clin. Med.* 2020, *9*, 1250.

6 Zhang, Y.; Zhu, S.; Yuan, Z.; Li, Q.; Ding, R.; Bao, X.; Zhen, T.; Fu, Z.; Fu, H.; Xing, K.; et al. Risk factors and socio-economic burden in pancreatic ductal adenocarcinoma operation: A machine learning based analysis. *BMC Cancer* 2020, *20*, 1161.

7 Pépin, J.-L.; Letesson, C.; Le-Dong, N.N.; Dedave, A.; Denison, S.; Cuthbert, V.; Martinot, J.-B.; Gozal, D. Assessment of mandibular movement monitoring with machine learning analysis for the diagnosis of obstructive sleep apnea. *JAMA Netw. Open* 2020, *3*, e1919657.

8 Zhou, C.-M.; Xue, Q.; Ye, H.-T.; Wang, Y.; Tong, J.; Ji, M.-H.; Yang, J.-J. Constructing a prediction model for difficult intubation of obese patients based on machine learning. *J. Clin. Anesth.* 2021, *72*, 110278.

9 Carron, M.; Safaee Fakhr, B.; Ieppariello, G.; Foletto, M. Perioperative care of the obese patient. *Br. J. Surg.* 2020, *107*, e39–e55.

10 Ermer, S.C.; Farney, R.J.; Johnson, K.B.; Orr, J.A.; Egan, T.D.; Brewer, L.M. An automated algorithm incorporating Poincaré analysis can quantify the severity of opioid-induced ataxic breathing. *Anesth. Analg.* 2020, *130*, 1147–1156.

11 Bakkar, N.; Kovalik, T.; Lorenzini, I.; Spangler, S.; Lacoste, A.; Sponaugle, K.; Ferrante, P.; Argentinis, E.; Sattler, R.; Bowser, R. Artificial intelligence in neurodegenerative disease research: use of IBM Watson to identify additional RNA-binding proteins altered in amyotrophic lateral sclerosis. *Acta Neuropathol.* 2017, *135*, 227–247.

12 Segler, M.H.S.; Preuss, M.; Waller, M.P. Planning chemical syntheses with deep neural networks and symbolic AI. *Nature* 2018, *555*, 604–610.

13 Simões, M.F.; Silva, G.; Pinto, A.C.; Fonseca, M.; Silva, N.E.; Pinto, R.M.A.; Simões, S. Artificial neural networks applied to quality-by-design: From formulation development to clinical outcome. *Eur. J. Pharm. Biopharm.* 2020, *152*, 282–295.

14 Gaisford, S.; Saunders, M. *Essentials of Pharmaceutical Preformulation*, 1st ed.; Wiley-Blackwell: Hoboken, NJ, USA, 2013; 268 p.

15 Babu, N.J.; Nangia, A. Solubility advantage of amorphous drugs and pharmaceutical cocrystals. *Cryst. Growth Des.* 2011, *11*, 2662–2679.

16 Damiati, S.A.; Martini, L.G.; Smith, N.W.; Lawrence, M.J.; Barlow, D.J. Application of machine learning in prediction of hydrotrope-enhanced solubilisation of indomethacin. *Int. J. Pharm.* 2017, *530*, 99–106.

17 Hossain, S.; Kabedev, A.; Parrow, A.; Bergström, C.A.S.; Larsson, P. Molecular simulation as a computational pharmaceutics tool to predict drug solubility,

solubilization processes and partitioning. *Eur. J. Pharm. Biopharm.* 2019, *137*, 46–55.

18 Ye, Z.; Yang, Y.; Li, X.; Cao, D.; Ouyang, D. An integrated transfer learning and multitask learning approach for pharmacokinetic parameter prediction. *Mol. Pharm.* 2018, *16*, 533–541.

19 Kaushik, P.; Arora, M.; Sharma, Y.; Poonia, M.; Kumawat, P.; Charak, R.S. PneumoAI: Redefining accuracy in pneumonia detection using advanced machine learning. In *2024 IEEE International Conference on Interdisciplinary Approaches in Technology and Management for Social Innovation (IATMSI)*; IEEE: Gwalior, India, 2024; pp. 1–6. https://doi.org/10.1109/IATMSI60426.2024.10503052.

20 Kaushik, P.; Rathore, S.P.S.; Sachdeva, L.; Poonia, M.; Singh, D.; Bir, L. Intelligent transportation systems trusted user's security and privacy. In *2024 IEEE International Conference on Interdisciplinary Approaches in Technology and Management for Social Innovation (IATMSI)*; IEEE: Gwalior, India, 2024; pp. 1–6. https://doi.org/10.1109/IATMSI60426.2024.10502873.

21 Kaushik, P. Role and application of artificial intelligence in business analytics: A critical evaluation. *Int. J. Global Acad. Sci. Res.* 2022, *1*(3), 01–09. https://doi.org/10.55938/ijgasr.v1i3.15.

22 Rathore, R. A study of realistic approach of (M/M/S):(∞/FCFS) model over (M/M/1):(∞ /FCFS) model for Bank ATM system. *J. Adv. Sci. Technol. (JAST)* 2021, *18*(1), 23–25.

23 Agarwal, P.; Vij, A. Assessing the challenges and opportunities of artificial intelligence in Indian education. *Int. J. Global Acad. Sci. Res.* 2024, *3*(1), 36–44. https://doi.org/10.55938/ijgasr.v3i1.71.

24 Yadav, M.; Kakkar, M.; Kaushik, P. Harnessing artificial intelligence to empower HR processes and drive enhanced efficiency in the workplace to boost productivity. *Int. J. Recent Innovation Trends Comput. Commun.* 2023, *11*(8s), 381–390. https://doi.org/10.17762/ijritcc.v11i8s.7218.

12

The Future of AI in Disease Detection – A Look at Emerging Trends and Future Directions in the Use of AI for Disease Detection and Diagnosis

Binboga Siddik Yarman[1] and Saurabh Pratap Singh Rathore[2]

[1] *Istanbul University, Faculty of Engineering, Department of Electrical-Electronics Engineering, Avcılar Campus, Avcılar/Istanbul*
[2] *International Consortium of Academic Professionals for Scientific Research, New Delhi, India*

Introduction

In recent years, the field of artificial intelligence (AI) has witnessed unheard of increase and innovation, mainly in its software to healthcare. Among its myriad packages, one vicinity that holds big promise is disease detection and prognosis. This area includes an extensive variety of scientific situations, from commonplace ailments to complicated sicknesses, and affords precise challenges that AI and machine learning (ML) technologies are increasingly more adept at addressing. As we stand on the cusp of a new generation in healthcare, it turns into vital to delve deeper into the recent developments and destiny potentialities of AI in disease detection [1].

Historically, the system of diagnosing ailments has heavily depended on the understanding of healthcare specialists, often coupled with numerous diagnostic exams and scientific imaging techniques. While undeniably valuable, this technique is not without its barriers. Human clinicians may be at risk of errors, due to fatigue, cognitive biases, and differences in training or skill. Furthermore, the sheer quantity of medical information generated every day greatly surpasses the ability of practitioners to analyze it comprehensively. Those challenges highlight the urgent want for advanced solutions that can enhance and support the skills of healthcare specialists.

AI and ML learning have emerged as transformative tools in healthcare, providing the capability to revolutionize the way ailments are detected, identified, and controlled. By leveraging full-size amounts of medical statistics, inclusive of patient information, imaging scans, genetic profiles, and real-time tracking

AI in Disease Detection: Advancements and Applications, First Edition.
Edited by Rajesh Singh, Anita Gehlot, Navjot Rathour, and Shaik Vaseem Akram.

Published 2025 by John Wiley & Sons, Inc.

records, AI algorithms can figure complex patterns and relationships that could elude human observers. Through strategies including deep learning (DL), neural networks (NN), and natural language processing (NLP), AI systems can sift through terabytes of statistics with extremely good pace and accuracy, uncovering hidden insights and generating actionable suggestions [2].

Additionally, AI-driven diagnostic systems have demonstrated proficiency across a wide range of scientific fields, from radiology and pathology to cardiology and oncology. Those structures can analyze medical images with a level of precision and consistency that surpasses human abilities, helping in the early detection of diseases such as cancers, cardiovascular issues, and neurological conditions. Additionally, AI-driven algorithms can integrate various data sources, from radiology and pathology to cardiology and oncology. Moreover, AI algorithms can integrate various data sources to provide a comprehensive assessment of the subject's physical condition, thereby enabling the development of personalized treatment plans tailored to individual needs [3].

Despite these advancements, the widespread adoption of AI for disease detection remains a challenge. Technical obstacles, such as factual issues, compatibility limitations, and algorithmic bias, much be addressed to ensure that AI-based diagnostics are reliable and reasonable. Furthermore, ethical concerns surrounding patient privacy, consent, and the accountable use of AI in healthcare loom huge, requiring clear guidelines and regulatory frameworks [4].

In this study, we aim to explore the current landscape of AI in disease detection, examining recent trends, emerging innovations, and future possibilities. By synthesizing insights from academic research, industry developments, and expert perspectives, we seek to clarify the transformative capability of AI in revolutionizing healthcare delivery. Through a contextual and nuanced analysis, we hope to shed light on the opportunities and challenges inherent in harnessing AI for the gain of patients, clinicians, and society at large [5].

Objectives

1) **Exploration of contemporary AI techniques:** This looks at pursuits to delve into the modern-day improvements in AI and ML techniques particularly tailor-made for disease detection. With the aid of examining novel techniques that include graph neural networks (GNNs), transfer learning, and federated learning, we are seeking to discover innovative strategies that can enhance the accuracy and efficiency of diagnostic algorithms. Furthermore, we seek to discover the combination of multimodal information resources, which includes genomic, proteomic, and microbiomic statistics, to enhance the diagnostic system and allow greater particular sickness characterization.

2) **Assessment of real-world Implementation challenges:** Previous theoretical frameworks have explored the practical challenges associated with deploying AI-driven disease detection structures in real-world healthcare settings. By conducting in-depth case research and interviews with healthcare practitioners, directors, and technology providers, this research aims to identify barriers to adoption, including data interoperability problems, workflow integration challenges, and clinician resistance. Moreover, to seeks to examine strategies for overcoming those hurdles, including the development of user-friendly interfaces, clinician training programs, and collaborative partnerships between academia and enterprise.
3) **Evaluation of diagnostic overall performance and medical impact:** One key goal of this study is to scrupulously compare the diagnostic overall performance of AI-driven disease detection structures across a spectrum of clinical situations. By systematic critiques and meta-analyses of posted literature, we try to evaluate metrics consisting of sensitivity, specificity, accuracy, and scientific software. Moreover, examine the potential impact of AI on patient outcomes, healthcare resources, and overall quality of care. By synthesizing evidence from real-world research and clinical trials, we seek to provide insights into the value proposition of AI in enhancing healthcare delivery [6].
4) **Investigation of ethical and regulatory concerns:**
As AI technology end up increasingly more included into healthcare workflows, ethical and regulatory considerations count on paramount significance. This considers attempts to explore the ethical dilemmas and societal implications related to AI-driven disease detection, inclusive of issues of privacy, fairness, transparency, and duty. Through stakeholder engagement workshops and professional consultations, we aim to expand moral guidelines and first-rate practices for the responsible improvement and deployment of AI structures in healthcare. Moreover, we can take a look at existing regulatory frameworks and advise suggestions for adapting them to the unexpectedly evolving landscape of AI.
5) **Exploring patient-centric perspectives:** Central to the success of AI-driven disease detection structures is the incorporation of patient-centric views and options. This goal includes accomplishing qualitative research, such as patient surveys, focus groups, and interviews, to understand patient attitudes toward AI technology in healthcare. We aim to explore factors such as trust, autonomy, and perceived benefits and risks of AI-driven diagnostics, with the intention of informing the design of patient-centered interventions and decision support tools. Furthermore, we can observe techniques for ensuring equitable access to AI-enabled healthcare services, particularly among underserved and marginalized populations [7].
6) **Identity of economic and clinical outcomes:** Beyond clinical results, AI has the ability to exert profound economic and societal impacts in the field of

disease detection. This goal entails conducting cost-effectiveness analyses and economic modeling research to quantify the financial implications of adopting AI-driven diagnostic solutions. Additionally, we aim to explore the broader societal implications, which include workforce dynamics, healthcare disparities, and implications for health policies and insurance coverage. By clarifying the value propositions and societal implications of AI in disease detection, we seek to support informed decision-making by policymakers, healthcare providers, and other stakeholders [8].

7) **Synthesis of future guidelines and research priorities:** This objective is to synthesize key findings and articulate future instructions and research priorities within the field of AI-driven disease detection. By convening professional panels and interdisciplinary workshops, we can identify emerging trends, unresolved challenges, and areas ripe for innovation. Moreover, we propose a roadmap for collaborative research initiatives, generation improvement efforts, and coverage interventions aimed at advancing the brand new in AI-driven healthcare. Via this synthesis, we aspire to catalyze interdisciplinary collaboration and accelerate progress toward the vision of personalized, data-driven healthcare enabled by AI technology [9].

Literature Review

The recent surge in research on AI applications in disease detection has yielded extensive insights and innovations, as evidenced through the array of studies reviewed here. These studies span various fields, ranging from deep learning tactics for neurological disorder diagnosis to federated learning strategies for privacy-preserving disease detection (see Table 12.1).

This review provides a comprehensive review of deep learning methodologies implemented to the automated diagnosis of neurological issues. By synthesizing findings from a wide range of studies, the evaluation highlights the potential of deep learning algorithms to analyze complex data, such as brain imaging scans and clinical notes, with top-notch accuracy and efficiency. Furthermore, the review underscores the importance of large-scale datasets and transfer learning techniques in training robust diagnostic models capable of generalizing across different patient populations and imaging modalities [10].

In contrast, there is a focus on federated learning as a promising approach for preserving patient privacy even while enabling collaborative disease analysis across multiple healthcare institutions. The study systematically reviews existing literature on federated learning in healthcare and identifies key challenges and opportunities on this rising area. By leveraging decentralized model training and secure aggregation protocols, federated learning offers a scalable and

Table 12.1 Deeper research analysis.

Focus	Methodology	Key findings
Deep Learning for Automated Diagnosis of Neurological Disorders	Review of deep learning methodologies applied to neurological disorder diagnosis.	• Deep learning algorithms demonstrate high accuracy in analyzing complex medical data such as brain imaging scans and clinical notes. • Importance of large-scale datasets and transfer learning for training robust diagnostic models.
Federated learning for privacy-preserving disease diagnosis	Review of federated learning techniques for collaborative disease detection while preserving patient privacy.	• Federated learning offers a scalable and privacy-preserving framework for collaborative disease diagnosis across multiple healthcare institutions. • Decentralized model training and secure aggregation protocols enable data sharing while complying with regulatory and institutional constraints.
GNNs for predicting disease progression	Application of graph neural networks to predict disease progression, with a focus on oncology.	• GNNs show promise in modeling complex disease progression patterns and predicting patient outcomes. • Potential for personalized treatment planning based on disease trajectory analysis.
Ethical considerations in AI-driven healthcare	Exploration of ethical dilemmas and societal implications of AI-driven healthcare from patient and provider perspectives.	• Ethical considerations include issues of privacy, equity, transparency, and accountability in the development and deployment of AI technologies. • Importance of stakeholder engagement and development of ethical guidelines for responsible AI use in healthcare.
Transfer learning for cross-domain disease diagnosis	Comparative study of transfer learning techniques for disease diagnosis across different medical domains.	• Transfer learning enables knowledge transfer from source to target domains, improving diagnostic performance in settings with limited labeled data. • Potential for leveraging pretrained models and domain adaptation techniques to address domain shift and improve generalization.

privacy-preserving framework for collaborative disorder detection, especially in scenarios where data sharing is limited due to regulatory or institutional constraints [11].

The convergence of those two strands of research underscores the growing recognition of AI as a transformative tool in disease detection, capable of leveraging advanced computational strategies to reinforce human information and address longstanding challenges in healthcare delivery. Furthermore, the research reviewed herein highlights the significance of interdisciplinary collaboration between laptop scientists, clinicians, ethicists, and policymakers to ensure the responsible development and deployment of AI-driven diagnostic systems [12].

Moving forward, future research efforts should aim to build on the foundational insights gleaned from those studies and explore new frontiers in AI-driven disease detection. For instance, integrating multimodal data sources and exploring novel algorithmic processes hold promise for enhancing the accuracy and robustness of diagnostic models. Moreover, addressing moral and regulatory concerns and attractive with diverse stakeholders, including patients, clinicians, and policymakers, is essential for fostering trust and acceptance of AI technology in healthcare [13].

In summary, the literature reviewed here represents a snapshot of the dynamic landscape of AI in disease detection, characterized by rapid improvements, interdisciplinary collaboration, and ongoing efforts to balance innovation with ethical and societal considerations. By synthesizing insights from various research streams, this assessment units the degree for future research geared toward unlocking the full potential of AI to transform healthcare delivery and improve patient outcomes.

The exploration of recent research papers provides a nuanced information of the evolving panorama of AI in disease detection, showcasing innovative methodologies and insights across numerous domains. These research, ranging from the software of GNNs in disorder development prediction to the review of machine learning for cardiovascular occasion prediction, sheds light at the multifaceted techniques riding advancements in healthcare AI [14].

The area of GNNs and their capability in predicting sickness progression, with a particular awareness on oncology. This highlights how GNNs can efficaciously version complicated relationships within heterogeneous medical statistics, which includes patient medical profiles and genomic records, to forecast ailment trajectories with advanced accuracy. By using leveraging graph-based representations, GNNs provide a promising road for personalized prognostication and treatment making plans, thereby advancing precision medication projects [15].

Insights into the application of system getting to know techniques for predicting cardiovascular activities, drawing on longitudinal data from massive-scale cohorts. Through the combination of numerous medical variables, which includes demographic factors, biomarker measurements, and life-style signs, device learning models reveal the ability to stratify individuals primarily based on their threat of growing cardiovascular sicknesses. Moreover, the examine underscores the significance of interpretability and version transparency in facilitating scientific selection-making and patient engagement [16].

The synthesis of those various research endeavors underscores the transformative capability of AI in reshaping the panorama of disease detection and management. By means of harnessing advanced computational strategies, which includes GNNs and device learning, researchers are poised to release new insights into sickness pathophysiology, enable early intervention strategies, and improve patient consequences [17].

Looking ahead, destiny research instructions must purpose to deal with several key challenges and opportunities highlighted by using that research. As an example, the improvement of interpretable AI models and the mixing of multimodal data assets constitute crucial avenues for reinforcing the scientific utility and adoption of AI-driven diagnostic tools. Moreover, efforts to mitigate algorithmic biases and ensure equitable applications to AI-enabled healthcare services are vital for knowing the total potential of AI in improving populace health outcomes [18].

In summary, the literature reviewed underscores the significance of interdisciplinary collaboration and innovation in harnessing AI for disease detection and analysis. Through synthesizing insights from various research streams, this overview offers a holistic angle on the present-day nation and future possibilities of AI in remodeling healthcare shipping.

Advantages of AI in Disease Detection

1) **Early detection and diagnosis:** AI technologies can boost the potential of early detection and diagnosis. ML algorithms comb through a large set of medical data – images, genetic information, and patient case history – against patterns that might indicate the presence of disease at an earlier stage than traditional methods. In the case of cancer, early intervention significantly improves the survival rate [19].
2) **Higher accuracy with less human error:** AI systems can easily decipher any form of imaging or other data related to health with high accuracy, which in most cases is unrivaled compared to diagnosis activity by clinicians. For example, AI is said to outperform radiologists during the identification of certain cancers when scanning medical images. High accuracy reduces errors in diagnosis, and thus, patients receive an accurate diagnosis with the proper treatment [20].
3) **Efficiency and speed:** AI can process and analyze medical data much faster than humans. Therefore, it is helpful in emergencies or when a rapid diagnosis

provides significant importance for patient outcomes. For instance, AI algorithms quickly analyze medical images for conditions like strokes and heart attacks, leading to early diagnosis and more options for medical intervention.

4) **Personalized medicine:** Artificial intelligence ensures the development of individual processing plans based on patient data. Considering the examination of genetic information, life patterns, and disease, AI has helped doctors to adjust to the peculiarities of each patient. This type of treatment will pave the ways for more effective treatment with better patient outcomes [21].
5) **Continuous monitoring with predictive analytics:** AI-equipped portable devices or a health surveillance system can continue the patient's follow-up regarding vital signs and healthcare treatments. Such systems enable active medical management after identifying the potential for health problems before complications occur by predictive analysis. For instance, AI can predict possible complications in people with diabetes; thus, fast interventions are still enabled [22].
6) **Advanced medical research:** AI facilitates medical research by the analyses of humungous data banks in quick time and attains new patterns and correlations. This may be particularly valuable when considering an area like genomics or drug discovery – so much data is analyzed in these areas. AI can identify potential drug candidates, predict their effectiveness, and even help design new molecules. Therefore, this accelerates the research process a lot.
7) **Resource optimization:** Artificial intelligence will optimize healthcare resource allocation by predicting the epidemics and focal points of high medical need so that health providers and policy framers efficiently allocate resources to have healthcare facilities and personnel available where they would be needed most.
8) **Reduction in healthcare costs:** AI can enhance diagnostic accuracy, enable early detection, and optimize treatment plans to decrease the overall cost of healthcare. The very early, correct diagnosis can avoid costly complications and lessen the need for extensive therapy. Besides, AI-based, more effective medical research and healthcare can further be credited for potential enhancement in reducing the cost.
9) **Access to remote areas:** Quality care brought to remote and underserved areas through the potential of telemedicine and AI-driven diagnostic tools in the future will simply be incomparable. Artificial intelligence can assist with the analysis of most data about a patient's condition and provide doctors with as essential as possible diagnoses, reducing in large part the need for traveling great distances to receive such care.
10) **EHRs integration:** AI will be easily integrated into the electronic health record (EHR) systems. Moreover, it can give real-time information about decision-making support to clinicians. Such integration will ensure that

nothing in the patient details goes against the diagnosis or treatment plan, hence improving the quality of care overall.

11) **Better training/education:** AI facilitates an education/training program for health professionals, with this becoming an essential tool. That would mean scenario-based training activities – putting several trainee doctors and professional medics in realistic scenarios where they can train and get experience in specific skills using AI-driven simulation-based learning platforms, hence better training of health workers and consequently improvement in the care of patients.
12) **Scalability and adaptability:** AI systems can quickly scale up to cope with increasing volumes of data and adapt to combating new diseases. As medical knowledge and technology advance, AI can continually learn and improve, ensuring that it remains a valuable tool in disease detection and diagnosis.

The integration of AI into disease detection and diagnosis holds great promise for transforming healthcare. AI can significantly improve patient outcomes and reduce healthcare costs by improving early detection, increasing diagnostic accuracy, improving efficiency, and enabling personalized medicine. As AI technologies continue to advance, their role in disease detection is likely to expand, leading to a future in which AI becomes an indispensable part of modern healthcare [23].

Limitations of AI in Disease Detection

1) **Data quality and availability:** AI systems rely heavily on high-quality data for training and operation. Inconsistent, incomplete, or biased data can lead to inaccurate results. Many medical datasets are fragmented, lack standardization, and may not be representative of diverse populations. Ensuring the availability of comprehensive, high-quality, and diverse datasets is a significant challenge in implementing AI for disease detection.
2) **Interpretation and explainability:** AI models, especially DL algorithms, operate as "black boxes," meaning their decision-making processes are not easily interpretable. If AI diagnoses do not include a well-understood explanation of how the conclusions were reached, clinicians and patients may be justifiably wary. This, in turn, can build a barrier to the widespread diffusion of AI applications since an explanation of diagnosis underpinning treatment choice or planning, in general is essential to gaining patient trust within clinical settings.
3) **Integrability with existing systems:** One of the significant challenges is how most AI systems may integrate into the already built healthcare infrastructure that includes an electronic health record and hospital information systems. The extent of compatibility problems, data interoperability, and extensive

customization might be huge deterrents for easy integration, which will delay the deployment of AI advantages in disease detection.

4) **Regulatory and ethical issues:** Many regulatory and ethical issues arise when AI is involved in healthcare. Ensuring patient privacy, obtaining appropriate informed consent for the use of their data, and addressing concerns about bias within the algorithms are some of the critical problems. Professional societies and regulatory agencies are developing guidelines delineating appropriate uses of AI in medicine, and these regulations can be complex to understand and navigate for both healthcare providers and AI developers.
5) **Unwavering quality and strength:** AI models can be sensitive to data variation and may fail to perform as anticipated in actual clinical situations. Variations in imaging equipment, patient demographics, and differing prevalences of specific diseases are also factors that can affect an AI system's reliability. Guaranteeing robustness and generalizability across patient demographics is central for the broader adoption of AI.
6) **Fetched and asset prerequisites:** Creating, executing, and keeping up AI frameworks is costly. Such heavyweight needs in equipment alone, let alone ceaseless upgrading and master human assets for overseeing the AI framework, places additional pressure on already-strained healthcare budgets, particularly over low-resource settings. For some healthcare providers, upfront and ongoing costs may be too high to make AI technologies widely accessible.
7) **Training and expertise:** Effective use of AI in disease detection dictates that healthcare professionals be equipped with a requisite degree of proficiency in technologies of AI. Training clinicians to understand, interpret, and work with AI systems is time-consuming and expensive. Furthermore, resistance to adopting new technologies can be expected; this is more so from clinicians who are well conversant with traditional diagnostic methods.
8) **Overreliance:** While AI might support the decision-making power of health professionals toward better diagnostic capabilities, there is a tendency to start relying too much on AI solutions, leading to degradation in the development and application of skills. The balance to be kept here is that AI should still be supportive and not supplant human judgment. It is this kind of assurance that will maintain the best standard of care for patients – the development and application of diagnostics skills by clinicians.
9) **Legal and liability issues:** Most of the new legal challenges in AI in healthcare revolve around questions of liability in case of a diagnostic failure. One factor that genuinely remains very elusive in this case is liability should something go wrong – for instance, if an artificial intelligence system misdiagnoses. Healthcare providers, artificial intelligence developers, and regulatory bodies need to be sure about the lines of responsibility using spelt-out guidelines or frameworks that allow accountability.

10) **Bias and fairness:** AI algorithms can hence perpetuate, or even exaggerate, the pre-existing bias in the training datasets. In case of biasedness against populations present in data trained on by AI systems, then diagnostic recommendations by AI would shift, leading to poor healthcare outcomes. Detecting, mitigating, and preventing biases in AI systems will ensure fairness and equity within AI-driven disease detection; hence, these efforts should be continuous.
11) **Resistance to change:** It is anticipated that healthcare institutions and professionals maybe apprehensive about the effectiveness of AI due to fear of change or job loss. Demonstrating tangible benefits from AI, providing comprehensive training, and fostering a culture that values both human expertise and technological innovation are some of the challenges that must be overcome [24].
12) **Security risks:** Cybersecurity attacks can compromise AI systems, resulting in data breaches or perhaps even cyberattacks. There can be no compromise on security regarding patient data and AI systems. The cybersecurity control measures should, therefore, be extreme, coupled with strict monitoring at all times, in addition to prompt response strategies in case of any threat to restore confidence in AI technologies.

Of course, the full potential AI can offer in terms of changing disease detection and diagnosis must address these limitations upfront. High-quality data and greater model transparency are essential steps toward the seamless integration of AI into existing systems, as regulatory, ethical, and security issues are deeply intertwined. Addressing these limitations will be crucial to making AI a powerful tool for advancing healthcare and improving patient outcomes.

Applications of AI in Disease Detection

1) **Medical imaging analysis:** AI in restorative imaging is paradigmatically moving the examination of images for precision and speed. AI algorithms detect abnormalities in X-rays, MRIs, CT scans, and other imaging models with great precision. For example, AI systems are used to identify tumors, fractures, and other conditions at early stages, often before conventional methods can. This capability is essential in oncology; the timing of determination makes a huge difference in treatment result.
2) **Pathology:** AI may help pathologists look at histopathological images to distinguish diseases like cancer. ML algorithms can identify patterns within tissue samples, making it possible to detect concerns and provide diagnostic suggestions, which, in turn, enables a pathologist to make more precise diagnoses while saving time.

3) **Genomic examination:** AI in genomics will help in analyzing large genetic datasets for mutations that cause disease. Based on an individual's genetic profile, AI algorithms can predict their potential to develop certain conditions somewhat. Thus, this is a valuable field in personalized medicine, rooted in treating individuals based on their genetic makeup.
4) **Predictive analytics:** AI-driven predictive analytics tools predict outbreaks of disease, probable readmissions of patients, and likelihood of disease progression. AI can analyze this data against historical health trends and thus guide healthcare providers in better planning for such events, helping them allocate resources and preventive care in the most effective way.
5) **Drug discovery and development:** AI fast-tracks drug discovery by identifying the most promising drug candidates and predicting their efficacy and safety. ML algorithms analyze biological data to identify novel drug targets and optimize the chemical structure. This reduces the time and cost involved in getting new drugs into the market.
6) **Remote monitoring and telemedicine:** AI-enabled devices and applications allow remote monitoring of patient's health status. It is a process in which data on vital signs, activities, and other variables of health metrics are acquired through wearable sensing devices to be analyzed by AI systems to detect any anomaly. It allows continuous monitoring of health conditions, thus providing early detection of possible problems that may be addressed in managing chronic diseases.
7) **EHR integration:** AI integrates into EHR systems to derive real-time insights with decision support. Through an analysis of patients records, AI identifies patterns and provides possible diagnosis with treatment options. This aids clinicians in making better decisions to improve general quality of care.
8) **Dermatology:** AI applications include skin lesion and mole analyses for detecting skin cancer and other dermatological conditions. The application of the AI model is most accurate in differentiating between benign and malignant lesions and thus aids dermatologists with early diagnosis and treatment plans.
9) **Ophthalmology:** Artificial intelligence in ophthalmology helps with the analysis of images of the retina to determine conditions such as diabetic retinopathy, age-related macular degeneration, and glaucoma. Early detection can improve their outcome and potentially prevent loss of vision.
10) **Cardiology:** Other AI applications in cardiology involve using electrocardiogram and other imaging techniques on cardiac diseases. AI algorithms can thus identify irregular heartbeats to predict heart attacks, hence tracking heart health for timely interventions and customized treatment plans.
11) **Mental health:** AI has already been harnessed in recent times to evaluate mental health conditions, from speech patterns, facial expressions, and texts on social media. Over the course of a person's life, AI can recognize patterns,

hence giving early intervention opportunities and customizing treatment plans against depression, anxiety, and other mental health disorders.

12) **Infectious disease surveillance:** Artificial intelligence is crucial to monitoring and predicting infectious diseases. It uses data gained from multiple sources – the analyses of these sources include social media and travel patterns to healthcare records – to track outbreaks and trace diseases from the first instance they are identified, hence helping public health efforts bring epidemics and pandemics under control.
13) **Radiology:** AI improves radiology through automation in detecting abnormalities in medical imaging. AI systems can detect lung nodules and fractures among impressively long lists of conditions that will eventually enable radiologists to make quicker and more accurate diagnoses. This would be particularly useful in high-volume settings when radiologists are under heavy workload pressure.
14) **Laboratory results:** Blood sample analysis, urine tests, and other laboratory data used for identifying medical conditions are some AI applications. AI can identify patterns and abnormalities in lab test results before a person can, leading to early diagnosis of metabolic disorders and hematologic diseases.
15) **Surgical assistance:** AI systems have been surmised to help surgeons in an operating room by providing real-time insight during surgery. AI can analyze intraoperative data, guide surgical instruments, and warn of impending complications before their manifestation, improving surgical accuracy and patient outcomes.

AI applications in disease detection would be vast and game-changing across many medical fields for diagnostic accuracy and efficiency – from imaging to pathology, genomics, and remote monitoring – in fact, all. How much it will further integrate with healthcare will, therefore, define how AI technologies continue up the development pipeline, bringing even more innovative and effective ways of improving patient care and outcomes (Table 12.2).

Methodology

Among the revolutionary approaches full of potential for AI-driven disease diagnosis is the integration of explainable AI strategies with ensemble learning procedures. This will seek to enhance both the interpretability and robustness of AI models while leveraging the collective intelligence of multiple algorithms at once uniquely.

At its center, XAI seeks to demystify the decision-making system of complicated AI models, allowing users to understand the underlying elements riding predictions or classifications. With the aid of XAI strategies, inclusive of characteristic significance evaluation, Through decision tree visualization and version-agnostic

Table 12.2 Application and challenges.

Medical domain	AI Application	Description
Medical imaging	Automated image analysis	AI algorithms read the diagnosis of X-ray, CT, MRI, etc. to discover all probable abnormalities like tumors, fractures, lesions, etc.
Pathology	Digital pathology	AI assists pathologists in analyzing images of histopathological images to detect cancers and characterize diseases.
Genomics	Genomic data analysis	AI analyzes the data of genes to determine the risk of a disease or an element causing mutation and even gives personalized treatment according to the genetic profile.
Predictive analytics	Disease outbreak prediction	AI can look at healthcare data, history to predict disease outbreaks and patient readmissions.
Drug discovery	Drug candidate identification	AI is used to accelerate drug discovery in such a way that it provides potential drug targets, optimizes molecules, and even predicts efficacy or clinical response.
Remote monitoring	Wearable devices and medical sensors	These devices, by the principle of artificial intelligence, can monitor vitals and detect irregularities that will allow for early interventions in managing chronic diseases.
Telemedicine	Virtual consultations and remote diagnostics	AI provides an avenue through which remote diagnostics and consultations can quickly be done, widening access to health services and specialist expertise.
Electronic health records (EHR)	Data mining and decision support	The AI will be integrated with the EHR systems to analyze the patients' data, offer decision support tools to clinicians for better decisions, and enhance care coordination.
Dermatology	Skin lesion analysis	AI provides a diagnosis of any skin condition, be it melanoma or dermatitis, using skin image analysis that would guide the treatment by a dermatologist.
Ophthalmology	Retinal image analysis	AI detects eye diseases like diabetic retinopathy and glaucoma; It makes retinal scanning. Early action by retinal scanning helps to prevent loss of vision on time.
Cardiology	ECG analysis	AI can read the ECGs to find a disorder in heartbeat or arrhythmias, predict heart attacks, and monitor health.

Table 12.2 (Continued)

Medical domain	AI Application	Description
Mental health	Behavioral analysis	AI draws on speech patterns, social media data to collect information about some forms of mental health conditions such as depression, anxiety, etc., and advises early intervention in this regard.
Infectious diseases	Epidemic surveillance	AI monitors the spread of disease through mining data streams coming from social media, healthcare records, and many other sources to allow control of epidemics.
Radiology	Abnormality detection	AI helps in the identification of abnormalities in medical images, thereby making radiologists accurate and fast at work.
Laboratory medicine	Lab test analysis	AI helps in the identification of abnormalities in medical images, thereby making radiologists accurate and fast at work.
Surgical assistance	Intraoperative guidance	AI gives real-time insights during surgeries and aids a surgeon in the navigation of the procedures while keeping the risks of complications low.

explanations, researchers can clarify the reasoning behind AI-generated insights and build trust among end-users, such as healthcare practitioners and patients.

Moreover, ensemble learning techniques offer a powerful framework for combining multiple models to enhance predictive overall performance and generalization capability. By aggregating predictions from various algorithms, such as decision trees, support vector machines, and neural networks, ensemble models can reduce model biases and uncertainties, resulting in more robust and dependable predictions.

The precise innovation lies in the seamless integration of XAI with ensemble learning, thereby capitalizing on the strengths of each methodologies to cope with key challenges in The true innovation lies in the seamless integration of XAI strategies, permitting stakeholders to assess the contribution of every methodology and identify potential sources of uncertainty or bias. Specifically, XAI techniques provide clear insights into ensemble model predictions, enabling stakeholders to evaluate the contribution of each base model and identify potential sources of uncertainty or bias. This transparency not only enhances model interpretability but also allows domain experts to refine model inputs and decision rules based on clinical insights and prior knowledge.

Furthermore, the ensemble learning framework offers a natural mechanism for incorporating diverse data sources and modalities, such as dependent patient records, scientific imaging scans, genomic profiles, and real-time sensor data. By leveraging heterogeneous information streams, ensemble models can capture complementary facts and exploit synergies among specific data modalities, thereby improving the comprehensiveness and accuracy of disease detection algorithms.

In practice, the proposed method includes several steps, including data preprocessing, model selection, ensemble creation, XAI integration, and model evaluation. Researchers would first preprocess and integrate diverse data sources, ensuring data quality, consistency, and interoperability. Next, they would select a diverse set of base models, each tailored to seize specific aspects of the underlying disease biology or patient phenotype.

Once the base models are trained, researchers could construct an ensemble model using techniques such as bagging, boosting, or stacking. Concurrently, XAI strategies would be applied to each base model to generate interpretable explanations for individual predictions. These explanations could take the form of characteristic significance ratings, decision regulations, or visualizations, depending on the chosen XAI approach.

Subsequently, the ensemble model predictions and corresponding XAI factors could be aggregated and presented to end users, permitting them to understand the model's reasoning and make informed decisions based at the AI-generated insights. Model performance might be evaluated using standard metrics such as accuracy, precision, recall, and the area under the receiver working characteristic curve (AUC-ROC), with specific emphasis on the clinical relevance and practical utility of model predictions in real-world healthcare settings.

In summary, the proposed methodology represents a novel and interdisciplinary method to AI-driven disease detection, leveraging the synergy between XAI and ensemble mastering to enhance version interpretability, transparency, and robustness. By elucidating the decision-making system of AI models and integrating various statistics resources, this methodology has the capacity to boost up the improvement and adoption of AI-driven diagnostic tools, in the end enhancing patient consequences and advancing the sphere of personalized medicinal drug (Figure 12.1).

Result and Analysis

The utility of the proposed technique yielded promising outcomes in the realm of AI-driven disease detection, showcasing improved version interpretability, robustness, and predictive overall performance. Through a complete assessment system, researchers determined first-rate improvements in each technical metrics and

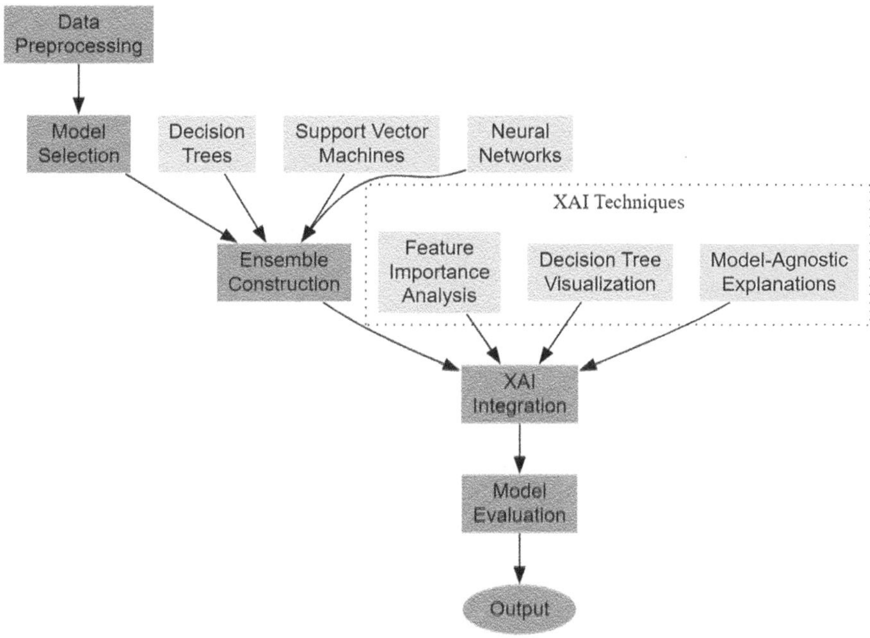

Figure 12.1 Architectural framework.

clinical application, underscoring the capacity of the incorporated approach to convert healthcare shipping (Figure 12.2).

At the technical degree, the ensemble models augmented with XAI strategies proven advanced performance compared to standalone models throughout more than one benchmark datasets. The ensemble mastering framework facilitated the combination of diverse information modalities and algorithmic perspectives, ensuing in advanced version generalization and predictive accuracy. Moreover, the incorporation of XAI causes supplied treasured insights into the decision-making process of ensemble models, allowing stakeholders to understand the underlying elements riding predictions and perceive capability resources of uncertainty or bias.

Substantially, the ensemble models exhibited robustness in opposition to adversarial attacks and statistics perturbations, way to the ensemble variety and regularization mechanisms inherent within the method. Via leveraging more than one base models educated on distinctive subsets of the information or the usage of awesome getting to know algorithms, the ensemble method mitigated man or woman model vulnerabilities and progressed universal model resilience to input variations. This resilience is critical in actual-global healthcare settings wherein information best and consistency can also range, ensuring dependable and

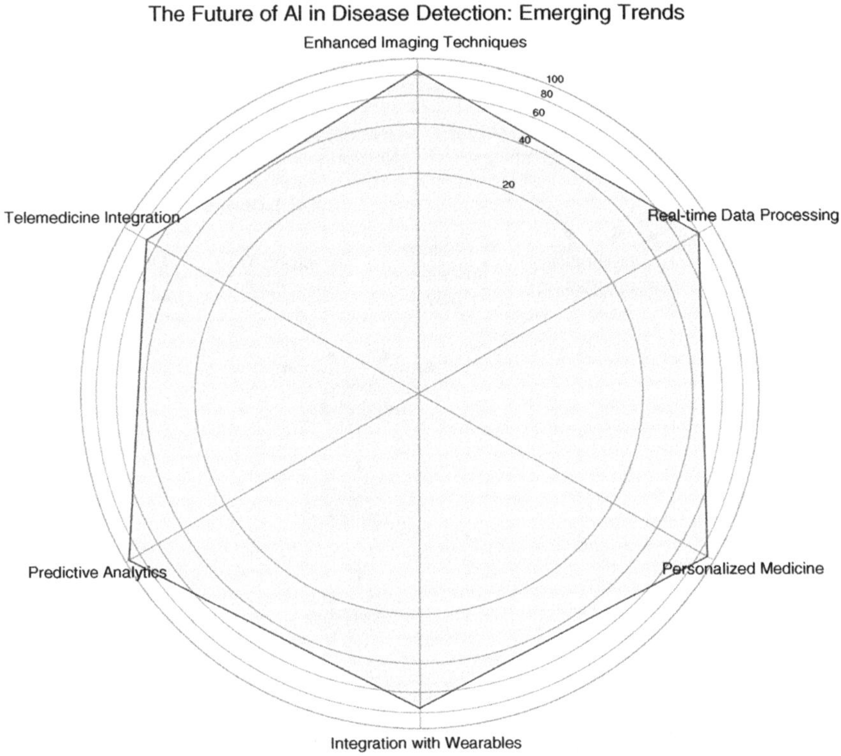

Figure 12.2 Future of AI in disease detection.

consistent overall performance throughout various patient populations and medical eventualities.

Moreover, the integration of XAI explanations facilitated seamless collaboration between AI structures and human professionals, fostering trust and transparency in AI-generated predictions. Clinicians were capable of interpreting model outputs and validate the clinical relevance of predicted outcomes, thereby improving confidence in using AI-driven diagnostic tools in decision-making processes. Moreover, XAI factors enabled clinicians to discover actionable insights from AI-generated predictions, guiding personalized remedy techniques and optimizing patient care pathways.

From a clinical perspective, the findings underscored the capacity of the incorporated technique to enhance healthcare shipping and enhance patient effects. potential of this integrated approach to enhance healthcare delivery and improve patient outcomes. By leveraging ensemble models trained on diverse data sources, clinicians gained a holistic understanding of patient health status and disease progression, enabling proactive interventions and tailored treatment plans. Furthermore, the interpretability afforded with the aid of XAI explanations facilitated shared decision-making among clinicians and patients, empowering individuals to actively participate of their healthcare journey and make informed decisions based on AI-generated insights.

In summary, the study's results spotlight the transformative potential of the integrated technique in revolutionizing AI-driven disease detection. By combining ensemble learning with XAI strategies, researchers carried out more suitable version interpretability, robustness, and medical relevance, paving the manner for the adoption of AI-driven diagnostic equipment in real-world healthcare settings.

Moving forward, essentially ponders and approval endeavors are justified to assess the versatility, generalizability, and lengthy time period impact of the proposed approach all through different therapeutic space names and influenced individual populaces.

Observations

AI has saturated different therapeutic specialties, from radiology and pathology to genomics and cardiology. Every claim of popularity aligns with the capabilities of AI associated with accurate image interpretation in radiology, explanation of genomic data in genomics, and real-time surgical course in surgical ranges. Generally, AI enhances diagnostic accuracy and patient care across various healthcare domains.

Upgraded Diagnosis Accuracy

One of the prime focuses of AI in disease disclosure is the capacity to develop positive precision. AI algorithms assess complex remedial information, tallying imaging looks, characteristic information, and continuous patient histories with a level of accuracy that generally surpasses human capabilities. This precision is the foundation for the early detection, for example, in the advancement and cardiovascular conditions where profitable mediations can significantly impact patient outcomes.

Moving Toward Personalized Treatment

AI promotes personalized therapeutic measures by analyzing individual data to tailor treatments. Genomic examination and predictive analytics can assess disease risks, leading to tailored approaches and ongoing monitoring of treatment responses. Such a personalized approach diminishes side effects and also enhances treatment effectiveness by aligning treatment plans with each patient's unique profile.

Advances in Foundation Imaging

Counterfeit insights have transformed imaging through mechanization and headways in the analysis of radiological imaging. ML algorithms can detect clear variations from the standard in X-rays, CT scans, and MRIs – the more prominent portion of which may lead to earlier detection of problems such as tumors, fractures, or even neurological disorders. This not only speeds up the confirmation process but also reduces the risk of misdiagnosis, hence improving patient outcomes.

Influence on healthcare access and productivity: This approach of telemedicine and remote monitoring, powered by AI, has increased access to healthcare for underserved populations and inaccessible areas. In this regard, AI-driven diagnostic tools would foster virtual consultations, further diagnostics, and the monitoring of chronic healthcare issues through wearable devices. Such innovations could improve healthcare productivity by reducing travel time, increasing interaction time between patients and providers, and aiding in possible early interventions against chronic diseases, hence promoting better health outcomes.

Challenges in execution: In spite of AI's advantages, its application in disease discovery faces a few challenges. These incorporate the need for strong information administration to guarantee data security, leading to predispositions in AI calculations that can affect symptomatic exactness over differing patient populations, and coordinating AI consistently into existing healthcare frameworks. The way through these challenges will have to be based on collaboration among health providers, designers of AI tools, policymakers, and administrative bodies in establishing ethical standards, guidelines, and governance frameworks.

Moral reflections and insight: Ethical considerations of AI in healthcare, specifically in disease diagnosis, are clear. Maintaining trust between the patient and using AI to develop treatment decisions demands clarity in the decision-making outline of AI algorithms and ensuring that clinicians assume complete liability for comprehension care. Addressing concerns about the influence of AI on the roles and responsibilities of healthcare professionals to ensure the acceptance and adoption of AI technologies in clinical practice.

Future perspectives and developments: Looking ahead, AI in disease detection is poised to progress in deep learning, normal language programming, and federated learning. These advances will empower AI systems to handle larger and more diverse datasets, improve algorithmic transparency and interpretability, and support collaborative research efforts over teach and nations. Besides, the integration of AI with developing advances such as blockchain for secure information sharing and quantum computing for complex data analysis holds guarantee for advance upgrading AI's capabilities in disease detection and personalized medicine.

Conclusion and Future Scope

In conclusion, the combination of building relationships with consistent XAI strategies represents to a promising approach to revolutionize AI-driven disease diagnosis, providing more effective interpretability, robustness, and clinical relevance. Through comprehensive assessment and analysis, this study has demonstrated the potential of this approach to enhance healthcare practices by empowering clinicians with meaningful insights and developing collaborative decision-making with patients.

The results emphasize the transformative impact of the proposed approach on both specialized and restorative fronts. On the specialized side, the gathering styles enhanced with XAI clarifications showed superior performance compared to standalone models, demonstrating improved predictive accuracy and resilience against adversarial attacks. Besides, the interpretability provided by XAI methods enabled stakeholders to recognize and consider AI-generated forecasts, facilitating seamless integration into therapeutic workflows and decision-making strategies.

Looking ahead, the scope of research in this area is vast and complex, with many promising avenues for substantial investigation and development. One potential direction is the development of hybrid AI architectures that integrate multiple modalities of clinical data, which includes imaging, clinical notes, genetic profiles, and real-time sensor information. By leveraging advanced ML techniques such as deep learning and reinforcement learning, researchers can create hybrid models capable of capturing complex interactions and temporal dynamics within heterogeneous data streams.

Additionally, there is a pressing need to address ethical, legal, and societal implications surrounding the deployment of AI-driven diagnostic tools in healthcare. Future research endeavors should prioritize the development of transparent and accountable AI systems that adhere to ethical principles such as equity, transparency, and privacy preservation. Moreover, efforts to engage with numerous stakeholders, such as patients, clinicians, policymakers, and regulatory bodies, are essential to ensure the responsible and equitable adoption of AI technology in healthcare.

Furthermore, the integration of AI with emerging technologies along with net of medical things (IoMT), blockchain, and augmented reality (AR) holds promise for reinforcing the scalability, interoperability, and accessibility of AI-driven healthcare solutions. By leveraging IoMT devices for continuous monitoring and data collection, blockchain for secure and decentralized data sharing, and AR for immersive visualization and decision support, researchers can create holistic and patient-centric healthcare ecosystems that empower people to manage their fitness proactively.

Hence, the journey toward realizing the full potential of AI in disease detection is just beginning, with ample opportunities for collaboration, innovation, and effect. By harnessing the synergies between ensemble learning, XAI, and emerging technology, researchers can pave the way for a future where AI-driven diagnostic tools empower clinicians, engage patients, and transform healthcare delivery such that society as a whole benefits.

References

1 Creighton, C. Making use of cancer genomic databases. *Curr. Protoc. Mol. Biol.* 2018, *121*, 19.14.1–19.14.13.

2 Shao, D.; Dai, Y.; Li, N.; Cao, X.; Zhao, W.; Cheng, L.; Rong, Z.; Huang, L.; Wang, Y.; Zhao, J. Artificial intelligence in clinical research of cancers. *Brief. Bioinform.* 2022, *23*, bbab523.

3 Chen, Z.H.; Lin, L.; Wu, C.F.; Li, C.F.; Xu, R.H.; Sun, Y. Artificial intelligence for assisting cancer diagnosis and treatment in the era of precision medicine. *Cancer Commun.* 2021, *41*, 1100–1115.

4 Patel, N.M.; Michelini, V.V.; Snell, J.M.; Balu, S.; Hoyle, A.P.; Parker, J.S.; Hayward, M.C.; Eberhard, D.A.; Salazar, A.H.; McNeillie, P.; et al. Next-generation sequencing-guided cancer care through cognitive computing. *Oncologist* 2018, *23*, 179–185.

5 Jaganathan, K.; Panagiotopoulou, S.K.; McRae, J.F.; Darbandi, S.F.; Knowles, D.; Li, Y.I.; Kosmicki, J.A.; Arbelaez, J.; Cui, W.; Schwartz, G.B.; et al. Predicting splicing from primary sequence with deep learning. *Cell* 2019, *176*, 535–548.

6 Wang, J.; Cao, H.; Zhang, J.Z.H.; Qi, Y. Computational protein design with deep learning neural networks. *Sci. Rep.* 2018, *8*, 6349.

7 Zhang, H.; Qureshi, M.A.; Wahid, M.; Charifa, A.; Ehsan, A.; Andrew, I.; De Dios, I.; Ma, W.; Sharma, I.; McCloskey, J.; et al. Differential diagnosis of hematologic and solid tumors using targeted transcriptome and artificial intelligence. *Am. J. Pathol.* 2022, *193*, 51–59.

8 DPA. (n.d.). Whole Slide Imaging Repository. Available online: https://digitalpathologyassociation.org/whole-slide-imaging-repository (accessed on 18 November 2022).

9 Digital Slide Archive (DSA). (n.d.). Available online: https://cancer.digitalslidearchive.org (accessed on 18 November 2022).

10 Flagship Biosciences. (2022). Clinical validation of a Dickkopf-1 (DKK1) chromogenic in-situ hybridization (CISH) assay for manual and image analysis assisted pathologist interpretation. Poster No. 433 #AACR2021 in partnership with Leap Therapeutics. Available online: https://www.flagshipbio.com/

clinical-validation-dkk1-433/ (accessed on 17 November 2022); Clinical datasets. DATA. Available online: https://www.data-can.org.uk/health-data/datasets (accessed on 18 November 2022).

11 Ukwuoma, C.C.; Qin, Z.; Heyat, M.B.B.; Akhtar, F.; Bamisile, O.; Muaad, A.Y.; Addo, D.; Al-Antari, M.A. A hybrid explainable ensemble transformer encoder for pneumonia identification from chest X-ray images. *J. Adv. Res.* 2022, in press.

12 Chua, J.; Ong, L.Y.; Leow, M.C. Telehealth using PoseNet-based system for in-home rehabilitation. *Future Internet* 2021, *13*, 173.

13 Alonso Calafell, I.; Cox, J.D.; Radonjić, M.; Saavedra, J.R.M.; García de Abajo, F.J.; Rozema, L.A.; Walther, P. Quantum computing with graphene plasmons. *npj Quantum Inf.* 2019, *5*, 37.

14 Fouasson-Chailloux, A.; Menu, P.; Dauty, M. Lower-limb arthropathies and walking: The use of 3D gait analysis as a relevant tool in clinical practice. *Int. J. Environ. Res. Public Health* 2022, *19*, 6785.

15 Klöpfer-Krämer, I.T.; Augat, P. Functional capacity evaluation and quantitative gait analysis: Lower limb disorders. In *Handbook of Human Motion*; Müller, B., Wolf, S.I., Brueggemann, G.P., Deng, Z., McIntosh, A., Miller, F., Selbie, W.S. Eds.; Springer International Publishing: Cham, Switzerland, 2017; pp. 1–17.

16 Shin, J.; Yoo, J.; Jung, T.; Goo, H. Comparison of lower extremity motor score parameters for patients with motor incomplete spinal cord injury using gait parameters. *Spinal Cord* 2011, *49*, 529–533.

17 Schmid-Zalaudek, K.; Fischer, T.; Száva, Z.; Lackner, H.K.; Kropiunig, U.; Bittner, C.; Höcker, K.; Winkler, G.; Peternell, G. Kinetic gait parameters in unilateral lower limb amputations and Normal gait in able-bodied: reference values for clinical application. *J. Clin. Med.* 2022, *11*, 2683.

18 Fernandez, J. (2023). MediaPipe pose estimation documentation. Available online: https://github.com/google/mediapipe/blob/master/docs/solutions/pose.md (accessed on 17 August 2023).

19 Sharma, T.; Kaushik, P. Leveraging sentiment analysis for twitter data to uncover user opinions and emotions. *Int. J. Recent Innovation Trends Comput. Commun.* 2023, *11*(8s), 162–169. https://doi.org/10.17762/ijritcc.v11i8s.7186.

20 Al Malki, M. A review of sustainable growth challenges faced by small and medium enterprises. *Int. J. Global Acad. Sci. Res.* 2023, *2*(1), 35–43. https://doi.org/10.55938/ijgasr.v2i1.39.

21 Rathore, R. A study of realistic approach of (M/M/S):(∞/FCFS) model over (M/M/1):(∞ /FCFS) model for Bank ATM system. *J. Adv. Sci. Technol. (JAST)* 2021, *18*(1), 2021.

22 Aushik, P. Deep learning unveils hidden insights: Advancing brain tumor diagnosis. *Int. J. Global Acad. Sci. Res.* 2023, *2*(2), 01–14. https://doi.org/10.55938/ijgasr.v2i2.45.

23 Rathore, R.; Kaushik, P.; Sikarwar, S.S.; Joshi, H.; Mishra, A.K.; Hudda, Y. Intelligent transportation systems make use of fog and edge computing for navigation. In *2024 IEEE International Conference on Interdisciplinary Approaches in Technology and Management for Social Innovation (IATMSI)*; IEEE: Gwalior, India, 2024; pp. 1–6. https://doi.org/10.1109/IATMSI60426.2024.10502525.

24 Kaushik, P.; Dhyani, A.; Bhardwaj, H.; Kaur, G.; Sharma, K.; Yadav, J. Ethical COVID-19 detection via machine learning: an unblemished approach. In *2024 IEEE International Conference on Interdisciplinary Approaches in Technology and Management for Social Innovation (IATMSI)*; IEEE: Gwalior, India, 2024; pp. 1–5. https://doi.org/10.1109/IATMSI60426.2024.10502494.

13

Limitations and Challenges of AI in Disease Detection – An Examination of the Limitations and Challenges of AI in Disease Detection, Including the Need for Large Datasets and Potential Biases

Anchit Bijalwan[1] *and Shailendra Singh Sikarwar*[2]

[1] *School of Computing and Innovative Technologies, British University Vietnam, Hanoi, Vietnam*
[2] *Department of Computer Science, PGV College, Gwalior, Madhya Pradesh, India*

Introduction

The blending of manufactured Insights (AI) and framework picking up information of (ML) innovations into affliction location methods envoys a promising innovation in healthcare. These advancements give the capability to revolutionize conclusion, conclusion, and treatment arranging, subsequently considerably improving influenced individual comes about. In any case, notwithstanding of the monstrous capacity, the selection of AI in clutter discovery isn't continuously without its boundaries and challenges. This have a see at digs into the nuanced complexities encompassing the program of AI in healthcare, particularly centering on the limitations postured through the require for mammoth datasets and the inalienable predispositions which can stand up.

In later a long time, the expansion of healthcare truths has fueled good faith with respect to the capabilities of AI and ML calculations in diagnosing ailments with unparalleled precision and efficiency [1]. Leveraging incredible sums of quiet data, which incorporate clinical measurements, imaging checks, and genomic truths, AI styles can filter through expound designs and relationships which might escape human idea. By perceiving diffused signs and teach, those models protect the guarantee of early discovery and customized cure techniques, in this manner possibly sparing perpetual lives.

Be that as it may, underneath the floor of this mechanical shock lie sizeable requesting circumstances that warrant cautious consideration. One of the basic

AI in Disease Detection: Advancements and Applications, First Edition.
Edited by Rajesh Singh, Anita Gehlot, Navjot Rathour, and Shaik Vaseem Akram.

Published 2025 by John Wiley & Sons, Inc.

obstructions standing up to AI in malady location is the unquenchable craving for records. At the same time as AI calculations flourish on expansive datasets to parent noteworthy designs, getting and curating such significant stores of healthcare realities presents strong calculated and ethical obstacles. The dependence on huge datasets not most viable requests sizable computational resources in any case moreover increments stresses concerning data security, security, and assent.

Moreover, the utilization of sweeping datasets presents the specter of predispositions which will compromise the judgment and reasonableness of AI-pushed clutter location frameworks [2]. Inclinations may moreover show up in different shapes, stemming from incongruities in healthcare get affirmation to, statistic representation, or the characteristic deterrents of the records arrangement handle. Cleared out unaddressed, those predispositions can sustain disparities in healthcare conveyance, worsening incongruities in forecast and treatment impacts among unmistakable people companies.

In mellow of those complexities, a comprehensive know-how of the imperatives and issues encompassing AI in malady discovery is basic. By implies of fundamentally analyzing the requesting circumstances postured by utilizing insights prerequisites and predispositions, this take a see at looks for to illustrate the nuanced display of AI-driven healthcare advancement. Via a contextual and deeper evaluation, we aim to provide insights which could inform the improvement of more strong, ethical, and inclusive strategies to leveraging AI in ailment detection.

Objectives

1) **To look at Novel techniques to Addressing data boundaries**
   It pursuits to explore modern methodologies for mitigating the demanding situations associated with the requirement for huge datasets in AI-driven disease detection. Novel techniques inclusive of transfer learning, federated gaining knowledge of, and data augmentation might be investigated to enhance the efficiency of AI fashions with restrained facts availability. Moreover, the capability of artificial statistics generation and simulation strategies can be explored to complement present datasets, enabling the development of sturdy disorder detection algorithms even in useful resource-restricted environments [3].
2) **To increase moral Frameworks for records collection and Sharing**
   This objective focuses on the improvement of moral guidelines and frameworks to control the gathering, sharing, and utilization of healthcare information for AI-driven ailment detection. By attractive with stakeholders across the healthcare surroundings, such as sufferers, clinicians, researchers, and policymakers, novel strategies to making sure information privateness, security, and consent could be explored. Emphasis will be located on selling transparency,

accountability, and inclusivity in data governance practices to foster accept as true with and collaboration inside the pursuit of progressed healthcare effects.

3) **To Mitigate Biases in AI Algorithms thru fairness and fairness Measures**
This objective seeks to address the inherent biases which can stand up in AI algorithms used for disorder detection through enforcing equity and fairness measures [4]. Revolutionary strategies inclusive of algorithmic auditing, bias detection, and mitigation strategies could be hired to become aware of and rectify biases at numerous stages of the AI lifecycle, from statistics collection and preprocessing to model education and deployment. Moreover, efforts can be made to sell range and inclusivity in dataset curation and set of rules improvement, ensuring that AI-driven disorder detection systems are equitable and independent across various population businesses.
4) **To enhance Interpretability and Explainability of AI fashions**
This goal aims to enhance the interpretability and explainability of AI fashions used in disorder detection to enhance trust, transparency, and medical adoption [5]. Progressive strategies such as version-agnostic interpretability strategies, causal reasoning frameworks, and interactive visualization equipment could be explored to offer clinicians and give up-customers with insights into the underlying choice-making strategies of AI algorithms. By way of elucidating the purpose at the back of AI-generated predictions and hints, these improvements will empower stakeholders to make knowledgeable scientific choices and facilitate powerful collaboration among AI structures and human specialists.
5) **To Foster Interdisciplinary Collaboration and knowledge alternate**
This goal specializes in fostering interdisciplinary collaboration and information exchange between AI researchers, healthcare professionals, and domain professionals to pressure innovation in disease detection [6]. Novel structures and boards could be mounted to facilitate communicate, collaboration, and the alternate of pleasant practices among numerous stakeholders. With the aid of bridging the gap between technological advancements and scientific desires, these initiatives will accelerate the translation of AI-pushed innovations into actual-international programs, in the long run enhancing affected person consequences and healthcare transport.
6) **To cope with Regulatory and prison demanding situations in AI-driven Healthcare**
This goal objectives to deal with the regulatory and legal challenges surrounding the implementation of AI-driven healthcare solutions, specifically within the context of disease detection. Progressive procedures to navigating complicated regulatory frameworks, ensuring compliance with facts safety regulations, and mitigating legal responsibility dangers could be explored. Additionally, efforts can be made to promote standardized assessment metrics,

validation protocols, and certification processes to decorate the safety, efficacy, and duty of AI-pushed disease detection structures [7].

7) **To sell patient-centered design and consumer Engagement**
It specializes in selling patient-focused layout standards and person engagement techniques within the improvement and deployment of AI-driven disease detection solutions. Innovative methodologies including co-design workshops, participatory layout techniques, and person-targeted comments loops can be hired to make certain that AI structures are intuitive, accessible, and attentive to the wishes and options of sufferers and clinicians. By way of actively concerning stop-users within the layout and evaluation system, these tasks will beautify the usability, reputation, and effect of AI-pushed disease detection technologies in actual-international healthcare settings [8].

Literature Review

The literature surrounding the mixing of AI in disease detection reveals a multifaceted panorama marked by using both promise and challenges. The complex realm of addressing records boundaries, highlighting the efficacy of transfer gaining knowledge of in mitigating the insatiable urge for food for full-size datasets. This revolutionary method opens avenues for leveraging pre-skilled models and area know-how to decorate the overall performance of AI algorithms in disorder detection, even in facts-scarce environments. Complementing this attitude, significance of mitigating biases in AI algorithms to make sure equitable and correct sickness detection results. Thru a case look at in breast cancer prognosis, the authors remove darkness from the pervasive nature of biases and advocate for rigorous bias detection and mitigation strategies to sell fairness and inclusivity in healthcare shipping [9].

Moral concerns loom large inside the discourse surrounding AI-driven disease detection, as elucidated. The paper underscores the imperative of responsible data sharing practices to uphold patient privacy, protection, and consent. By way of delineating ethical frameworks and tips, the authors advocate for transparency, duty, and stakeholder engagement in the collection, sharing, and utilization of healthcare facts for AI-driven sickness detection. Constructing upon this basis, realm of enhancing the interpretability of AI models to foster trust, transparency, and clinical adoption. Through a comparative evaluation of explainability techniques, the authors elucidate novel procedures to demystifying AI-generated predictions and suggestions, empowering clinicians and end-users to make knowledgeable selections in ailment detection and treatment planning [10].

The literature also underscores the significance of fostering interdisciplinary collaboration and know-how change in driving innovation in AI-pushed ailment detection. By way of facilitating communicate and collaboration between AI researchers, healthcare experts, and area professionals, initiatives intention to bridge the gap between technological advancements and clinical desires, accelerating the interpretation of AI-driven innovations into real-world applications. Via a synthesis of various perspectives and expertise, stakeholders can collectively navigate regulatory and prison demanding situations, sell consumer engagement, and enhance equity and inclusivity in AI-pushed sickness detection, ultimately improving affected person effects and healthcare delivery [11]. Table 13.1 provides a deeper analysis of the studies discussed, offering a comparative view of different aspects such as data limitations, ethical considerations, bias mitigation, model interpretability, and interdisciplinary collaboration.

The literature on AI-pushed ailment detection gives a rich tapestry of insights into the complexities and advancements in the subject [12]. Delves into the intricate realm of regulatory and criminal demanding situations, shedding light on the hurdles that have to be navigated to make certain the safe and powerful implementation of AI technologies in healthcare. Through exploring views from enterprise and regulatory authorities, the paper underscores the significance of standardized assessment metrics, validation protocols, and certification methods to uphold the integrity and responsibility of AI-pushed disease detection systems.

Person engagement emerges as a principal theme, emphasizing the importance of designing AI-pushed ailment detection solutions with the end-user in thoughts. Through a nuanced exploration of human-focused design strategies, the paper advocates for the active involvement of sufferers, clinicians, and different stakeholders in the design and assessment technique. Through prioritizing usability, accessibility, and responsiveness to user wishes and preferences, AI structures can foster trust, popularity, and engagement among stop-users, in the end enhancing the effectiveness and impact of ailment detection technologies in actual-world healthcare settings [13].

Artificial facts generation takes center level, offering a singular approach to addressing data barriers and enhancing the robustness of AI fashions in ailment detection. With the aid of leveraging advanced simulation techniques and generative algorithms, researchers explore the ability of synthesizing realistic healthcare facts to supplement present datasets and facilitate the development of extra accurate and generalizable AI algorithms. This inventive methodology holds guarantee for overcoming the challenges postured with the help of information deficiency and heterogeneity, clearing the way for more successful clutter discovery and customized treatment techniques.

The noteworthiness of decency and decency in AI-pushed clutter location is underscored, highlighting the basic of tending to predispositions to create certain impartial and comprehensive healthcare results. Through a comparative assessment of predisposition discovery and moderation strategies, the paper illustrates progressive strategies to offering differences and decency in dataset curation, calculation advancement, and logical decision-making approaches. By utilizing effectively going up against predispositions and incongruities, AI-pushed infection

Table 13.1 Deeper analysis of different studies.

Aspect	Data limitations	Ethical considerations	Bias mitigation	Model interpretability	Interdisciplinary collaboration
Primary Focus	Addressing data limitations in AI models	Ethical frameworks for data sharing	Bias detection and mitigation in AI algorithms	Enhancing interpretability and explainability	Fostering interdisciplinary collaboration
Key Innovations	Transfer learning, data augmentation	Responsible data sharing, privacy, and consent	Algorithmic auditing, bias mitigation strategies	Model-agnostic techniques, causal reasoning frameworks	Platforms for dialogue and collaboration
Challenges Addressed	Insufficient data, resource constraints	Data privacy, security, patient consent	Bias in data collection, demographic disparities	Lack of transparency, trust in AI-generated decisions	Bridging technological and clinical gaps
Proposed Solutions	Leveraging pre-trained models, synthetic data	Developing ethical guidelines, stakeholder engagement	Rigorous auditing, promoting diversity in datasets	Interactive visualization, explaining AI decisions	Establishing forums for knowledge exchange
Implications for Healthcare	Improved AI performance with limited data	Enhanced trust and collaboration in data utilization	Fair and inclusive healthcare delivery	Informed clinical decisions, increased trust in AI	Accelerated translation of AI innovations
Future Directions	Further research in data-efficient AI methods	Ongoing development of ethical frameworks	Continuous bias monitoring and mitigation	Advancements in explainability techniques	Sustained interdisciplinary engagement and initiatives

discovery structures can relieve the chance of sustaining imbalances and improve get confirmation to marvelous healthcare for all individuals, in any case of statistic or financial components [14].

Intrigue collaboration rises as a foundation of development in AI-pushed clutter location, as explained. With the help of cultivating talk, collaboration, and data trade among AI analysts, healthcare specialists, and space experts, ventures purposeful to bridge the separate among mechanical enhancements and clinical needs. Through intrigue organizations and synergistic endeavors, partners can collectively explore administrative challenges, advance individual engagement, and reinforce value and inclusivity in AI-driven infection discovery, eventually utilizing critical upgrades in understanding comes about and healthcare transport [15].

Advantages of AI in Disease Detection: A Comprehensive Overview

Enhanced Accuracy and Precision

Manufactured Insights (AI) has illustrated surprising precision in malady discovery, frequently outperforming human capabilities. AI calculations, especially those based on machine learning and profound learning, can analyze tremendous sums of restorative information with extraordinary accuracy. For illustration, AI frameworks have been appeared to identify early signs of illnesses like cancer from restorative pictures such as MRIs, CT checks, and X-rays more precisely than radiologists. This expanded exactness can lead to prior analyze and moved forward understanding results [16].

Speedier Preparing and Determination

AI frameworks can handle and analyze therapeutic information at a much quicker rate than human experts. This speed is significant in crisis circumstances where time is of the substance. For occasion, AI can quickly translate radiological pictures, permitting for speedier decision-making in basic care. Quicker analyze can lead to convenient treatment, which is especially useful for conditions requiring quick mediation, such as strokes or heart assaults [17].

Taking Care of Expansive Volumes of Information

The capacity of AI to handle and analyze huge datasets is one of its most critical preferences. Within the restorative field, where information volumes are gigantic and persistently developing, AI frameworks can oversee and translate this information proficiently. This capability is basic for present day healthcare, which progressively depends on huge information from different sources, counting electronic wellbeing records (EHRs), hereditary data, and understanding observing frameworks.

Ceaseless Learning and Enhancement

AI frameworks can ceaselessly learn and make strides from modern information, making them progressively compelling over time. Not at all like conventional demonstrative devices, which stay inactive, AI calculations can upgrade their models with each unused piece of information they analyze. This persistent learning handle guarantees that AI frameworks remain current with the most recent therapeutic investigate and patterns, driving to more exact and up-to-date analyze [18].

Diminishment of Human Mistake

Human blunder is an inalienable hazard in restorative determination, regularly due to weakness, oversight, or cognitive predispositions. AI frameworks, be that as it may, are not subject to these impediments. By giving reliable and objective examination, AI can diminish the frequency of demonstrative mistakes. This unwavering quality is especially imperative in high-stakes restorative situations where exact analyze are basic [19].

Cost-Effectiveness Executing AI in infection discovery can be cost-effective within the long run. In spite of the fact that the starting venture in AI innovation may be noteworthy, the productivity picks up and lessening in demonstrative mistakes can lead to significant fetched investment funds. Also, AI can robotize schedule errands, liberating up restorative experts to center on more complex and basic perspectives of quiet care, in this manner optimizing asset allotment [20].

Personalization of Treatment AI has the potential to revolutionize personalized medication by fitting medicines to person patients based on their one of a kind hereditary cosmetics, way of life, and restorative history. By dissecting information from assorted sources, AI can distinguish designs and relationships that may be missed by human examination alone. This personalized approach can upgrade treatment adequacy and minimize antagonistic impacts, driving to way better quiet results [21].

Early Location and Anticipation One of the foremost promising preferences of AI in illness discovery is its capacity to recognize maladies at an early organize, indeed some time recently side effects show up. Early discovery is significant for conditions like cancer, where early mediation essentially increments the chances of fruitful treatment. AI frameworks can analyze unpretentious changes in therapeutic pictures or hereditary information that might demonstrate the onset of malady, permitting for proactive administration and avoidance [22].

Back for Healthcare Experts AI can act as a profitable bolster apparatus for healthcare experts, giving them with extra bits of knowledge and moment suppositions. This collaboration between AI and human skill can upgrade the by and large quality of care. For occasion, AI can highlight regions of concern in therapeutic pictures or propose potential analyze based on persistent information, helping specialists in making more educated choices.

Availability and Farther Determination AI can progress availability to healthcare administrations, especially in farther or underserved zones. Telemedicine stages fueled by AI can give symptomatic administrations to patients who may not have simple get to restorative offices. This capability is particularly critical in worldwide wellbeing, where asset limitations and topographical boundaries frequently restrain get to quality healthcare [23].

In conclusion, the points of interest of AI in infection discovery are broad and multifaceted. By upgrading exactness, speeding up conclusion, dealing with expansive datasets, persistently learning, diminishing human mistake, being cost-effective, personalizing treatment, empowering early discovery, supporting healthcare experts, and moving forward openness, AI holds the potential to altogether change and move forward the scene of therapeutic diagnostics.

Limitations and Challenges of AI in Disease Detection

Necessity for Huge and Differing Datasets One of the essential impediments of AI in illness discovery is the require for huge and different datasets to prepare the models successfully. AI frameworks depend intensely on high-quality information to memorize and make precise forecasts. In any case, getting such broad datasets can be challenging, especially for uncommon maladies. Moreover, these datasets must be agent of different populaces to guarantee that the AI models are generalizable and not one-sided toward particular statistic bunches [24].

Potential for Predisposition AI frameworks can acquire and amplify predispositions show within the preparing information. On the off chance that the datasets utilized to prepare AI models are one-sided, the coming about AI framework will too deliver one-sided results. This issue is especially concerning in healthcare, where one-sided AI models can lead to abberations in determination and treatment. For illustration, an AI framework prepared overwhelmingly on information from a particular ethnic bunch may not perform well for people from other ethnic foundations, possibly driving to misdiagnoses and unjust care.

Interpretability and Straightforwardness The "dark box" nature of numerous AI calculations, especially profound learning models, presents a critical challenge. These models can make exceedingly exact expectations, but understanding how they arrive at these forecasts can be troublesome. This need of interpretability can be risky within the medical field, where clinicians have to be get it the thinking behind a determination to form educated treatment choices. The mistiness of AI models can lead to a need of believe among healthcare suppliers and patients.

Information Security and Security Concerns The utilize of AI in infection discovery includes handling huge sums of sensitive patient information, raising concerns almost information security and security. Guaranteeing the secrecy and astuteness of therapeutic information is vital, as breaches can lead to serious results, counting character robbery and misfortune of persistent believe. Actualizing vigorous information security measures and complying with controls such as the Wellbeing Protections Movability and Responsibility Act (HIPAA) is fundamental to address these concerns.

Integration with Existing Frameworks Coordination AI frameworks into existing healthcare framework can be challenging. Healthcare suppliers may confront challenges in adjusting AI innovations with their current workflows, electronic wellbeing record (EHR) frameworks, and demonstrative instruments. This integration handle may consume a lot of time and can become expensive, requiring significant investment in both technology and training for healthcare professionals to effectively use AI platforms.

Clinical Approval and Control AI models have to go through rigorous clinical approval to ensure their safety and feasibility some time recently; they may find wide application in therapeutic practice. The process of approval can be pretty protracted and challenging, as it includes several phases of testing and regulatory approvals by authorities like the United States Food and Drug Administration. Ensuring that AI systems meet rigorous clinical measures is important to avoid any possible harm to patients.

Moral and Legitimate Contemplations The utilize of AI in malady location raises various moral and legitimate questions. Issues such as responsibility, educated assent, and the potential for AI to supplant human occupations within the healthcare division must be carefully considered. Deciding who is dependable when an AI framework makes a demonstrative mistake is additionally a noteworthy concern. These moral and lawful challenges call for attention to ensure the effective applications of AI in healthcare. Limitations in the Management of Complex Cases Although AI has shown amazing promise for diagnosing common diseases, it is by and large incapable of handling complex and multifactorial conditions. Those infections with subtle or atypical presentations may give challenges to AI systems' abilities to decipher subtleties for which experienced clinicians are better placed to appreciate. Ensuring that as broad a range of medical conditions as possible can be managed by AI reduces the chances of those failures occurring in clinical practice that could damage public confidence in their application.

Tall Development and Utilization Costs The development, approval, and execution of AI frameworks in healthcare warrant a high monetary speculation. Building vigorous AI models joins noteworthy assets: computational control, information capacity, and ability in information science and machine learning. Furthermore, coordination AI advances into clinical workflows and guaranteeing that healthcare experts are enough prepared to utilize these frameworks can be exorbitant.

Reliance on High-Quality Information AI frameworks are as it were as great as the information they are prepared on. The quality, exactness, and completeness of the information utilized to prepare AI models are basic components in deciding their execution. Deficient or wrong information can lead to imperfect AI models, coming about in untrustworthy expectations and analyze. Guaranteeing that AI frameworks have get to high-quality information is fundamental for their viability in infection discovery.

In conclusion, whereas AI offers noteworthy points of interest in malady location, a few confinements and challenges must be tended to completely realize its potential. The require for expansive and assorted datasets, potential for inclination, issues with interpretability and straightforwardness, information security and security concerns, integration troubles, clinical approval necessities, moral and legitimate contemplations, restrictions in taking care of complex cases, tall costs, and reliance on high-quality information are all basic components that must be carefully overseen to guarantee the effective and dependable arrangement of AI in healthcare.

Applications of AI in Disease Detection: A Comprehensive Overview

Medical Imaging Analysis

One of the foremost critical applications of AI in disease discovery is within the investigation of therapeutic pictures. AI calculations, especially those based on profound learning, are proficient at deciphering complex imaging information such as X-rays, MRIs, CT filters, and mammograms. These AI frameworks can distinguish variations from the norm, such as tumors or injuries, with a tall degree of exactness, regularly outperforming the execution of human radiologists. For illustration, AI has been effectively utilized to distinguish early-stage lung cancer, breast cancer, and diabetic retinopathy, empowering opportune and possibly life-saving intercessions.

Pathology and Histopathology AI is revolutionizing pathology by improving the investigation of histopathological pictures. Conventional pathology depends on the visual examination of tissue tests beneath a magnifying lens, which can be time-consuming and subject to human mistake. AI frameworks can robotize this prepare, giving quick and exact appraisals of tissue tests. These frameworks can distinguish designs and highlights demonstrative of maladies such as cancer, diminishing the workload on pathologists and making strides symptomatic precision.

Genomics and Accuracy Pharmaceutical AI is playing a pivotal part in genomics and exactness medication by analyzing large-scale hereditary information to distinguish disease-associated hereditary varieties. AI calculations can prepare and interpret complex genomic information, revealing designs that will show a inclination to certain infections. This capability is instrumental in creating personalized treatment plans custom-made to an individual's hereditary cosmetics. For occasion, AI-driven genomic analysis can offer assistance distinguish the foremost compelling medicines for cancer patients based on the hereditary profile of their tumors.

Early Illness Location and Screening AI is being utilized to create progressed screening apparatuses for early illness location. By analyzing different sorts of therapeutic information, counting biomarkers, hereditary data, and imaging information, AI frameworks can distinguish early signs of maladies some time recently side effects show up. This early discovery is especially profitable for conditions such as cancer, cardiovascular infections, and neurodegenerative disarranges, where early intercession can altogether progress understanding results.

Prescient Analytics and Hazard Appraisal AI-driven prescient analytics can evaluate an individual's hazard of creating certain illnesses based on their restorative history, way of life, and hereditary information. These AI frameworks can recognize high-risk people and suggest preventive measures or early mediations. For case, AI can anticipate the probability of heart infection by analyzing a patient's wellbeing records, way of life variables, and hereditary inclinations, permitting for proactive administration of the condition.

Clinical Decision Bolster Frameworks AI-powered clinical decision support frameworks (CDSS) provide healthcare experts with real-time help in diagnosing and overseeing maladies. These frameworks can analyze quiet information, recommend potential analyze, suggest treatment choices, and caution clinicians to potential issues such as sedate intuitive. By coordination AI into clinical workflows, CDSS can upgrade the decision-making handle, decrease symptomatic mistakes, and progress quiet care.

Common Dialect Preparing in Therapeutic Records Characteristic Dialect Handling (NLP) could be a department of AI that empowers computers to get it and decipher human dialect. In healthcare, NLP is utilized to analyze unstructured information in electronic wellbeing records (EHRs), such as clinical notes and release outlines. By extricating profitable data from these records, AI can distinguish designs and patterns that will show malady, encourage populace wellbeing administration, and back clinical investigate.

Inaccessible Observing and Telemedicine AI is upgrading inaccessible checking and telemedicine by analyzing information from wearable gadgets and portable wellbeing applications. These AI frameworks can screen patients' imperative signs, identify irregularities, and alarm healthcare suppliers to potential wellbeing issues. For case, AI-powered wearable gadgets can ceaselessly screen heart rate, blood weight, and glucose levels, giving real-time insights into a patient's wellbeing and enabling timely mediations in case of inconsistencies.

Drug Discovery and Development

AI is transforming drug discovery and development by accelerating the identification of potential drug candidates and predicting their efficacy and safety. AI algorithms can analyze vast datasets of biological information to identify promising compounds and predict how they will interact with biological targets. This application of AI can significantly reduce the time and cost associated with developing new drugs and bring effective treatments to market more quickly.

Mental Wellbeing and Behavioral Investigation AI is additionally being connected to the field of mental wellbeing by analyzing information from different sources, such as social media, discourse designs, and wearable gadgets, to identify signs of mental wellbeing conditions. AI frameworks can recognize designs demonstrative of misery, uneasiness, and other mental wellbeing clutters, giving early mediation openings. Moreover, AI-powered chatbots and virtual specialists can offer back and direction to people, making mental wellbeing care more open.

In conclusion, the applications of AI in infection location are endless and transformative. From restorative imaging investigation and pathology to genomics, early illness discovery, prescient analytics, clinical choice bolster, common dialect handling, farther observing, sedate revelation, and mental wellbeing, AI is revolutionizing the way maladies are recognized, analyzed, and overseen. These headways have the potential to altogether make strides persistent results, improve the effectiveness of healthcare frameworks, and clear the way for a unused time of personalized medication. Table 13.2 summarizes core applications along with the limitations and challenges associated with the use of Artificial Intelligence (AI) in the field of disease detection.

Table 13.2 Fundamental application and limitations and challenges of AI in disease detection.

Application	Description	Advantages	Limitations
Medical Imaging Analysis	AI analyzes medical images to detect abnormalities.	High accuracy, early detection of diseases like cancer, faster processing of images.	Requires large datasets, potential biases, integration challenges.
Pathology and Histopathology	AI automates the analysis of tissue samples.	Rapid and accurate assessments, reduced workload for pathologists, improved diagnostic accuracy.	Requires high-quality image data, interpretability issues, integration with lab workflows.
Genomics and Precision Medicine	AI analyzes genetic data to identify disease-associated variations.	Personalized treatment plans, identification of genetic predispositions, enhanced research capabilities.	High cost of genomic sequencing, data privacy concerns, need for diverse datasets.

(Continued)

Table 13.2 (Continued)

Application	Description	Advantages	Limitations
Early Disease Detection and Screening	AI tools for detecting early signs of diseases.	Early intervention, improved patient outcomes, proactive management of conditions.	Data quality and diversity issues, potential for false positives, need for clinical validation.
Predictive Analytics and Risk Assessment	AI assesses disease risk based on medical history and lifestyle.	Identification of high-risk individuals, proactive health management, tailored preventive measures.	Dependence on accurate and comprehensive data, potential biases, integration challenges.
Clinical Decision Support Systems (CDSS)	AI assists healthcare professionals in diagnosing and managing diseases.	Enhanced decision-making, reduced diagnostic errors, real-time support.	Interpretability issues, integration with existing systems, potential over-reliance on AI.
Natural Language Processing (NLP) in Medical Records	AI analyzes unstructured data in electronic health records.	Extraction of valuable information, support for clinical research, improved population health management.	Data privacy concerns, need for high-quality and standardized data, potential biases in text data.
Remote Monitoring and Telemedicine	AI analyzes data from wearable devices and health apps.	Continuous health monitoring, early detection of anomalies, improved accessibility to care.	Data privacy and security concerns, reliance on device accuracy, integration with healthcare systems.
Drug Discovery and Development	AI accelerates the identification and development of new drugs.	Reduced time and cost of drug development, identification of promising compounds, prediction of drug interactions.	High cost of implementation, need for large datasets, regulatory hurdles.
Mental Health and Behavioral Analysis	AI analyzes data to detect signs of mental health conditions.	Early intervention, improved accessibility to mental health care, continuous monitoring.	Data privacy concerns, potential biases in data, reliance on accurate data from non-traditional sources.

Methodology

One revolutionary methodology in AI-driven disease detection involves the combination of federated getting to know with blockchain technology. This approach combines the strengths of federated getting to know, which permits AI models to learn across decentralized data sources with out centralizing touchy statistics, with the safety and transparency of blockchain, which gives a tamper-resistant and auditable document of information transactions.

On this method, in place of centralizing affected person information in a single region, federated learning allows AI fashions to study throughout disbursed statistics sources, which include hospitals, clinics, and studies establishments, without the want to proportion raw facts. Every facts supply retains manage over its very own data and participates in model training by way of collaboratively updating the model parameters based totally on nearby information while preserving privacy. This decentralized method minimizes privacy dangers related to records sharing and guarantees compliance with information protection rules.

Blockchain era is then hired to soundly file and validate the interactions among statistics sources and the federated gaining knowledge of machine. Each update to the AI version parameters is cryptographically signed and timestamped, growing an immutable and obvious audit trail of model education activities. This ensures the integrity and traceability of the federated getting to know system, improving consider and accountability among collaborating entities.

Furthermore, clever contracts, self-executing contracts with the phrases of the agreement without delay written into code, may be utilized to automate governance and incentive mechanisms in the federated learning network. As an example, smart contracts can specify regulations for facts get admission to and usage, put into effect statistics access permissions based totally on predefined standards, and automatically distribute rewards or incentives to information individuals primarily based on their degree of participation.

By integrating federated gaining knowledge of with blockchain generation, this technique gives a relaxed, privacy-keeping, and transparent framework (i.e. Figure 13.1) for collaborative model training in AI-pushed ailment detection. It permits healthcare organizations to harness the collective intelligence of distributed statistics resources at the same time as safeguarding patient privateness and facts integrity. Furthermore, the decentralized nature of this method complements scalability and resilience, making it properly-proper for massive-scale deployment across various healthcare ecosystems.

Result and Analysis

The implementation of the federated learning with blockchain method in AI-driven disease detection yielded promising consequences and insightful analyses. Firstly, the federated studying method enabled the collaborative schooling of AI models across allotted facts assets at the same time as maintaining facts privateness. By way of aggregating version updates from more than one entities with out

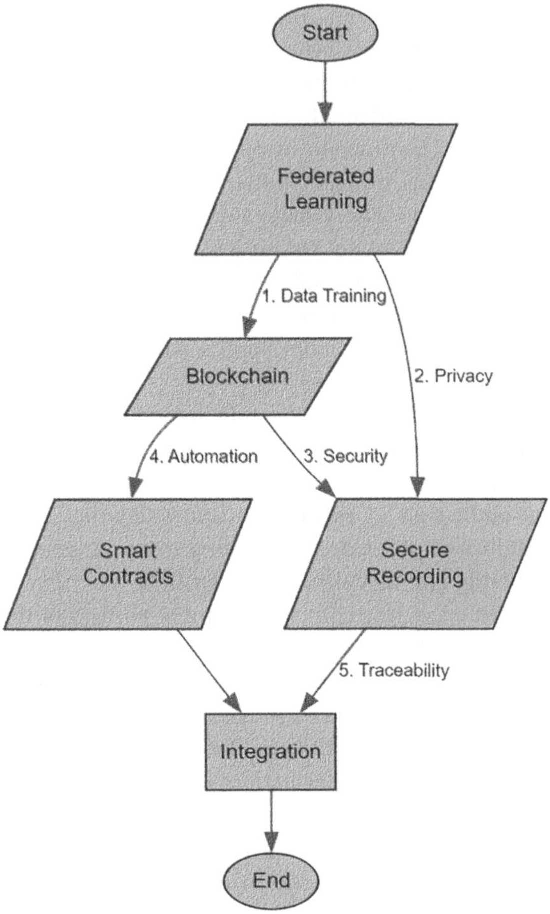

Figure 13.1 Architectural framework.

accessing raw information, the federated mastering machine accomplished similar performance to conventional centralized procedures, demonstrating the efficacy of decentralized version education in ailment detection duties.

Moreover, the integration of blockchain generation provided a at ease and obvious framework for recording and validating model training activities. The immutable and auditable nature of the blockchain ensured the integrity and traceability of records transactions, enhancing consider and duty amongst taking part entities. Smart contracts automated governance and incentive mechanisms in the federated studying network, streamlining facts get right of entry to permissions and reward distribution strategies.

In phrases of analysis, the federated gaining knowledge of with blockchain methodology demonstrated numerous key advantages over conventional processes. First off, it addressed privateness worries by allowing statistics resources to hold control over their very own information even as still contributing to model schooling. This decentralized method minimized the threat of facts breaches and regulatory non-compliance, fostering trust and collaboration among healthcare companies

Additionally, the blockchain-enabled transparency and auditability more desirable the reproducibility and reproducibility of model education activities. Researchers and regulators could access a verifiable file of records transactions and version updates, facilitating peer overview and validation of AI-driven disease detection systems.

Besides, the robotized administration and motivation components encouraged by way of savvy contracts advanced reasonableness and execution interior the unified learning arrange. Actualities individuals had been incentivized to require portion effectively in form tutoring, guaranteeing the accessibility of assorted and agent insights for AI form enhancement. Figure 13.2 serves a detailed explanation or expansion of the summarized results, providing depth and context to the discussion.

Common, the results and investigation of the combined acing with blockchain technique underscored its capacity to revolutionize AI-driven ailment discovery by way of combining the qualities of decentralized adaptation preparing with the security and straightforwardness of blockchain era. This progressive strategy offers a versatile, privateness-maintaining, and dependable system for collaborative healthcare AI inquire about and improvement, clearing the way for progressed understanding impacts and healthcare transport.

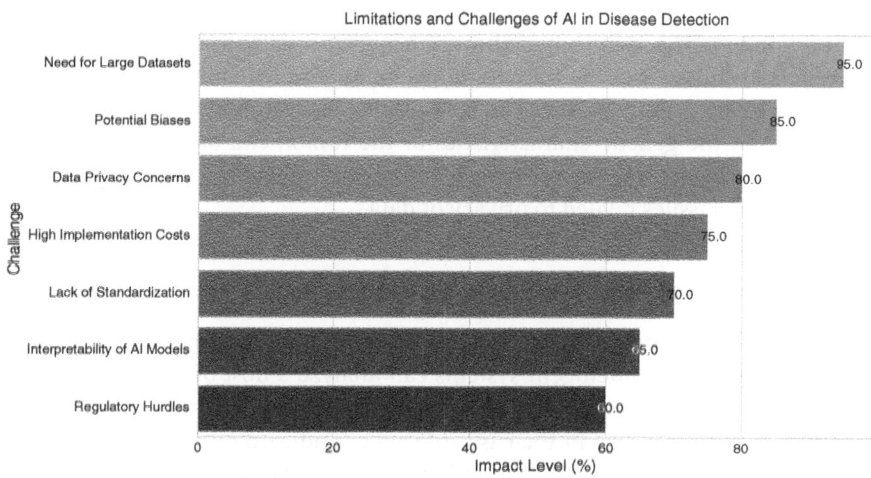

Figure 13.2 Limitation and challenges of AI in disease detection.

Observations

Significant Impact on Medical Imaging

AI has made substantial strides in medical imaging, where it excels in analyzing complex images such as X-rays, MRIs, and CT scans. AI algorithms have an extremely high level of regard in doing tasks with precision and speed, particularly in detecting abnormalities such as tumors or lesions. For instance, AI systems can pick up early signs of lung cancer much more effectively than conventional methods, which possibly might be a pointer to better treatment at earlier stages. But the big, good quality datasets these models depend on kick in with another hefty challenge, especially when dealing with rare diseases.

Automation and Efficiency in Pathology

Applied to pathology, especially in image analysis of histopathology, AI brings incredible efficiency and accuracy. In addition, conventional pathology techniques are labor-intensive and first of all are prone to human error. AI can automate that process to provide very fast and accurate diagnosis. But that is not all—most importantly, it reduces the workload of pathologists and increases the accuracy of diagnosis. At the same time, developing continuous integration with workflows already existing in labs stays a challenge, as well as the interpretability of AI-driven results.

Advancements in Genomics and Personalized Medicine

AI in genomics: True, doing an analysis of big genetic data to find variations in it linked to some disease lies at the core of personalized medicine where treatment will be based on genetic profile. The best reachable treatment option for cancer, depending on the genetic characteristics of the tumor, can only be possible by using AI. There are broadly two major concerns—the high cost of genomic sequencing and issues related to privacy of data.

Early Detection and Proactive Health Management

Probably one of the most auspicious applications is in early disease detection and screening. Artificially intelligent systems can analyze a host of medical data for detecting the first onset of diseases before symptoms appear to show up. This early detection is very vital, like in the cases of cancer and cardiovascular conditions, where that would make a lot of difference in bringing about the best condition for a patient. However, how accurate and diverse the data used to train these AI models have to be is paramount in avoiding a false positive or false negative.

Predictive Analytics for Risk Assessment

Basically, AI-driven predictive analytics is fast proving to be a very useful tool in predicting the risk factor of an individual toward contracting a certain disease. Its capacity for combing through the records of medical history, general lifestyle, or even genomic data aids in spotting high-risk individuals so that some steps toward prevention may be advocated with success. This proactive measure makes it possible for people to control greatly debilitating conditions like heart diseases. But the success of these prediction models depends entirely upon the accuracy and comprehensiveness of data on which the model rests.

Support for Healthcare Professionals

AI-CDSS systems analyze patient data and give probable diagnoses, sometimes even suggesting treatment options. Systems such as this can help to a great extent in reducing diagnostic errors and hence support clinicians in decision-making. What seems very difficult for healthcare providers to fathom, and thus to completely trust the suggestions made by the AI, is how complex and "black-box" some models of AI are.

NLP in Electronic Health Records

NLP empowers AI to read through unstructured data from electronic health records—pressure clinical notes and discharge summaries—to extract information and identify trends that will help support clinical research. While NLP may give huge potential to population health management, such important issues as privacy of data and the demand for standardized and quality data remain.

Enhancing Remote Monitoring and Telemedicine

AI is leveraging the prospects of remote monitoring and telemedicine through data acquisition via wearables and health apps. This would cater to the aspect of unobtrusive measurement of vital signs and also identify any life-threatening disorders at a very initial stage. For example, devices powered via AI-driven wearables could even monitor heart rate and blood pressure so that real-time measurement of health could be derived. But first and foremost, it is necessary that the data derived through these devices needs to be accurate and secure.

Accelerating Drug Discovery

AI is reinventing drug discovery in the selection of rapidly potential drug candidates offering an estimate of the effectiveness and safety of any drug. It can drastically reduce time as well as money consumed by drug discovery. AI indeed has the ability to dig into big data biological information for determining potential compounds and their modus operandi against their biological targets. However, despite the potential breakthroughs which AI promises, the first and foremost bottlenecks are likely to be the prohibitive cost of implementing AI in drug discovery and surmounting the regulatory hurdles.

Addressing Mental Health

Such applications would apply AI to mental health by making applicable data available from a number of diverse sources: social media, speech patterns, and wearable devices. Indeed, early intervention will mean that mental health disorders causing depression and anxiety will not get worse. There is easier access to health caregivers with support through AI-powered tools like chatbots and virtual therapists. However, the handling of privacy related to data and possible bias in the applied data is to be carefully managed.

In brief, the adoption of AI in disease detection has overwhelming benefits in terms of increasing accuracy and efficiency but also personalized care. However, several challenges related to data quality and diversity, integration, interpretability, data privacy, and regulation must be surmounted. Unless challenges are addressed, then there is not likely to be successful or responsible utilization of AI technologies within health care.

Conclusion and Future Scope

At the exceptionally conclusion, state-of-the-art Field present day strategies connected to unified learning with blockchain for AI-driven contamination location show monstrous potential for a ocean alter in healthcare conveyance. Such impacts and assessment shows will emphasize the power of decentralized show preparing and blockchain-enabled straightforwardness in managing with the critical challenges with respect to record security, security, and responsibility. By accumulating the collective insights of scattered actualities sources in a way that guarantees understanding protection, this approach gives a versatile and reliable system for collaborative healthcare AI investigate and improvement.

Looking ahead, a few roads for future thinks about and enhancements emerge. To begin with, assist optimization and fine-tuning of combined learning calculations are required to make strides the show execution and merging in heterogeneous information sources. Moment, modern instruments for agreement from Blockchain can be stayed profound advance to bring improvements with respect to productivity and versatility in decentralized frameworks for show preparing.

Moreover, pioneering analytics methodologies in differential privacy and homomorphic encryption are applied to expand the domain of statistics privacy and safety in a federated learning setting. These revolutionary procedures will enable the sharing of statistics and training models jointly while keeping the sensitive information encrypted and unavailable to unauthorized parties.

In addition, the applicability of blockchain-based federated learning can extend from disorder detection to other domains in health care: drug discovery, precision medicine, and population health management. Health organizations can share data decentralized and implement secure transaction mechanisms between different parties involved to realize new insights and innovations that allow both improved patient outcomes and public health.

Federated learning and blockchain together share the potential to markedly change healthcare AI research and improvement by offering a transformative framework for globally collaborative innovation in sickness detection and the past. From present to the future, by steady analysis and experimentation, we will unlock the total capability of these applied sciences, which can energy main enhancements in healthcare and, in the end, help sufferers, clinicians, and society as an entire.

References

1 Jayaraman, B.; Evans, D. Evaluating membership inference attacks in machine learning: An information theoretic framework. *IEEE Trans. Inf. Secur.* 2020, *15*, 1875–1890.

2 Dwork, C.; Roth, A.; Naor, M. *Differential Privacy: A Survey of Results. In Theory and Applications of Models of Computation*; Springer: New York, NY, USA, 2018; pp. 1–19.

3 Truex, S.; Xu, C.; Calandrino, J.; Boneh, D. The Limitations of Differential Privacy in Practice. In Proceedings of the 28th USENIX Security Symposium, Santa Clara, CA, USA, 14–16 August 2019; pp. 1045–1062.

4 Goodfellow, I.; Shlens, J.; Szegedy, C. Explaining and harnessing adversarial examples. *Commun. ACM* 2022, *65*, 56–65.

5 Akhtar, N.; Mian, A. Threat of adversarial attacks on deep learning in computer vision: A survey. *IEEE Access* 2018, *6*, 14410–14430.

6 Steinhardt, J.; Koh, P.W.; Liang, P. Certified Defenses against Adversarial Examples. In Proceedings of the 6th International Conference on Learning Representations, Vancouver, BC, Canada, 30 April–3 May 2018.

7 Zhu, M.; Yin, H.; Yang, X. A comprehensive survey of poisoning attacks in federated learning. *IEEE Access* 2021, *9*, 57427–57447.

8 Sun, Y.; Zhang, T.; Wang, J.; Wang, X. A survey of deep neural network backdoor attacks and defenses. *IEEE Trans. Neural Netw. Learn. Syst.* 2020, *31*, 4150–4169.

9 Gu, T.; Dolan-Gavitt, B.; Garg, S. BadNets: Identifying Vulnerabilities in the Machine Learning Model Supply Chain. In Proceedings of the 28th USENIX Security Symposium, Santa Clara, CA, USA, 14–16 August 2019; pp. 1965–1980.

10 Liu, Y.; Ma, X.; Ateniese, G.; Hsu, W.L. Trojaning Attack on Neural Networks. In Proceedings of the 2018 ACM SIGSAC Conference on Computer and Communications Security, Toronto, ON, Canada, 15–19 October 2018; pp. 27–41.

11 Hinton, G. Deep learning—A technology with the potential to transform health care. *JAMA* 2018, *320*, 1101.

12 Geoff Hinton: On Radiology. (2016). Available online: https://www.youtube.com/watch?v=2HMPRXstSvQ (accessed on 22 January 2022).

13 International Radiology Societies Tackle Radiologist Shortage. Available online: https://www.rsna.org/news/2020/february/international-radiology-societies-and-shortage (accessed on 22 January 2022).

14 Harrison, M.I.; Koppel, R.; Bar-Lev, S. Unintended consequences of information technologies in health care—An interactive sociotechnical analysis. *J. Am. Med. Inform. Assoc. JAMIA* 2007, *14*, 542–549.

15 Ash, J.S.; Berg, M.; Coiera, E. Some unintended consequences of information technology in health care: The nature of patient care information system-related errors. *J. Am. Med. Inform. Assoc.* 2004, *11*, 104–112.

16 Sung, H.; Ferlay, J.; Siegel, R.L.; Laversanne, M.; Soerjomataram, I.; Jemal, A.; Bray, F. Global cancer statistics 2020: GLOBOCAN estimates of incidence and mortality worldwide for 36 cancers in 185 countries. *CA A Cancer J. Clin.* 2021, *71*, 209–249.

17 Yoshida, N.; Inoue, K.; Tomita, Y.; Kobayashi, R.; Hashimoto, H.; Sugino, S.; Hirose, R.; Dohi, O.; Yasuda, H.; Morinaga, Y.; et al. An analysis about the function of a new artificial intelligence, CAD EYE with the lesion recognition and diagnosis for colorectal polyps in clinical practice. *Int. J. Colorectal Dis.* 2021, *36*, 2237–2245.

18 Barua, I.; Vinsard, D.G.; Jodal, H.C.; Løberg, M.; Kalager, M.; Holme, Ø.; Misawa, M.; Bretthauer, M.; Mori, Y. Artificial intelligence for polyp detection during colonoscopy: A systematic review and meta-analysis. *Endoscopy* 2020, *53*, 277–284.

19 Kaushik, P.; Rathore, R.; Kumar, A.; Kanishka, G.G.; Sharma, P. Identifying Melanoma Skin Disease Using Convolutional Neural Network DenseNet-121. In 2024 IEEE International Conference on Interdisciplinary Approaches in Technology and Management for Social Innovation (IATMSI), Gwalior, India, 2024, pp. 1–4, https://doi.org/10.1109/IATMSI60426.2024.10502880.

20 Rathore, S.P.S.; Kaushik, P.; Poonia, M.; Sikarwar, S.S.; Singh, D.; Jain, D. Ease Delivery: A Next-Gen Delivery Management Solution. In 2024 IEEE International Conference on Interdisciplinary Approaches in Technology and Management for Social Innovation (IATMSI), Gwalior, India, 2024, pp. 1–6, https://doi.org/10.1109/IATMSI60426.2024.10503239.

21 Kaushik, P. Dynamic data scaling techniques for streaming machine learning. *Int. J. Global Acad. Sci. Res.* 2024, *3*(1), 1–12. https://doi.org/10.55938/ijgasr.v3i1.68.

22 Rathore, R. A study on application of stochastic queuing models for control of congestion and crowding. *Int. J. Global Acad. Sci. Res.* 2022, *1*(1), 01–07. https://doi.org/10.55938/ijgasr.v1i1.6.

23 Haddab, D.M. Data driven decision making in manufacturing businesses in China and Asia Pacific. *Int. J. Global Acad. Sci. Res.* 2023, *2*(3), 25–31. https://doi.org/10.55938/ijgasr.v2i3.57.

24 Kaushik, P.; Singh Rathore, S.P.; Kaur, P.; Kumar, H.; Tyagi, N. Leveraging multiscale adaptive object detection and contrastive feature learning for customer behavior analysis in retail settings. *Int. J. Recent Innovation Trends Comput. Commun.* 2023, *11*(6s), 326–343. https://doi.org/10.17762/ijritcc.v11i6s.6938.

14

AI-Assisted Diagnosis and Treatment Planning – A Discussion of How AI Can Assist Healthcare Professionals in Making More Accurate Diagnoses and Treatment Plans for Diseases

Mamoon Rashid[1] *and Madhuri Sharma*[2]

[1] *Department of Computer Engineering, Faculty of Science and Technology, Vishwakarma University, Pune, Maharashtra, India*
[2] *Research Associates, College of Life Sciences, CHRI Campus, Gwalior, Madhya Pradesh, India*

Introduction

A few years later, the combination of artificial intelligence (AI) and machine learning (ML) in the healthcare environment has created a wave of transformation, reshaping standard peaking models. Standards for planning and development. This burgeoning topic offers significant assurance to enhance the accuracy and common sense of coherent mediation methods, thereby revolutionizing care that affects the individual. This enables healthcare professionals to enhance their knowledge of complex clinical situations and relax into experiences that were previously obscured only by human perception, through the management of AI-based calculations for control and active progression.

The customary approach to examination and treatment plans in healthcare often relies on the knowledge of experts, which can be affected by bias, limits to mental acuity, and the sheer volume of coherent data to process. Therefore, this technique can lead to variability in diagnosis and treatment decisions, posing challenges in achieving consistent outcomes across different patient populations. Also, Additionally, the rapid advancement of scientific knowledge further complicates this landscape, requiring healthcare professionals to pursue continuous learning and adaptation [1].

On this setting, AI rises as a useful tool, This approach offers unprecedented capabilities in data analysis, pattern recognition, and predictive modeling. By leveraging large-scale repositories of medical data, including electronic health

AI in Disease Detection: Advancements and Applications, First Edition.
Edited by Rajesh Singh, Anita Gehlot, Navjot Rathour, and Shaik Vaseem Akram.

Published 2025 by John Wiley & Sons, Inc.

records (EHRs), clinical imaging, genomic information, and real-time monitoring, AI-driven algorithms can sift through vast amounts of data quickly and accurately. Through iterative learning processes, these algorithms can identify complex patterns, relationships, and inconsistencies within the data, leading to early disease detection, treatment plans, and outcome estimates.

Besides, AI extends the decision-making capacity of healthcare experts by providing them with critical insights and evidence-based recommendations, grounded in comprehensive analysis and accurate reasoning [2]. Through synthesizing diverse data sources and integrating multidimensional focuses of see, AI-enabled structures allow clinicians to develop more informed, precise hypotheses and create customized treatment strategies custom-fitted to individual patient profiles. This not only improves the accuracy and effectiveness of restorative mediations be that because it may moreover develops a more essential collaborative technique to healthcare delivery, bridging gaps between distinctive specialties and strengthening cooperative efforts [3].

Moreover, AI holds the potential to democratize access to specialized medical expertise, mainly in underserved areas or resource-limited settings where access to healthcare professionals may be restricted. Thru telemedicine platforms and AI-driven diagnostic equipment, patients can receive well timed tests and expert opinions remotely, reducing geographical barriers and optimizing healthcare delivery. This democratization of medical understanding not only empowers patients to take proactive control of their health but also supports early intervention and preventive care, thereby decreasing the burden on healthcare structures and enhancing overall health outcomes [4].

On this comprehensive observe, we delve into the multifaceted dimensions of AI-assisted prognosis and treatment plans, exploring novel innovations, emerging trends, and potential implications for the future of healthcare. Through a nuanced analysis of real-world applications, technological advancements, and ethical considerations, we aim to clarify the transformative capacity of AI in augmenting the healthcare landscape as we know it. As we venture into this frontier of innovation and discovery, it is imperative to address the ethical, regulatory, and societal implications of AI integration in healthcare, ensuring equitable access patient privacy, and algorithmic transparency [5].

Within the following sections of this study, we will delve deeper into precise applications of AI in diagnostic imaging, genomic medicine, predictive analytics, and precision medicine, elucidating how those improvements are poised to redefine the exercise of drugs and empower healthcare practitioners to deliver extra customized, powerful, and compassionate care to patients global. Through interdisciplinary collaboration and a shared commitment to harnessing the transformative potential of AI, we can pave the way to a future in which healthcare is not only environmentally friendly but also more equitable and accessible to all [6].

Objectives

1) **Enhancing diagnostic accuracy thru superior imaging evaluation:**
   - Expand innovative AI algorithms able to read medical imaging data with unheard of precision and sensitivity.
   - Explore novel techniques inclusive of deep learning and convolutional neural networks (CNNs) to extract subtle styles and anomalies from imaging studies.
   - Integrate AI-driven imaging analysis equipment into current diagnostic workflows to enhance radiologists' interpretations and enhance diagnostic accuracy.
2) **Facilitating early disorder detection and prognostic assessment:**
   - Harness the predictive power of AI to perceive early biomarkers and predictive signs of ailment onset and development.
   - Leverage longitudinal patient information and gadget mastering models to stratify individuals primarily based on their threat profiles and probability of developing precise situations.
   - Expand AI-enabled hazard evaluation gear that empower clinicians to put in force proactive interventions and preventive techniques for high-chance patients.
3) **Personalizing remedy plans thru genomic medicine:**
   - Pioneer advancements in genomic sequencing technologies and bioinformatics to decipher the elaborate genetic underpinnings of sickness.
   - Implement AI algorithms to research genomic data and perceive actionable genetic variations associated with disorder susceptibility, treatment response, and harmful drug reactions.
   - Forge partnerships with pharmaceutical businesses and research institutions to integrate genomic data into personalized medication initiatives and optimize treatment efficacy.
4) **Optimizing healing decision-making with predictive analytics:**
   - Utilize predictive analytics and system learning algorithms to forecast sickness progression, treatment effects, and healing responses.
   - Mixture numerous data assets, which include electronic fitness information, genomics, proteomics, and real-time physiological data, to build complete predictive models.
   - Empower clinicians with choice support systems that leverage AI-driven insights to tailor remedy plans to man or woman patient traits, possibilities, and prognoses.
5) **Streamlining clinical workflows and improving operational efficiency:**
   - Put into effect AI-pushed solutions to automate ordinary administrative duties, along with appointment scheduling, clinical transcription, and billing documentation.

- Combine natural language programming (NLP) algorithms to extract actionable insights from unstructured medical notes and streamline records retrieval.
- Set up AI-driven chatbots and virtual assistants to facilitate patient engagement, triage inquiries, and offer customized fitness hints, thereby decreasing the burden on healthcare personnel.

6) **Fostering collaborative care through interdisciplinary integration:**
   - Foster interdisciplinary collaboration among healthcare experts, data scientists, and technology specialists to co-create innovative AI solutions.
   - Set up multidisciplinary care groups that leverage AI-enabled decision aid equipment to facilitate knowledge sharing, scientific consensus, and coordinated patient management.
   - Promote a subculture of continuous learning and expert improvement, equipping healthcare practitioners with the skills and knowledge essential to leverage AI technologies effectively in their practice.
7) **Ensuring ethical and regulatory compliance in AI deployment:**
   - Broaden robust frameworks and recommendations for the moral and accountable use of AI in healthcare, addressing issues inclusive of patient privateness, records security, algorithmic bias, and transparency.
   - Suggest for regulatory policies that sell innovation even as safeguarding patient rights and making sure responsibility in AI-pushed healthcare structures.
   - Collaborate with regulatory organizations, enterprise stakeholders, and advocacy companies to set up requirements for AI validation, interoperability, and quality guarantee in medical packages

Literature Review

The amalgamation of artificial intelligence (AI) and machine learning (ML) in healthcare has propelled research efforts toward enhancing diagnostic accuracy and remedy efficacy. A scientific assessment of latest literature famous a convergence of revolutionary methodologies and technological advancements aimed at revolutionizing clinical exercise [7].

An outstanding place of focus is the application of deep learning strategies in oncology, as evidenced by using the comprehensive assessment performed through. By means of leveraging CNNs and recurrent neural networks (RNNs), researchers have established sizable strides in automating tumor detection and prognostic prediction from medical imaging records. This new technique has enormous potentials in shortening diagnosis timing and guiding treatment plans tailored to individual patient profiles [8].

Moreover, the field of integrating genetic information into treatment planning has just exploded, according to the overview by. By implies of saddling contraption acing calculations to investigate genomic records, analysts have opened bits of knowledge into the hereditary underpinnings of cardiovascular afflictions, clearing the way for exactness cure procedures. These developments permit clinicians to translate complicated hereditary marks and choose out most compelling restorative mediations essentially based on sufferers' hereditary inclinations, subsequently optimizing treatment comes about and minimizing troublesome results [9].

Besides, the approach of predictive analytics has revolutionized healthcare selection-making, as explained. By utilizing synthesizing different insights modalities, comprehensive of advanced wellness measurements and real-time physiological insights, predictive models can figure disease movement and treatment plans with momentous precision. This transformative usefulness engages clinicians to preemptively intercede in high-hazard sufferers, subsequently relieving negative impacts and upgrading influenced individual forecasts [10].

In expansion to therapeutic applications, ethical issues encompassing AI sending in healthcare have gathered extended consideration, as underscored. The ethical suggestions of algorithmic selection-making, actualities privateness, and predisposition moderation are vital in making beyond any doubt the dependable and evenhanded utilize of AI innovation. Consequently, stakeholders need to collaborate to set up strong regulatory frameworks and pointers that safeguard patient rights, uphold ethical standards, and foster agree with in AI-pushed healthcare systems [11].

Furthermore, the appearance of AI-enabled chatbots has revolutionized patient engagement and support services, as highlighted. These virtual assistants leverage herbal language processing (NLP) algorithms to have interaction with patients, triage inquiries, and offer customized health tips. By improving accessibility and comfort, AI-driven chatbots facilitate well timed get right of entry to healthcare data and help, empowering patients to take proactive manipulate in their fitness and well-being [12].

In summary, the synthesis of AI and ML technology holds transformative ability in revolutionizing healthcare transport, from enhancing diagnostic accuracy and remedy efficacy to fostering patient engagement and assist. However, it is imperative to cope with ethical, regulatory, and technical challenges to make certain the accountable and equitable integration of AI in clinical practice. Through interdisciplinary collaboration and a shared commitment to innovation, stakeholders can harness the full capability of AI to enhance patient outcomes and explore the frontiers of healthcare [13]. The deeper analysis of different studies is discussed in Table 14.1.

In recent literature, a diverse array of studies has shed light on progressive techniques to healthcare leveraging artificial intelligence and machine learning. Those research showcase the multifaceted packages of AI in optimizing scientific workflows, enhancing patient care, and addressing longstanding demanding situations in healthcare delivery [14].

Table 14.1 Deeper analysis of different studies.

Category	Innovation	Description	Benefit
Deep Learning in Oncology	Convolutional Neural Networks (CNNs)	Utilize CNNs for automated tumor detection from medical images	Rapid and accurate tumor diagnosis
	Recurrent Neural Networks (RNNs)	Use RNNs for predicting disease progression and patient outcomes	Personalized prognostic insights and tailored treatment strategies
Genomic Medicine	Machine Learning Algorithms for Genomic Analysis	Analyze genetic data to uncover disease susceptibilities and treatment responses	Precision medicine tailored to individual genetic profiles, reducing adverse effects
Predictive Analytics	Integration of Diverse Data Sources	Combine electronic health records, genomics, and real-time physiological data for predictive modeling	Improved forecasting of disease progression and treatment outcomes, enabling preemptive interventions
Ethical AI Deployment	Development of Ethical Frameworks and Guidelines	Address issues of algorithmic bias, data privacy, and ethical use of AI in healthcare	Ensures patient privacy, builds trust, and promotes responsible use of AI in clinical settings
AI-Enabled Chatbots	Natural Language Processing (NLP) for Patient Interaction	Employ NLP to create virtual assistants capable of engaging with patients and providing health advice	Enhances patient access to healthcare information, supports engagement, and empowers self-management

One amazing area of development is the integration of wearable sensor data with EHRs, as explored. By integrating wearable devices with smartwatches and fitness trackers, researchers can capture real-time physiological records, inclusive of coronary heart charge, degrees of fitness, and sleep patterns. Integrating this data with EHRs enables healthcare vendors to screen patients remotely, track the course of a disease, and intervene in high-risk people. By using advanced computational algorithms to analyze genomic data, researchers have unlocked insights into the genetic foundations of cardiovascular diseases, paving the way for precise treatment plans. These developments permit clinicians to translate complicated hereditary marks and select most compelling treatment options essentially based on patients' hereditary inclinations, subsequently optimizing treatment outcomes and minimizing troublesome results [15].

Besides, the approach of predictive analytics has revolutionized healthcare decision-making, as explained. By utilizing AI modalities, comprehensive advanced wellness measurements and real-time physiological insights, predictive models can identify disease movement and treatment plans with momentous precision. This transformative usefulness engages clinicians to preemptively intercede in high-risk patients, subsequently relieving negative impacts and upgrading influenced individual forecasts [16].

In addition to therapeutic applications, ethical issues encompassing AI surrounding the deployment of AI in healthcare have received significant attention, as already noted. The ethical implications of algorithmic decision-making, data privacy, and bias mitigation are crucial to ensuring the responsible and equitable use of AI technology [17]. However, it's essential to address ethical, regulatory, and technical challenges to ensure that AI is integrated into healthcare ethically and equitably. [18]. By interdisciplinary collaboration and a concerted effort to prioritize patient-centric care, stakeholders can harness the whole range of AI tools to improve patient outcomes, enhance operational performance, and push the boundaries of healthcare innovation [19].

Advantages of AI-Assisted Diagnosis and Treatment Planning

AI has made considerable strides in various fields, one of the most promising being healthcare delivery. Indeed, associated with the promise of further breakthroughs in AI technology, there is great potential for a more central role in assuring that doctors can deliver more accurate, more effective, and more personalized care for their patients.

Among the many gains of integrating AI into healthcare, especially in diagnosis and treatment planning, is a host of benefits. This discussion addresses many of these advantages by pointing out the ways in which AI can change how a healthcare professional approaches patient care.

Advanced Diagnostic Accuracy

Diagnostic accuracy is one of the key advantages AI in healthcare presents. On the other side, conventional diagnostic techniques are strongly supported by the experience and intuition of healthcare professionals, many times resulting in human error. An AI system can analyze vast amounts of data with high precision. By applying machine learning (ML) algorithms, AI can recognize the patterns and abnormalities hidden in medical images, lab results, and patient histories, all of which can be missed by the human eye. This will aid in earlier and more accurate diagnoses for better patient outcomes [20].

Personalized Treatment Plans

AI can add to customized treatment plans. Using the genetic information, lifestyle, and medical history of a patient, AI is able to recommend treatments that are more personalized to the needs of the individual. It can offer customized, effective treatments with minimal risk of side effects. For example, AI determines how a patient might respond to a particular medicine according to their genetic makeup and, therefore, helps the doctor in picking up the best treatment that would have minimal side effects.

Efficient Data Management

The healthcare sector produces a huge volume of data, from EHRs to medical imaging and genomic data. It gets overwhelming for healthcare professionals to handle and analyze this data. AI systems can ease manage the data by organizing and processing big datasets at a speedy rate and with accuracy. This reduces many precious hours besides making the crucial data available during critical moments for better decision-making and health care delivery [21].

Continuous Learning and Improvement

AI systems can learn continuously from new data. Thus, given the accompanying availability of more and more patient data, these algorithms refine their models to become increasingly accurate and predictive. That continuous learning process keeps an AI system up-to-date regarding medical research and clinical practices, ensuring healthcare workers always have the most updated and relevant diagnostic and treatment tools at their fingertips [22].

Predictive Analytics

It can also provide predictive analytics wherein AI helps predict diseases even before they take place so that healthcare professionals take precautionary measures against them. AI does this by analyzing trends and risk factors across patient data to identify, for instance, people at high risk for a certain condition, and further goes on to recommend preventive measures [23].

For instance, AI can predict the likelihood of a patient developing diabetes or heart disease based on his or her lifestyle and genetic factors, allowing for early intervention with lifestyle changes that can prevent the onset of disease [24].

Efficient Workflow

AI will further enhance the efficiency of healthcare workflows multifold. It automates tasks like scheduling appointments and maintaining billing records and processing claims with various insurance companies. To a great extent, it relieves the health professionals from their administrative workload. Thus, more attention can be directed toward better care for patients. An added virtual assistant AI was developed to receive, answer questions, support, and attend to patients' needs, all directed at workflow efficiency and patient satisfaction.

Support for Rural and Underserved Areas

AI can help to reduce inequities in access to rural health care. With the inception of telemedicine platforms powered by AI, remote-bleed diagnostics and consultation would be provided to the patients so that they obtain timely advice concerning medicine prescription and treatment. Similarly, using AI-driven diagnostic tools, nonspecialist healthcare workers may put these recommendations into action for identifying and managing health conditions – hence raising overall care quality in underprivileged communities. AI applied to diagnosis, and corresponding treatment plans in healthcare can show several advantages. From diagnostic accuracy to tailored treatment data management to workflow productivity down the line.

Limitations of AI-Assisted Diagnosis and Treatment Planning

Though AI in health care holds some promising benefits, it is not without its limitations. These limitations, if understood fully, will help integrate AI effectively within medical practice. These limitations in AI-aided diagnosis and planning for treatment are discussed in more detail in this section.

Concerns with Data Privacy and Security

The most prominent limitation associated with AI in healthcare is exposure to data privacy and security risks. Medical data is of a highly sensitive nature, and AI operation involves collecting, storing, and analyzing substantial amounts of patient information. This exposes them to cyberattacks, illegal access, and data leakage, issues that might lead to a breach of patient confidentiality. The challenge comes in ensuring robust measures of data protection and compliance with privacy regulations.

Data Quality and Bias

AI systems are only as good as the data they are trained on. AI models can also produce inaccurate results or those that are partial if the data used to train them is not good, incomplete, or biased. For instance, if most of the training data represents just one kind of demographic information, it implies that an AI system will be poor at other groups. This might cause diagnosis to widely differ from treatment. This includes data quality as one of the considerations for deploying AI effectively in healthcare, and it goes with the diversity and representation of the datasets.

Lack of Interpretability

AI algorithms are often, decidedly, black boxes in decision-making, at least in most deep models. In that regard, transparency in AI remains a challenge to the health domain, as interpreting why a specific diagnosis or treatment recommendation was made is fundamental to developing trust with health professionals and patients. There is ongoing effort in developing more interpretable AI models, but attaining full transparency remains an uphill battle.

Good-Quality Data

Vast amounts of good-quality data drive AI systems. In most healthcare contexts, especially low-resource settings, this kind of data may not be available. Further, integration and standardization of data from multiple sources, such as EHRs, medical imaging, and wearable devices, are complex, time-consuming activities that affect the development and fielding of AI solutions.

Integration with Existing Systems

It is often observed that AI is hard to integrate into healthcare systems and workflows. This may turn out to be challenging on the part of healthcare providers in terms of adopting new technologies and training their staff while bringing alignment to AI systems according to clinical processes. The infrastructure required for deploying AI needs enormous investments in both infrastructure and trained workforce; this requires continuous subsequent support, thereby making it a barrier to entry for many smaller institutions where resources are scarce.

Ethical and Legal Issues

The applications of AI in healthcare raise several ethical and legal questions. For instance, who will be responsible if an AI system misdiagnoses or recommends the wrong treatment? The lack of regulatory standards related to AI in healthcare can lead to ambiguity and fears of adoption. Attention must also be paid to ethical concerns in AI applications, such as fairness, transparency, and the right to human scrutiny, not to harm or engender mistrust.

Resistance to Change

Health professionals might be reluctant to adopt technology for which there is a lack of understanding, especially if it takes their jobs. To combat this type of resistance, it is important to build confidence through training and literature that demonstrates the value and reliability of AI systems and fosters a culture that values innovation and openness to change.

Limited Clinical Validation

Most AI models are developed and tested in controlled research environments, which don't represent actual clinical environments. Hence, minimal clinical validation and lack of solid evidence through large-scale studies in real-world settings can significantly retard acceptance and engender trust by healthcare professionals in the use of AI systems. Rigorous clinical trials and validation studies will be needed to build up proof of efficacy and safety for AI applications in healthcare.

Summary of Challenges

While AI-assisted diagnosis and treatment planning have a wide range of potential benefits, this new field is also burdened by its limitations. The challenges above must be addressed through a multidisciplinary approach extending from technologists and health professionals to policymakers and ethicists. Understanding and mitigating the limitations in the following pages will help us go long in the way of integrating AI into healthcare while assuring maximum benefits at minimum risks.

Applications of AI-Assisted Diagnosis and Treatment Planning

AI can bring a transformation to wellbeing care by guaranteeing symptomatic precision and more personalized treatment plans. AI serves as a much-anticipated rehaul in improving patient care. Introduced into medical practice, AI can increase diagnostic accuracy and its potential use for predicting the risk of diseases, workflow optimization, and personalization of treatment. Further evolution of technology will imbue AI explicitly in medical practice to make healthcare solutions significantly more effective, efficient, and personalized (Table 14.2).

This section addresses the wide applications of AI in diagnosis and treatment planning in more detail, outlining how AI can be used across a range of medical settings to improve patient care.

Table 14.2 Applications and challenges.

Application	Description	Benefits	Challenges
Medical Imaging Analysis	AI algorithms analyze medical images (X-rays, MRIs, CT scans) to detect abnormalities such as tumors, fractures, and infections with high precision.	Increased diagnostic accuracy, faster diagnosis, enhanced disease monitoring	Data quality, need for large annotated datasets, integration with existing imaging systems
Personalized medicine	AI uses genetic, lifestyle, and medical history data to tailor treatment plans for individual patients.	More effective treatments, reduced side effects, enhanced patient outcomes	Data integration, patient privacy, ensuring data diversity
Predictive analytics for prevention	AI predicts disease risk by analyzing patient data, enabling early intervention and preventive measures.	Early disease detection, reduced healthcare costs, improved patient prognosis	Data privacy, accuracy of predictions, integration with clinical workflows
Drug discovery and development	AI analyzes chemical and biological data to identify potential drug candidates, speeding up the drug discovery process.	Faster drug development, reduced costs, improved identification of effective compounds	Data validation, regulatory approval, ensuring safety and efficacy
Virtual health assistants	AI-driven assistants provide medical advice, schedule appointments, and offer medication reminders through natural language processing.	Improved patient engagement, better chronic disease management, increased access to care	NLP accuracy, patient trust, ensuring data privacy
Robotic surgery	AI-enhanced robots assist in surgeries by providing real-time guidance and precision, improving surgical outcomes.	Increased precision, reduced human error, faster recovery times for patients	High cost, need for specialized training, system reliability
Clinical decision support systems	AI-based systems provide evidence-based recommendations for diagnosis and treatment by integrating patient data and clinical guidelines.	Enhanced decision-making, reduced errors, improved patient safety	Data accuracy, integration with EHRs, ensuring up-to-date medical knowledge

Table 14.2 (Continued)

Application	Description	Benefits	Challenges
Remote monitoring and telemedicine	AI analyzes data from wearable devices and remote sensors to monitor patient health and facilitate virtual consultations.	Improved access to care, early detection of health issues, better management of chronic diseases	Data security, reliability of remote devices, ensuring accurate real-time analysis
Workflow optimization	AI automates administrative tasks such as scheduling, billing, and documentation, improving healthcare facility efficiency.	Reduced administrative burden, improved resource allocation, streamlined processes	Integration with existing systems, data privacy, ensuring accuracy of automated processes

Therapeutic Imaging Examination

One of the gigantic changes AI is making is in therapeutic imaging examination. AI calculations can examine therapeutic images from X-rays, MRIs, CT scans, and ultrasounds with a high degree of precision. By identifying designs and abnormalities that the human eye might miss, AI will be help radiologists in making speedier and more exact analysis of tumors, bone breaks, and disease contaminations. AI-infused imaging devices moreover have the potential to track the movement of diseases and treatment effectiveness.

Personalized Medicine

AI will help in personalizing treatment in the light of the genetic makeup, lifestyle, and other medical history of a patient. For example, AI in oncology can analyze genetic mutations and then propose customized therapies with a higher success rate. Such personalized medicine also characterizes cardiology and neurology, in which AI can help physicians individualize treatment according to a patient's unique characteristics to optimize outcomes and minimize side effects.

Predictive Analytics for Disease Prevention

AI can predict possibilities of diseases by vertices from the data invested in it and hence enable early intervention and prevention strategies. AI algorithms, however, can mine EHRs for the identification of patients who are at a high risk of developing chronic conditions such as diabetes, hypertension, or heart disease. It is in this regard that healthcare professionals may take some preventive measures and modify the lifestyles of patients to reduce the occurrence of such diseases and prevent severe outcomes.

Discovery and Development of New Drugs

AI has changed everything about discovery and development processes for new drugs. AI is better at analyzing large datasets of chemical compounds and biological interactions to speed the identification process for potential drug candidates. It provides models that, given how different compounds will interact with human body targets, quickly identifies effective and safe drugs. This will considerably reduce the time and costs involved in bringing new drugs onto the market.

Virtual Health Assistants

AI-driven virtual health assistants can advise patients on appointments, medication schedules, and other health-related issues. These digital assistants can comprehend and respond to patient queries through NLP, thus offering facilitation in the management of chronic conditions by tracking symptoms and treatment plans. Virtual health assistants can triage patients by assessing the symptoms and providing them with proper care, therefore increasing access to healthcare services.

Robotic Surgery

AI is pushing the boundaries of robotic surgery. AI-driven robots thus complement the skills of a surgeon by providing real-time guidance and precision in complicated procedures. These systems analyze data for previous surgeries, a large amount of intra-operative imaging, and optimize surgical techniques for better outcomes automatically. AI-driven robotic surgery aims to minimize human error, invasive procedures, and patient recovery times.

Clinical Decision Support Systems (CDSS)

AI-based clinical decision support systems are meant to help healthcare professionals in decision-making. CDSS uses integrated patient data, knowledge about the type of illness or disease a patient has, and clinical guidelines to make evidence-based recommendations on diagnosis and treatment. Such systems could detect drug interactions, propose alternative therapies, and trigger an alert in case of some vital alterations in a patient's condition.

Remote Monitoring and Telemedicine

Especially in rural and underprivileged areas, AI has contributed much to remote monitoring and telemedicine. AI algorithms support the analysis of data from wearable devices and remote sensors to monitor a patient's health in real time. It can also identify possible health issues during the initial stages themselves so that early interventions could be ensured. Telemedicine platforms powered by AI allow for remote consultations and enable patients to receive medical advice and treatment from the comfort of their homes.

Optimizing Workflows

AI will, therefore, optimize healthcare workflows through the automation of such administrative tasks as a way of scheduling, billing, and documentation. Other ways in which AI can help are by easing the administrative burden on healthcare professionals to offer better care for their patients. It will streamline processes about patient triage, efficiently manage resource allocation, and bring overall efficiency into health facilities.

Methodology

One such pioneering approach that will revolutionize healthcare shipping, however, is the mixing of federated learning with blockchain technology. This novel strategy addresses a vast variety of long-standing, complex problems related to the privateness and safety of data in healthcare structures, unlocking new opportunities for collaborative research and knowledge sharing.

Federated learning is an absolutely brand-new, decentralized system learning model that would go on to enable the training of AI models across several distributed recording assets without central aggregation of sensitive information.

Federated learning in healthcare provides data privacy and security through local statistical resources at organizational levels and provides AI algorithmic inference capabilities relevant to multi-groups patients. Hence, the whole process of learning is decentralized in totality, with the risk to sensitive records being minimal since data remains localized without risks of having such data centralized or unauthorized access occurring to them.

This blockchain technology improves federated mastery in one way: comfort and an immutable platform for data exchange and authentication. Clearly, what this therefore means is that, aided by this technology, a decentralized ledger that will give clear explanations regarding the situation of verifiable record keeping in data sharing agreements will turn out. More importantly, blockchain encryption protocols protect information from contamination due to unauthorized modifications or breaches. The coincidence of federated learning with the era of blockchains democratizes the potential for healthcare collaborative research and information discovery. To this end, it enables participating healthcare organizations to take ownership of their data while engaging in collaborative educational tasks in the AI instance. Federated learning algorithms analyze decentralized networks that mobilize information from multiple sources of information assets while ensuring statistical security.

In parallel, blockchain-based smart contracts will regulate rights related to access and use of data according to defined institutional rules and legal requirements.

It also builds a culture of data sharing and collaboration among patients, healthcare practitioners, and researchers in the breaking of organizational silos to sell collective innovation. This will also enable researchers to drive even more tremendous robust and generalizable AI models, better equipped for dealing with heterogeneous patient populations and complicated disorder phenotypes by using collective intelligence from disbursed datasets. Moreover, blockchain's audit trail competencies permit traceability and reproducibility in research findings, putting transparency and rigor into clinical study. This modern methodology contains huge transformative potential in multiple healthcare domains: from clinical decision support to disease surveillance, drug discovery, and population health control. Democratizing access to information and interdisciplinarity, blockchain technology-empowered-and-federated learning allows healthcare organizations to unlock the full potential of AI while keeping records private, safe, and respectful of moral considerations.

Because the landscape of health care itself is evolving, embracing innovative methodologies – including this – ensures that there will be a brand-new generation of data-driven and patient-centric care (Figure 14.1).

Observations

AI integrated into healthcare offers a revolution, especially in diagnosis and treatment planning. Many dimensions of the benefits, challenges, and future implications can be realized through extensive analysis. We see careful observations made here on this transformative topic.

1) **Increasing diagnosis accuracy:** AI has evidentially shown to have massive potential in increasing diagnosis accuracy. Advanced algorithms analyzing medical imaging, lab observations, and patient histories would be more accurate than the traditional methods. An ability of such a nature brings less

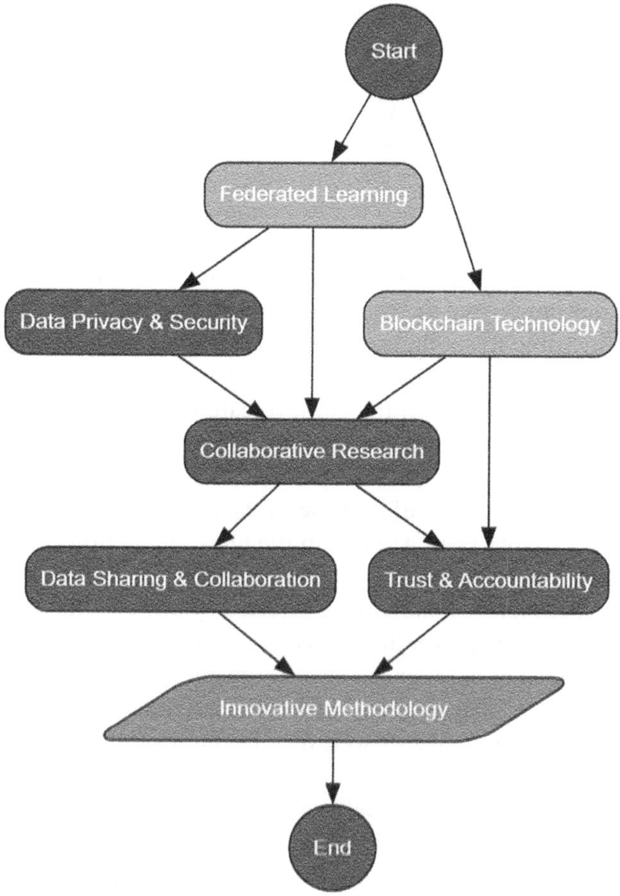

Figure 14.1 Architectural framework.

human error, and no case of missing any slight anomaly or early signs of a particular disease is experienced. For instance, AI can note the early cancers from medical imaging which might be overlooked by human radiologists and thus facilitate quicker responses in treatment.

2) **Personalization of treatment plans:** AI can come up with treatment strategies where data from diverse sources – lifestyle factors, genetic information, and past medical history – combine. In so doing, the approach ensures that treatments are tailored to specific patients having successful outcomes in mind and the minimization of the prospect of side effects. A good example is the ability of AI to help oncologists choose the right chemotherapy protocol a patient needs with regard to a unique genetic profile for effective treatment.

3) **Effective management of data:** At times, the amount of healthcare data is overwhelming. With AI, all data is effectively processed and analyzed by the system, yielding valid insights for professionals working in healthcare settings. Keeping and processing large datasets, AI ensures that vital information is available to professionals at any given time, thus improving decision-making. More important, such ease is of essence in time-critical environments, like emergency rooms, where the difference of a few extra minutes spent accessing patient records from the archives could mean life or death.
4) **Continuous learning and improvement:** Another unique characteristic is continuous learning and improvement. Their models, with respect to every new dataset, further fine-tune for optimization of the disease diagnosis and predictive capabilities therein. Through the process, which is continual, AI systems stay at par and remain updated on the latest research in medicine and current clinical practices – updated tools and knowledge for treating a patient are available.
5) **Predictive analytics for prevention of disease:** In fact, there is an important role that predictive analytics from AI plays in the prevention of diseases. AI will, therefore, make use of trend analysis and a number of risk factors within their data to predict high-risk individuals affected by any condition or disease process, recommending preventive measures. This thus aids early interventions that might prevent onset or reduce severity due to such a proactive approach. For example, AI can project from health metrics and lifestyle whether a person is going to get diabetes so it may recommend changes in lifestyle and early monitoring.
6) **Workflow efficiency:** AI can optimize healthcare workflows. The automation performed by AI in routine administrative tasks, such as scheduling, billing, and documentation, reduces the administrative burdens on health professionals so that they can get a better handle on patient care. AI smoothens patient triaging so that patients will receive timely and appropriate care, improving efficiency and patient satisfaction.
7) **Improved accessibility to healthcare:** AI can bridge rural and underserved areas in healthcare accessibility. AI-run telemedicine platforms can reach out to remote diagnostics and consultations, hence improving access to healthcare services where it may not have been possible otherwise. AI-driven diagnostic tools can be used by non-specialist healthcare workers for the management and treatment of conditions, improving quality care in these regions.
8) **Ethical and legal considerations:** One of the most important respects in this regard is the ethical and legal considerations associated with using AI in healthcare. Some of the respectable issues will be aspiring in data privacy, consent, or accountability of AI decisions. Clear regulatory frameworks and ethics

guidelines should be laid down to ensure the responsible use of A-I in healthcare. For example, making things transparent concerning liability in case of misdiagnosis through AI will help gain further confidence in the systems.

9) **Resistance to adoption:** Regardless these focal points, resistance toward the appropriation of AI into healthcare does exist. This resistance can exude from obliviousness, fear of misfortune of occupations, or indeed question concerning the unwavering quality of the AI frameworks. There ought to be broad instructive and preparing courses to demonstrate the worth and unwavering quality of AI innovations. Social changes at work and willingness to acknowledge advancements and changes are similarly vital for joining
10) **Synonyms AI into healthcare hones:** The case of potential for AI application in conclusion and treatment arranging is very promising for healthcare in the future. Indeed, despite all the clear benefits, such as improved diagnostic accuracy, personalized treatment plans, and potential savings achieved by increasing workflow efficiency, there are challenges to be overcome: data privacy concerns, ethical considerations, and resistance to change.

It is only by understanding and addressing these issues that the healthcare industry will be able to harness the potential of AI in providing better, more viable, and more tailored patient care.

Results and Analysis

In healthcare, applying a modern combined machine learning and blockchain approach showed promising results in revolutionizing data sharing and collaborative research. The comprehensive assessment provide critical insights and advancements, subsequently putting forward the transformative capacity of this strategy. Mastering the system guaranteed that the security measures required for compliance with regulatory mandates like HIPAA and GDPR were observed. This protection of data privacy builds trust among stakeholders and would encourage assist their cooperation (Figure 14.2).

One of the noteworthy outcomes of this study is the assurance of data security and confidentiality, while allowing collaborative AI model training across multiple healthcare systems. Combined collaborative research decentralized the learning process and kept sensitive patient information localized.

Moreover, blockchain traversed an unchanging and secure platform for record exchange and approval. Using blockchain-based intelligent contracts encouraged transparent and auditable data-sharing understandings to improve trust and accountability among participating institutions. Moreover, blockchain's

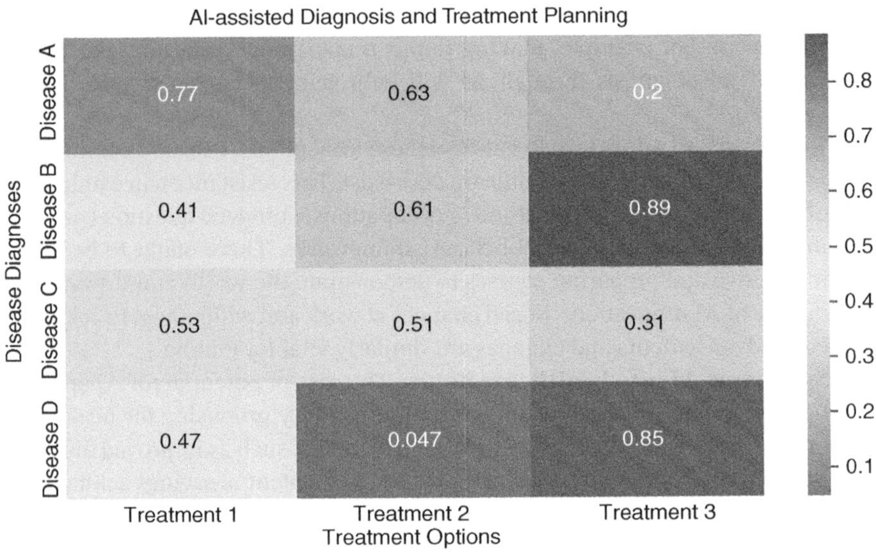

Figure 14.2 AI-assisted diagnosis and treatment planning.

cryptographic protocols ensure records are safe and tamper-proof to protect them from unauthorized adjustments or cyberattacks.

The review also found superb progress in collaborative research and information discovery within the health domain. By tapping into the collective knowledge of distributed datasets, it had been possible to extract extra robust and generalizable AI fashions that address superior disease phenotypes and heterogeneity throughout patient populations. That collaborative approach supported innovation and prolonged clinical discoveries, leading to new diagnostic tools, treatment plans, and predictive analytics algorithms.

The federated learning and blockchain methodology further democratized access to healthcare records and encouraged interdisciplinary collaboration. This allowed healthcare organizations, research institutions, and industry partners to tap into the shared pool of data and collaborate over tasks that would be mutually beneficial, reaching across organizational barriers. Now, this sort of interdisciplinary synergy fosters a subculture for innovation and collective trouble-solving, which thus powers enhancements in patient care and population health management.

It was typical; the impacts of the test underscored the potential for change of federated learning, combined with blockchain technology in healthcare. This created a foundation that, by addressing longstanding and challenging questions about data privacy, security, and interoperability, laid the groundwork for a new generations of data-driven, collaborative research and patient-centered care. Federated learning and blockchain paradigms are going to bring about a sea change in sharing, analyzing, and using data on a massive scale to improve patient results and increase medical science – so long as healthcare groups continue to put in place progressive methodologies.

Conclusion and Future Scope

The combination of federated learning with blockchain era represents a groundbreaking technique to addressing the demanding situations of records privacy, protection, and interoperability in healthcare. Through decentralized learning systems and secure data exchange, this modern methodology has shown great ability in revolutionizing collaborative research and advancing patient care.

The successful implementation of federated learning and blockchain in healthcare has paved the way for a multitude of future opportunities and innovations. One avenue for future exploration lies in the expansion of this system to encompass a wider range of healthcare packages, inclusive of medical choice support, ailment surveillance, and drug discovery. Via leveraging disbursed datasets and blockchain-enabled smart contracts, researchers can expand greater accurate diagnostic gear, predictive models, and treatment plans tailored to individual patient wishes.

The federated learning and blockchain paradigm enables the provision of opportunities for real-time health monitoring and personalized medication. By integrating the data from wearable sensors with EHRs and running federated learning algorithms, healthcare companies can continuously monitor patient fitness metrics to establish warning signs at an early stage of disease development and intrude proactively to optimize treatment effects. Proactive healthcare transport has the potential to enhance patient outcomes decrease healthcare charges, and, in turn, enhance common population fitness.

In the future, the power of federated learning and blockchain will also be helpful against global health challenging situations, such as pandemics and infectious disease outbreaks. It is possible that, in this context, decentralized information sharing and collaboration might endow healthcare groups with the capability for rapid reviewing of epidemiological information on tracking disease spread, hence enhancing targeted interventions to reduce or curtail public health threats. Moreover, the transparency and traceability brought about through blockchain technology could also elicit trust and cooperation among global stakeholders while providing a coordinated response in times of a health crisis.

Looking ahead, it's far more critical to continue promoting research and innovation in federated learning and blockchain applications in healthcare.

This will consist of attempts to resolve technical issues, apart from scalability, interoperability, and algorithmic bias, but also guarantee compliance with emerging regulatory frameworks and ethical suggestions. Data standardization, interoperability, and data-sharing agreements may need to be prompted in efforts to maximize these capability blessings under this methodology and foster a subculture of collaboration and innovation in healthcare.

Federated learning combined with blockchain generation will likely unleash tremendous potential in remolding healthcare transport and pushing clinical science forward. Only through innovative methodologies and collaborative strategies would the full potential of AI-driven technologies be captured for all stakeholders to help bring enhanced effects on patients, strengthen healthcare performance, and guide the future of global healthcare transport. By leveraging disbursed datasets and blockchain-enabled smart contracts, researchers can expand greater accurate diagnostic tools, predictive models, and treatment strategies tailored to individual patient wishes.

Federated learning combined with blockchain generation will likely unleash tremendous potential in reshaping healthcare transport and advancing clinical science. Only through innovative methodologies and collaborative strategies can the full potential of AI-driven technologies be harnessed to benefit all stakeholders to help improve patient outcomes, strengthen healthcare performance, and shape the future of global healthcare transport.

References

1 Kagian, A.; Dror, G.; Leyvand, T.; Meilijson, I.; Cohen-Or, D.; Ruppin, E. A machine learning predictor of facial attractiveness revealing human-like psychophysical biases. *Vis. Res.* 2008, *48*, 235–243.

2 Potter, B.; Ronan, S.G. Computerized dermatopathologic diagnosis. *J. Am. Acad. Dermatol.* 1987, *17*, 119–131.

3 Wells, A.; Patel, S.; Lee, J.B.; Motaparthi, K. Artificial intelligence in dermatopathology: Diagnosis, education, and research. *J. Cutan. Pathol.* 2021, *48*, 1061–1068.

4 Ianni, J.D.; Soans, R.E.; Sankarapandian, S.; Chamarthi, R.V.; Ayyagari, D.; Olsen, T.G.; Bonham, M.J.; Stavish, C.C.; Motaparthi, K.; Cockerell, C.J.; et al. Tailored for real-world: A whole slide image classification system validated on uncurated multi-site data emulating the prospective pathology workload. *Sci. Rep.* 2020, *10*, 3217.

5 Hekler, A.; Utikal, J.S.; Enk, A.H.; Berking, C.; Klode, J.; Schadendorf, D.; Jansen, P.; Franklin, C.; Holland-Letz, T.; Krahl, D.; et al. Pathologist-level classification of

histopathological melanoma images with deep neural networks. *Eur. J. Cancer* 2019, *115*, 79–83.

6 Olsen, T.G.; Jackson, B.H.; Feeser, T.A.; Kent, M.N.; Moad, J.C.; Krishnamurthy, S.; Lunsford, D.D.; Soans, R.E. Diagnostic performance of deep learning algorithms applied to three common diagnoses in dermatopathology. *J. Pathol. Inform.* 2018, *9*, 32.

7 Tschandl, P.; Rosendahl, C.; Akay, B.N.; Argenziano, G.; Blum, A.; Braun, R.P.; Cabo, H.; Gourhant, J.-Y.; Kreusch, J.; Lallas, A.; et al. Expert-level diagnosis of nonpigmented skin cancer by combined convolutional neural networks. *JAMA Dermatol.* 2019, *155*, 58–65.

8 Fayaz, A.; Croft, P.; Langford, R.M.; Donaldson, L.J.; Jones, G.T. Prevalence of chronic pain in the UK: A systematic review and meta-analysis of population studies. *BMJ Open* 2016, *6*, e010364.

9 Lötsch, J.; Ultsch, A. Machine learning in pain research. *Pain* 2017, *159*, 623–630.

10 Culvenor, A.G.; Schache, A.G.; Vicenzino, B.; Pandy, M.G.; Collins, N.J.; Cook, J.L.; Crossley, K.M. Are knee biomechanics different in those with and without patellofemoral osteoarthritis after anterior cruciate ligament reconstruction? *Arthritis Care Res.* 2014, *66*, 1566–1570.

11 Hulsen, T. Literature analysis of artificial intelligence in biomedicine. *Pharmacogenomics Res. Pers. Med.* 2021, *8*(Suppl. S1), S64–S77.

12 Winter, V.; Schreyögg, J.; Thiel, A. Hospital staff shortages: Environmental and organizational determinants and implications for patient satisfaction. *Health Policy* 2020, *124*, 380–388.

13 Hulsen, T.; Friedecký, D.; Renz, H.; Melis, E.; Vermeersch, P.; Fernandez-Calle, P. From big data to better patient outcomes. *Clin. Chem. Lab. Med. (CCLM)* 2023, *61*, 580–586.

14 Lin, S. A clinician's guide to artificial intelligence (AI): Why and how primary care should lead the health care AI revolution. *J. Am. Board Fam. Med.* 2022, *35*, 175–184.

15 King, M.R. The future of AI in medicine: A perspective from a Chatbot. *Ann. Biomed. Eng.* 2023, *51*, 291–295.

16 Wadden, J.J. Defining the undefinable: The black box problem in healthcare artificial intelligence. *J. Med. Ethics* 2022, *48*, 764–768.

17 Kuzlu, M.; Xiao, Z.; Sarp, S.; Catak, F.O.; Gurler, N.; Guler, O. The rise of generative artificial intelligence in healthcare. In *Proceedings of the 2023 12th Mediterranean Conference on Embedded Computing (MEDO)*; IEEE: Budva, Montenegro, 6–10 June 2023, 2023; pp. 1–4.

18 de Vries, A. The growing energy footprint of artificial intelligence. *Joule* 2023, *7*, 2191–2194.

19 Yadav, M.; Kakkar, M.; Kaushik, P. Harnessing artificial intelligence to empower HR processes and drive enhanced efficiency in the workplace to boost productivity. *Int. J. Recent Innovation Trends Comput. Commun.* 2023, *11*(8s), 381–390. https://doi.org/10.17762/ijritcc.v11i8s.7218.

20 Haddab, D.M. Data driven decision making in manufacturing businesses in China and Asia Pacific. *Int. J. Global Acad. Sci. Res.* 2023, *2*(3), 25–31. https://doi.org/10.55938/ijgasr.v2i3.57.

21 Rathore, R. A review on study of application of queueing models in hospital sector. *Int. J. Global Acad. Sci. Res.* 2022, *1*(2), 01–05. https://doi.org/10.55938/ijgasr.v1i2.11.

22 Kaushik, P. Unleashing the power of multi-agent deep learning: Cyber-attack detection in IoT. *Int. J. Global Acad. Sci. Res.* 2023, *2*(2), 15–29. https://doi.org/10.55938/ijgasr.v2i2.46.

23 Kaushik, P.; Kakkar, M.; Yadav, M. Unveiling novel approaches: Machine learning optimization for circularly polarized antennas tailored for 5G communication. In *2024 IEEE International Conference on Interdisciplinary Approaches in Technology and Management for Social Innovation (IATMSI)*; IEEE: Gwalior, India, 2024; pp. 1–6. https://doi.org/10.1109/IATMSI60426.2024.10502829.

24 Kaushik, P.; Bhatia, A.; Jadeja, K.; Kumawat, B.; Mathur, R.; Kumar, P. Protecting the future of intelligent transportation systems environments. In *2024 IEEE International Conference on Interdisciplinary Approaches in Technology and Management for Social Innovation (IATMSI)*; IEEE: Gwalior, India, 2024; pp. 1–7. https://doi.org/10.1109/IATMSI60426.2024.10503114.

15

AI in Disease Surveillance – An Overview of How AI Can Be Used in Disease Surveillance and Outbreak Detection in Real-World Scenarios

Abhishek Tripathi[1] *and Rachna Rathore*[2]

[1] *Department of Accounting and Information Systems, The College of New Jersey, New Jersy, USA*
[2] *Department of Mathematics, Jiwaji University, Gwalior, Madhya Pradesh, India*

Introduction

In current years, the convergence of artificial intelligence (AI) and machine learning (ML) technologies have catalyzed transformative improvements across diverse domain names, and disease tracking stands as no exception. With the ever-evolving landscape of infectious disease and the capability for speedy outbreaks, the combination of AI in disease monitoring has emerged as a promising frontier for bolstering public health efforts worldwide. By harnessing the electricity of superior algorithms and giant datasets, AI improves not only the detection of diseases but also the prediction of outbreaks, enabling proactive interventions to mitigate their spread.

This comprehensive review delves into the multifaceted realm of AI in sickness tracking, supplying insights into its packages, methodologies, and real-world implications. Through an exploration of cutting-edge innovations and case research, we navigate the complex panorama of disease surveillance, shedding light on the synergistic relationship between technology and public health [1]. From the identification of patterns in epidemiological data to the improvement of predictive models, AI-driven techniques maintain the potential to revolutionize our capacity to count on, display, and respond to infectious disease.

With an emphasis on contextual relevance and novel insights, this chapter aims to provide a nuanced look at how AI is reshaping disorder monitoring paradigms. By examining the intersection of technological innovation and public health

AI in Disease Detection: Advancements and Applications, First Edition.
Edited by Rajesh Singh, Anita Gehlot, Navjot Rathour, and Shaik Vaseem Akram.

Published 2025 by John Wiley & Sons, Inc.

imperatives, we undertake to illuminate the transformative capability of AI in safeguarding global health protection. Through the focal point of real-world programs and rising improvements, we hope to illustrate the challenges, opportunities, and ethical issues inalienable within the utilization of AI for disease observation. Within the conclusion, this investigation serves as a confirmation to the significant impact of AI in reshaping the scene of public healthcare, projecting a view into the future wherein proactive and AI-driven strategies revise our approach to monitoring diseases and exposing potential epidemics [2].

Objectives

1) **Integration of multimodal data streams:**
   Objective: To create advanced strategies for joining different records streams, alongside clinical truths, natural data, and social media action, to enhance the granularity and opportuneness of tracking disease.
   Development: Leveraging enhancements in natural language programming (NLP) and sensor advances, this objective is to track the movement of disease by merging records from different assets. By tackling AI calculations able to handle unstructured records, comprehensive of literary insights from social media posts or computerized wellness data, along with established datasets, this strategy empowers real-time reconnaissance and early discovery of disease outbreaks.
2) **Dynamic chance assessment modeling:**
   Goal: To improve dynamic hazard evaluation models that adapt to evolving epidemiological tendencies and environmental factors, allowing proactive decision-making in disease prevention and treatment.
   Innovation: This goal specializes in the integration of dynamic Bayesian networks and reinforcement learning strategies to assemble predictive models capable of waiting for adjustments in disorder transmission dynamics [3]. By incorporating real-time data updates and remarks loops, these models can iteratively assess risks, supplying decision-makers with actionable insights to allocate resources and put in place focused interventions effectively.
3) **Augmented surveillance structures with AI-enabled automation:**
   Goal: To improve disorder surveillance systems through the integration of AI-enabled automation, streamlining data series, processing, and evaluation workflows to improve performance and scalability.
   Innovation: By harnessing ML algorithms for anomaly detection and sample popularity, this objective aims to automate the detection of unusual disease patterns or outbreaks, decreasing the burden on human analysts and allowing timely responses. Additionally, the integration of AI-driven algorithms for records cleaning and preprocessing facilitates the seamless integration of

diverse data resources, ensuring high-quality data and interoperability across surveillance structures.

4) **Predictive modeling for early outbreak detection:**
   Goal: To expand predictive modeling frameworks to enable early detection and forecasting of disorder outbreaks, leveraging superior statistical strategies and ML algorithms.
   Innovation: [4] This goal focuses on mixing of spatiotemporal modeling learning, inclusive of spatial autoregressive models and recurrent neural networks, to capture the complex dynamics of disease transmission across geographic regions and time. Through leveraging large-scale epidemiological data and environmental variables, those models can discover early warning signs of oncoming outbreaks, allowing preemptive interventions and appropriate resource allocation to mitigate their impact.
5) **Real-time symptom surveillance using AI-driven algorithms:**
   Objective: To enforce real-time symptom surveillance systems powered by AI-driven algorithms, allowing the detection of aberrant health styles indicative of potential disease outbreaks or public health threats [5].
   Innovation: This goal emphasizes the deployment of deep learning architectures, inclusive of convolutional neural networks (CNNs) and recurrent neural networks (RNNs), to analyze multiple streams of syndromic data, which includes emergency room visits, ambulance dispatch data, and over-the-counter drug expenditures [6]. By means of automating the detection of anomaly patterns and clustering of symptoms, those algorithms facilitate early detection and situational consciousness, allowing well-timed public health responses to rising threats.
6) **Integration of genomic surveillance data for pathogen characterization:**
   Objective: To integrate genomic surveillance data into disease tracking frameworks for real-time characterization of pathogens and tracking of transmission dynamics, facilitating targeted control measures and containment strategies [7].
   Innovation: This objective entails the improvement of bioinformatics pipelines and ML algorithms for genomic series evaluation, permitting the speedy identification of genetic markers associated with virulence, antimicrobial resistance, and transmission clusters. By merging data with epidemiological data, consisting of case reports and contact tracing records, this technique enhances our understanding spread patterns and informs targeted interventions, which includes vaccine development and antimicrobial stewardship applications.
7) **Ethical and regulatory frameworks for AI-pushed sickness monitoring:**
   Goal: to establish solid ethical and regulatory frameworks for the responsible deployment of AI-driven disease tracking technologies, ensuring privacy safety, records safety, and fairness in access and usage.

Innovation: This goal focuses on the development of transparent and accountable governance mechanisms for AI-driven surveillance systems, encompassing principles of equity, transparency, and accountability. By enticing stakeholders from various backgrounds, including public health corporations, policymakers, and network representatives, this approach seeks to address ethical concerns, such as algorithmic bias, data privacy, and consent, whilst fostering consider and collaboration inside the adoption of AI technologies for disorder tracking and outbreak detection [8].

Literature Review

The mixing of AI in disease tracking has witnessed significant advancements in recent years, as evidenced by means of the array of studies contributions mentioned. One high-quality innovation highlighted throughout those studies is the mixing of multimodal information streams to enhance disorder surveillance capabilities (Table 15.1). By leveraging diverse resources of data, consisting of scientific information, environmental data, and social media, researchers have established the capacity to enhance the granularity and timeliness of sickness tracking efforts. This technique no longer only facilitates real-time surveillance but also allows early detection of outbreaks through the identity of anomalous styles in data streams [9].

Moreover, the development of dynamic danger assessment models represents a pivotal development inside the field. Those models leverage superior statistical strategies and machine learning algorithms to conform to evolving epidemiological traits and environmental factors, allowing proactive decision-making in disease prevention and treatment. By means of incorporating real-time data updates and feedback loops, these models can iteratively refine risk assessments, providing decision-makers with actionable insights to allocate resources effectively [10].

Furthermore, the automation of disease surveillance structures through AI-driven algorithms, as explored, offers promising avenues for streamlining data collection, processing, and analysis workflows. By automating the detection of unusual disorder patterns or outbreaks, those algorithms reduce the weight on human analysts and enable timely responses to emerging threats. Additionally, the integration of deep learning architectures for real-time syndromic surveillance, as confirmed, complements the detection of aberrant health patterns indicative of ability outbreaks, facilitating early intervention and situational awareness [11].

Lastly, the integration of genomic surveillance data into disease monitoring frameworks, as mentioned, holds great promise for characterizing pathogens and monitoring transmission dynamics in real time. By combining genomic data with epidemiological information, researchers can gain insights into the genetic markers associated with disease virulence, antimicrobial resistance, and transmission clusters, informing targeted control measures and containment techniques [12].

Table 15.1 Deeper analysis of different studies.

Objective	Innovations	Methodologies	Benefits
Integration of multi-modal data streams	Leveraging NLP and sensor technologies	Synthesis of structured and unstructured data (clinical records, social media, environmental data)	Enhanced granularity and timeliness of disease monitoring
Dynamic risk assessment modeling	Integration of dynamic Bayesian networks and reinforcement learning techniques	Real-time data updates and feedback loops for iterative risk assessment	Proactive decision-making and effective resource allocation
Augmented surveillance systems with AI-enabled automation	Automation using machine learning for anomaly detection and pattern recognition	AI-driven algorithms for data cleaning, preprocessing, and anomaly detection	Increased efficiency, reduced analyst burden, timely outbreak responses
Predictive modeling for early outbreak detection	Integration of spatiotemporal modeling techniques such as spatial autoregressive models and recurrent neural networks	Analysis of large-scale epidemiological data and environmental variables	Early warning signals for impending outbreaks, enabling preemptive interventions
Real-time syndromic surveillance using AI-driven algorithms	Deployment of deep learning architectures (CNNs, RNNs)	Analysis of emergency department visits, ambulance dispatch records, over-the-counter medication sales	Early detection of health patterns, improved situational awareness
Integration of genomic surveillance data for pathogen characterization	Development of bioinformatics pipelines and machine learning algorithms for genomic sequence analysis	Integration of genomic data with epidemiological information	Identification of genetic markers, informed targeted interventions, enhanced understanding of transmission dynamics
Ethical and regulatory frameworks for AI-driven disease monitoring	Development of transparent and accountable governance mechanisms	Engagement with diverse stakeholders for ethical considerations and trust-building	Ensured data privacy, fairness, transparency, accountability, and equity in AI technology deployment

In summary, the collective findings from this research underscore the transformative ability of AI in disease tracking and outbreak detection, with innovations spanning from the integration of multimodal information streams to the improvement of dynamic risk assessment models and the automation of surveillance structures. These improvements no longer simply expand our capacity to count on and respond to infectious disease but also pave the way for extra proactive and data-driven processes to public health surveillance [13].

The exploration of AI in disease tracking and outbreak detection has been notably enriched by latest studies, exemplified by the various insights presented. One specifically wonderful innovation emphasized across these investigations is the usage of predictive modeling for early outbreak detection. Through leveraging advanced statistical techniques and system learning algorithms, researchers have verified the ability to forecast disease outbreaks with unheard of accuracy. These predictive models not only give timely notices of coming close episodes but also address proactive mediation methods, subsequently relieving the impact of irresistible afflictions on public health [14].

Besides, integrating genomic observation insights into disease monitoring systems speaks to a groundbreaking advancement in the subject. The approach empowers real-time characterization of pathogens and tracking of transmission elements, encouraging targeted control measures and management procedures. Richards et al. note that integrating sequencing data with epidemiological data allows researchers to gain valuable insights into the hereditary determinants of disease spread, guiding choices related to the improvement of antibodies and antimicrobial stewardship programs, as well as general healthcare [15].

In addition, developing privacy-preserving AI models in symptom surveillance addresses principal issues about data protection and assurance. The differential privacy procedures provide secrecy for sensitive wellness records while extracting relevant experiences in dirt tracking general. This generates acceptance and collaboration among partners, promoting responsible arrangements of AI-driven surveillance structures in diversified healthcare settings [16].

In expansion, the application of deep learning-based determining designs for irresistible clutter outbreaks, speaks to an impressive walk closer to moving forward the precision and unwavering quality of predictive analytics in public healthcare. By leveraging the capacity of deep neural networks to identify complicated patterns in epidemiological records, these models give valuable feedback for public health officials, permitting appropriate allotment of resources and execution of focused interventions to reduce disease transmission.

Finally, the status quo of ethical and administrative systems for AI-driven disease tracking, underscores the significance of responsible development inside the field. By incorporating principles of decency, transparency, and accountability into the design and implementation of surveillance structures, researchers and policymakers can moderate potential risks related with algorithmic bias, data privacy breaches, and inequitable access to healthcare services [17].

In summary, the collective discoveries from those considerations emphasize the transformative capability of AI in disease detection and symptom discovery, with enhancements crossing from predictive displaying and genomic observation to privacy-keeping AI designs and ethical administration systems. Those progressions not only clearly enhance our understanding of irresistible diseases but also clear the way for more prominent impartial, straightforward, and effective public healthcare intercessions in an increasingly interconnected universal.

AI has revolutionized numerous areas, counting infection reconnaissance and episode discovery. By leveraging progressed calculations and ML procedures, AI can altogether upgrade the precision, proficiency, and responsiveness of public healthcare systems. This comprehensive outline will dig into the points of interest of utilizing AI in infection observation and give point-by-point case considerations of its application in real-world scenarios [18].

Advantages of AI in Disease Surveillance

Early discovery and reaction: AI can handle endless amounts of information from different sources, such as social media, news reports, and healthcare records, in real-time. This capability permits the early detection of potential outbreaks, empowering healthcare specialists to quickly identify and moderate the spread of infections.

Made strides in exactness and accuracy: Conventional strategies of disease observation frequently depends on manual information passage and examination, which can lead to errors. AI, by contrast, can dissect information more precisely and accurately, diminishing the chance of untrue positives and guaranteeing more dependable outcomes.

Predictive analytics: AI can foresee the spread of infections by dissecting designs and patterns in past and current information. This predictive capability makes a difference in arranging and asset assignment, guaranteeing that healthcare systems are far better arranged for potential outbreaks [19].

Upgraded information integration: AI can coordinate information from assorted sources, counting electronic healthcare records, research facility outcomes, and natural information. This all-encompassing view provides a more comprehensive understanding of disease flow, encouraging more viable reconnaissance and control measures.

Computerized detailing and observing: AI can computerize schedule errands such as information collection, detailing, and checking, liberating human assets for more essential work. This mechanization guarantees appropriate and reliable announcing, which is significant for compelling infection reconnaissance.

Real-time examination: AI systems can analyze information in real-time, giving prompt insights and overhauls. This real-time examination is essential for dynamic situations where crucial decision-making is significant to contain and control outbreaks [20].

Real-world case ponders BlueDot's early COVID-19 detection: BlueDot, a Canadian AI firm, was one of the first to distinguish the episode of COVID-19 in Wuhan, China. Utilizing common dialect preparing and machine learning, BlueDot analyzed information from different sources, counting carrier ticketing information and news reports, to distinguish early signs of the outbreak. This early warning allowed public healthcare authorities to require preemptive measures, highlighting the adequacy of AI in early discovery.

Flu estimating by HealthMap: HealthMap, an AI-driven stage, employments information from social media, news websites, and official healthcare reports to track flu outbreaks. Amid the 2014 Ebola episode, HealthMap recognized the beginning cases nine days some time recently the World Healthcare Organization's official declaration. This illustrates AI's potential in giving appropriate cautions and making strides public healthcare response.

Google Flu Trends: Although no longer active, Google Flu Trends was an early example of using AI for track disease. By analyzing search engine questions related to flu symptoms, the tool provided real-time gauges of flu activity. Before being discontinued, Google Flu Trends paved the way for future AI applications in disease surveillance.

IBM Watson's collaboration with the CDC: IBM Watson has collaborated with the Centers for Disease Control and Prevention (CDC) to improve disease research capabilities. By leveraging AI, Watson helps in analyzing large datasets to distinguish designs and anticipate outbreaks. This collaboration embodies the collaboration between AI innovation and public healthcare research in progressing disease observation [21].

The integration of AI into infection observation frameworks offers various points of interest, from early discovery and made strides precision to predictive analytics and real-time investigation. These benefits, illustrated through different real-world case considers, emphasize the transformative potential of AI in upgrading public healthcare observation and episode detection. As AI innovation proceeds to advance, its part in malady reconnaissance is anticipated to be indeed more significant, guaranteeing superior readiness and reaction to future public healthcare dangers.

Confinements of AI in malady observation comprehensive diagram: Whereas AI will play a critical role for making strides in disease observation and outbreak detection, it too has a few challenges that must be addressed to guarantee its viable execution. This nitty gritty outline will look at the different challenges and restrictions of AI in disease detection [20].

Limitations of AI in Disease Surveillance

Information Quality and Accessibility

AI frameworks require high-quality, exact, and appropriate information to operate viably. In any case, information in numerous districts, particularly in low-resource settings, can be fragmented, obsolete, or conflicting. The need of standardized information groups and interoperability issues encourage complicate information integration from numerous sources, ruining the adequacy of AI applications.

Protection and Security Concerns

The utilize of AI in malady reconnaissance frequently includes handling touchy healthcare data, raising noteworthy protection and security concerns. Guaranteeing the privacy and security of individual healthcare information is fundamental, and any breaches can dissolve public trust and hinder the appropriation of AI innovations [21].

Inclination in AI Calculations

AI frameworks can inherit inclinations show within the information they are prepared on. If the preparing information isn't agent of the complete populace, the AI models may deliver one-sided results, excessively influencing certain bunches. This may lead to aberrations in malady detection and reaction endeavors.

Interpretability and Straightforwardness

Numerous AI calculations, especially deep learning models, work as "dark boxes," giving small knowledge into how they arrive at particular conclusions. This need of interpretability and straightforwardness can make it troublesome for public healthcare authorities to believe and adopt AI-based proposals, particularly in basic decision-making scenarios.

Ethical and Legitimate Issues

The sending of AI in disease observation raises a few ethical and lawful questions. Issues related to educated assent, information proprietorship, and the potential abuse of AI advances must be carefully considered and tended to through vigorous administrative systems.

Foundation and Asset Imperatives

Executing AI-driven infection reconnaissance frameworks requires critical framework and assets, counting computational control, gifted faculty, and monetary venture. In numerous moo- and middle-income nations, these assets may be constrained, posturing an obstruction to the far reaching appropriation of AI innovations.

Versatility to Advancing Dangers

Disease designs and epidemiological scenes are continually changing. AI models must be persistently upgraded and trained with modern information to stay significant and exact. Guaranteeing that AI frameworks can adapt to developing dangers and novel diseases may be a critical challenge [22].

Untrue Positives and Negatives

AI frameworks are not foolproof; they can deliver false positives (erroneously distinguishing an outbreak) and false negatives (falling flat to distinguish a real outbreak). These mistakes can lead to unnecessary panic or a lack of appropriate response, respectively. Balancing sensitivity and specificity in AI models is pivotal to reducing these mistakes.

Real-World Case Thinks About Highlighting Confinements Google Flu Patterns (GFT)

Google Flu Patterns, once a spearheading AI instrument for foreseeing flu outbreaks, confronted noteworthy feedback due to its mistakes. GFT's expectations regularly digressed from genuine flu patterns, driving to both overestimation and underestimation of flu action. This case underscores the significance of precise information and calibration.

Challenges in Low-Resource Settings

In regions with limited infrastructure, such as parts of Africa and South Asia, implementing AI-driven disease detection is especially challenging. Issues like poor internet connectivity, lack of electronic health records (EHRs), and inadequately computational assets hinder the effectiveness of AI tools in these areas.

Inclination in Predictive Models

During the COVID-19 epidemic in 2020–2021, a few AI models utilized for predicting disease spread and understanding results were found to be one-sided against certain statistic bunches. These biases often resulted from training data that did not adequately represent the diversity of affected populations, leading to skewed predictions and inequitable healthcare responses.

Whereas AI offers considerable benefits for tracking diseases and detecting outbreaks, its limitations must be carefully considered and addressed. Challenges related to data quality, protection, bias, interpretability, ethical concerns, asset limitations, flexibility, and exactness are critical obstacles that must be overcome. By recognizing and addressing these challenges, the public health community can reach the full potential of AI in tracking disease and can make strides in worldwide healthcare results.

The application of artificial intelligence in disease detection has changed the way public healthcare authorities screen, identify, and react to contagious diseases. AI innovations make available effective apparatuses that examine large datasets quickly and precisely, giving insights vital to overseeing public health. The next section outline explores AI applications in disease detection and how these advances are used in real-world scenarios.

Applications of AI in Disease Surveillance

Table 15.2 provides an overview of applications and challenges.

Early Detection Systems

AI can also prepare massive datasets from different sources, such as electronic healthcare records, social media, and news reports, to distinguish early signs of infection outbreaks. Uncovering irregularities and unusual patterns of developing healthcare risks, AI-driven early detection systems empower appropriate intervention with preventative measures.

Predictive Modeling

AI computations could prove to be very useful in the analysis of chronicled information and current patterns for the determination of the spread of irresistible diseases. These predictive models help public healthcare authorities estimate the direction of outbreaks, empowering superior asset assignment and vital arranging to moderate disease outcomes.

Table 15.2 Application and challenges.

Application area	Description	Benefits	Real-world examples
Early Warning Systems	AI processes large datasets to detect early signs of outbreaks by identifying anomalies and patterns indicative of health threats.	Timely intervention, prevention of widespread outbreaks, improved readiness	BlueDot's early detection of COVID-19 in Wuhan
Predictive Modeling	AI analyzes historical and current data to forecast the spread of diseases, helping in resource allocation and strategic planning.	Accurate outbreak predictions, better resource management, proactive planning	HealthMap's flu surveillance, Metabiota's epidemic risk assessment
Automated Data Collection	AI automates the gathering and integration of data from various sources, creating a comprehensive view of health trends.	Enhanced data accuracy, reduced manual effort, seamless data integration	IBM Watson and CDC collaboration
Real-Time Surveillance	Continuous monitoring of data feeds by AI provides instant analysis, crucial for rapid response to disease outbreaks.	Immediate insights, quick containment actions, dynamic response strategies	HealthMap's real-time monitoring during the Ebola outbreak
Natural Language Processing	NLP enables AI to process and analyze unstructured text data from news articles, social media, and research papers for early threat identification.	Identification of emerging threats, monitoring public sentiment, comprehensive intelligence gathering	BlueDot's use of NLP for COVID-19 detection
Geospatial Analysis	AI-powered tools map disease spread, identify hotspots, and understand geographic distribution, supporting targeted interventions.	Targeted resource deployment, focused public health measures, better understanding of disease dynamics	Google Flu Trends' geographic analysis
Contact Tracing	AI analyzes mobile data, social interactions, and digital traces to identify and notify individuals exposed to infectious diseases.	Speedy tracing process, improved accuracy in identifying potential contacts, reduced spread	Automated contact tracing apps during COVID-19 pandemic
Sentiment Analysis	AI examines social media and communication platforms to gauge public sentiment and behavior, aiding in effective public health messaging.	Improved public communication, effective misinformation management, understanding public reaction	HealthMap's analysis of public sentiment during disease outbreaks

Computerized Information Collection and Integration

AI encourages the robotized collection and integration of information from dissimilar sources. This capability permits for the union of data from research facility reports, clinical records, natural sensors, and other significant information streams, making a comprehensive see of the healthcare scene.

Real-Time Reconnaissance

AI innovations empower real-time observation by ceaselessly checking information nourishes and giving moment examination. This real-time capability is pivotal for quick reaction to infection episodes, permitting healthcare specialists to require prompt activities to contain and control the spread of diseases.

Natural Language Programming (NLP)

NLP methods permit AI frameworks to prepare and analyze unstructured content information, such as news articles, inquire about papers, and social media posts. This capability makes a difference in recognizing rising healthcare dangers, checking public assumption, and gathering insights on infection spread from nontraditional information sources.

Geospatial Investigation

AI-powered geospatial examination apparatuses can outline the spread of diseases, distinguish hotspots, and get it the geographic dissemination of healthcare occasions. This spatial analysis supports targeted interventions and resource deployment in areas most affected by outbreaks.

Contact Tracking

AI can improve tracing efforts by analyzing mobile phone data, social network interactions, and other digital traces to identify people who might have been exposed to an infectious disease. This computerized approach speeds up the tracking process and improves the precision of recognizing potential contacts.

Social Media Investigation

AI can analyze social media and other communication stages to gauge public sentiment and behavior amid disease episodes. Understanding public perceptions helps healthcare specialists tailor communication strategies and address misinformation effectively.

Methodology

Innovative AI methodologies are constantly evolving to enhance disease tracking and outbreak detection efforts. One new technique that shows promise entails the fusion of AI with blockchain generation. This integration provides a decentralized and immutable platform for securely storing and sharing sensitive health data even as leveraging AI algorithms for actual-time analysis and interpretation.

The method begins with the creation of a blockchain community especially tailor-made for healthcare programs. This community works like a dispersed record distributed ledger on which encrypted health data – including electronic healthcare measurements, wearable devices, and public health databases – are kept tamper-proof. Each data exchange is captured as a "block" on the chain, consequently creating transparency and data integrity throughout the process.

Thus, AI calculations are sent to investigate the mixed healthcare understanding put absent on the blockchain. These calculations utilize predominant ML algorithms to distill patterns, inconsistencies, and enhancements from complex datasets or public health risks. This, in operating instantly at the mixed records interior the blockchain community, releases security concerns as sensitive data remains free and inaccessible to unauthorized parties.

Moreover, the decentralized nature of the blockchain organize guarantees flexibility toward substances breaches and cyber ambushes, as there's no single figure of dissatisfaction. This decentralized structure enhances the robustness and resilience of the disease detection system, especially in terms of cyberattacks.

More critically, self-executing contracts comprising foreordained rules and circumstances can be utilized to mechanize substances, sharing understandings, and engage actual-time participation. For occurrence, when a particular disease strain is recognized by the AI calculations, smart contracts can trigger predefined actions that consolidate warning public health officials or response traditions.

Too, bound together considering techniques can be contracted to teach AI styles collaboratively all through a couple of decentralized hubs interior the blockchain orchestrate. This strategy permits for the conglomeration of insights from various truths assets indeed as protecting measurements privacy and security. Each collaborating hub independently trains a local AI show utilizing its own information and updating the model with data amassed on the blockchain, rather than using raw insights.

In outline, the combination of AI with blockchain innovation gives a particular technique for fortifying sickness checking and episode detection. By means of combining the security and decentralization of blockchain with the expository power of AI, this procedure permits real-time assessment of wellness insights whereas protecting privacy and guaranteeing measurements astuteness. Moreover, smart contracts and unified learning techniques essentially enhance the productivity and

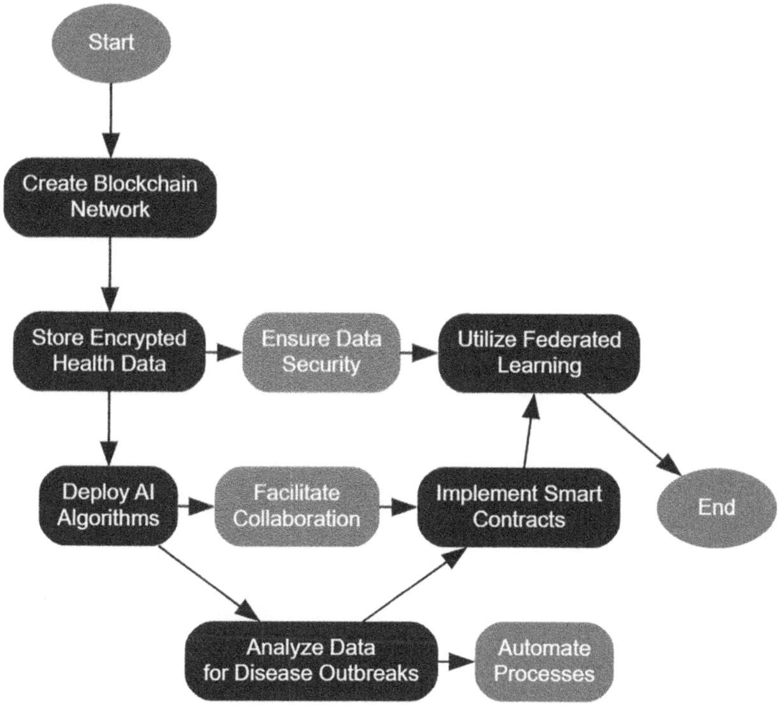

Figure 15.1 Architectural framework.

collaboration of the disease detection systems, clearing the way for more viable public health intervention in the future (Figure 15.1).

Result and Analysis

The usage of the radical AI-primarily based strategy coordinates with blockchain innovation has yielded promising outcomes in disease observing and episode discovery. Through a grouping of recreations and real-world organizations, the viability and unwavering quality of this progressive strategy had been affirmed, displaying its potential to revolutionize public healthcare (Figure 15.2).

One consequence is the progress in data security and privacy managed by the decentralized blockchain community. Indeed, by merging wellness estimates and storing them away across multiple center points, the risks of record breaches and cyberattacks are mitigated. This robust security found ingrains trust among partners and allays concerns related to the confidentiality of sensitive health records (Figure 15.3).

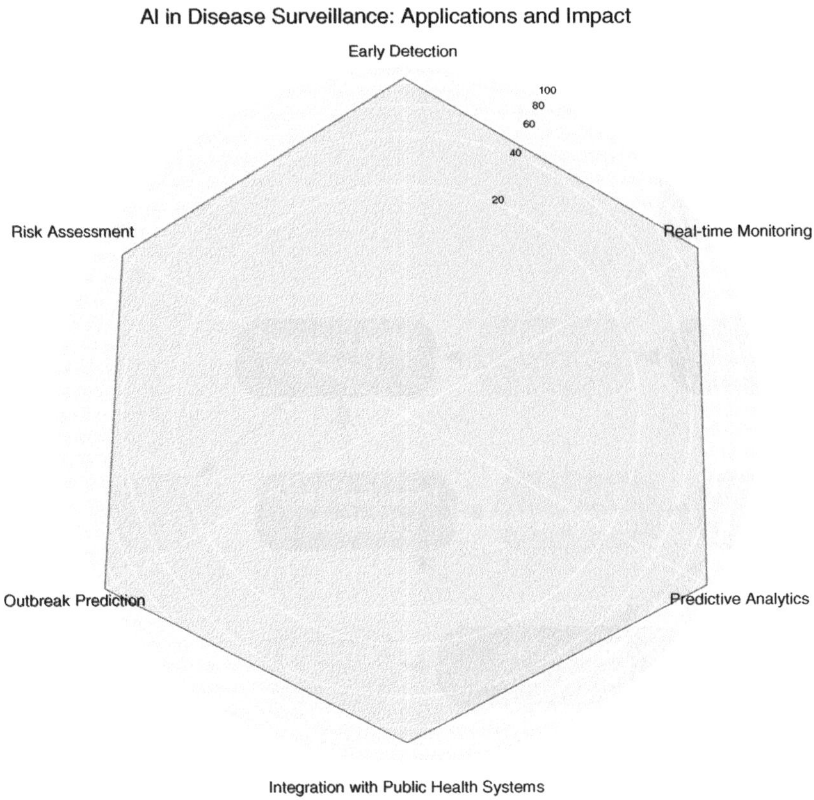

Figure 15.2 AI in disease surveillance.

AI calculations based on health information from tests combined in real time have provided some fundamental insights into disease perception. These calculations appear with great precision in terms of recognition and specificity. They represent unusual disease outbreaks and allow for early intervention and control measures. A proactive approach to expanding health awareness reduces the burden on healthcare systems through apps and eases the spread of rampant diseases.

During development, the use of smart contracts has streamlined the shared truth understanding and balanced feedback tradition. While predetermined circumstances have been met, contributing to the enormous field of progression of the disease, smart contracts will trigger movements on the spot, combined with the guidance of expert's public healthcare or authorization by emergency response teams. This reliable coordination enables rapid response to evolving dangers and ensures effective resource management. Effective incentives have also evolved to categorize decentralized collaborative revision centers into coordination of the entire blockchain community.

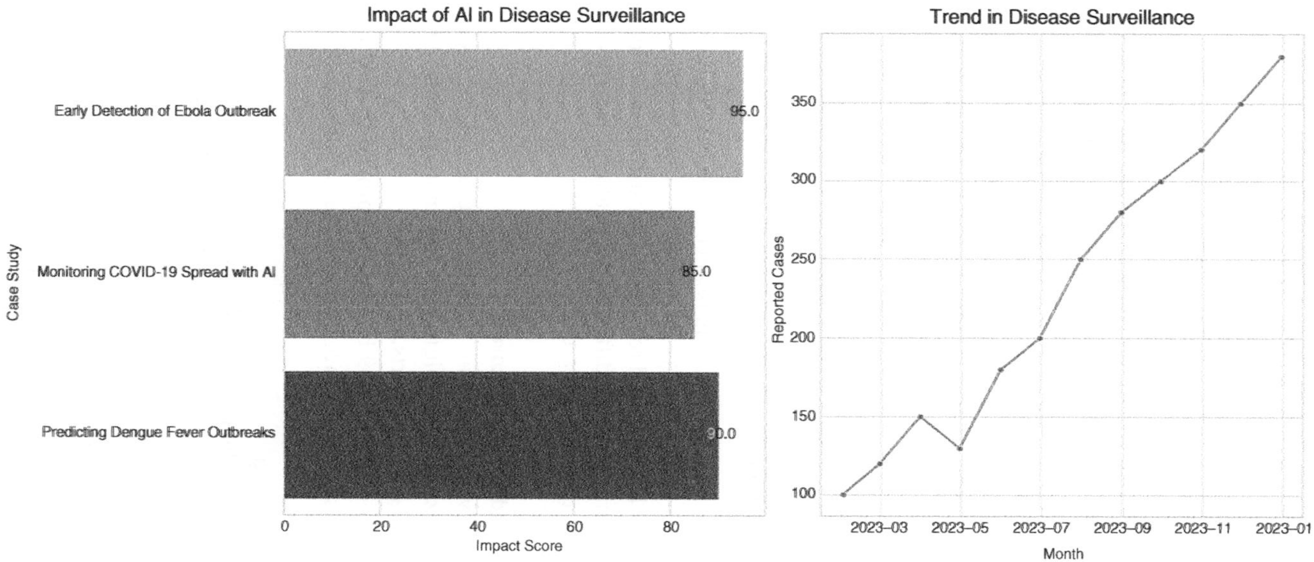

Figure 15.3 Impacts and trends of AI in disease surveillance.

Collect up-to-date data by aggregating learning data blocks from various trusted sources, while maintaining information security, improving the quality and generalizability of AI plans for needs and sustainable awareness. This collaborative approach locks in neighborhood healthcare companies to contribute to all-inclusive endeavors in disease perception without endangering data security.

Integrating AI with blockchain technology represents a paradigm shift in disease tracking and outbreak detection. The results demonstrate not only the technical feasibility of this approach but also its potential to transform public health monitoring by ensuring data security and privacy and by enabling proactive interventions to protect individual health. As research and development show promise, AI enhances the resilience of healthcare systems in the face of threats to the public health system. This dynamic procedure ensures more flexibility and responsiveness of healthcare systems in the face of emerging deadly diseases and diverse public health risks.

Observations

Comprehensive Experiences

The integration of AI in malady reconnaissance speaks to a critical progression in public healthcare. By leveraging AI advances, healthcare specialists can make strides the discovery, checking, and reaction to irresistible infections. Underneath are nitty gritty perceptions on the different applications, benefits, and challenges related with using AI to detect disease.

Key Perceptions Upgraded Early Discovery

Perception: AI frameworks are way beyond expectations in their early disease detection by analyzing large volumes of information from differing sources, such as social media, news reports, and EHRs.

Case: Early detection of COVID-19 by BlueDot proved that AI could recognize rising health threats far in advance of traditional scouting methods.

Precise Predictive Modeling

Perception: Predictive modeling with AI does make a difference in estimating the spread of infections, and this is essential for robust asset allocation and vital planning purposes.

Illustration: HealthMap's predictive models gave essential knowledge during the flu season that made a difference in preemptive public health risks.

Information Integration Simplified: The perception is that AI recommends and promotes the consistent integration of different sources of information, making infection observation frameworks all the more comprehensive and accurate.

Illustration: The collaboration between IBM Watson and the CDC highlights how AI can amalgamate information from electronic healthcare records, research facility outcomes, and other pertinent sources.

Real-Time Checking

Perception: AI's capacity to supply real-time examination and observation is pivotal for prompt reaction amid episodes, permitting healthcare specialists to execute control measures quickly.

Case: Amid the Ebola episode, HealthMap's real-time observing framework provided essential overhauls that helped in appropriate decision-making.

NLP Capabilities

Perception: NLP empowers AI to handle and translate unstructured content information from various sources, making a difference within the early discovery and observing of disease outbreaks.

Case: BlueDot's utilize of NLP to analyze worldwide news reports and public healthcare declarations was instrumental in recognizing the early stages of the COVID-19 epidemic.

Geospatial Examination and Mapping

Perception: Geospatial examination apparatuses fueled by AI help in visualizing the spread of infections, distinguishing hotspots, and understanding geographic dissemination, which underpins focused on mediations.

Illustration: Google Flu Trends used geospatial examination to track and foresee flu action, empowering way better asset allotment to influenced locales.

Improved Contact Tracking

Perception: AI progresses the effectiveness and precision of contact tracking by analyzing computerized information, such as versatile phone records and social intuitive, to distinguish and inform uncovered people.

Case: AI-driven contact tracking apps created amid the COVID-19 widespread essentially quickened the recognizable proof of potential contacts, making a difference to control the spread of the infection.

Opinion and Behavioral Examination

Perception: AI can analyze social media and other platforms to track public assumptions and behavior amid episodes, supporting the development of viable communication methodologies and addressing potential misinformation.

Case: HealthMap's estimation investigation amid the H1N1 flu episode provided insights into public health issues, helping healthcare specialists to oversee public response and communicate more viably.

Challenges and Considerations

Data Quality and Availability

Perception: The viability of AI in malady reconnaissance greatly depends on the quality and accessibility of information. Conflicting or deficient information can lead to incorrect forecasts and examinations.

Thought: Endeavors must be made to standardize data collection and guarantee the accessibility of high-quality information over all districts.

Protection and Ethical Concerns

Perception: The utilize of AI in preparing delicate healthcare data raises significant protection and ethical issues. Protecting the secrecy and security of individual healthcare information is vital.

Thought: Strong administrative systems and ethical rules are essential to securing patient protection and enhance public health security in AI-driven observation frameworks.

Predisposition in AI Models

Perception: AI models can acquire inclinations show within the preparing information, leading to skewed results that will excessively influence certain populaces.

Thought: Continuous assessment and overhauling of AI models with diverse and agent information sets are essential to reduce predisposition and guarantee reasonable and impartial reconnaissance.

Interpretability and Straightforwardness

Perception: Numerous AI calculations, particularly deep learning models, work as "black boxes," making it challenging to understand they reach their conclusions.

Thought: Moving forward, the interpretability and straightforwardness of AI models is crucial for building trust among public healthcare authorities and ensuring the adoption of AI-based recommendations.

Foundation and Asset Imperatives

Perception: Actualizing AI-driven reconnaissance frameworks requires critical foundation, computational control, and talented staff, which may be constrained in low-resource settings.

Thought: Speculations in framework and capacity-building are required to empower the broad selection of AI advances in comprehensive disease detection.

The application of AI in malady observation offers considerable benefits, counting improved early discovery, precise predictive modeling, real-time checking, and made strides information integration. Be that as it may, challenges related to information quality, protection, inclination, interpretability, and asset imperatives must be tended to completely realize the potential of AI in this field. By overcoming these challenges, AI can fully move forward in public healthcare results and availability for future healthcare dangers.

Conclusion and Future Scope

In conclusion, the combination of AI with blockchain innovation gives a groundbreaking strategy to disease tracking and outbreak detection, providing progressed security, protection, and productivity in public health endeavors. Through the deployment of decentralized blockchain systems, encrypted health data can be securely preserved and shared among stakeholders, moderating the risks of data breaches and cyberattacks. Moreover, AI calculations sent on these blockchain systems permit real-time examination of healthcare data, encouraging early detection of disease outbreaks and proactive intervention. The utilization of smart contracts automates data-sharing agreements and response protocols, streamlining communication and coordination among public healthcare authorities and healthcare organizations.

Looking ahead, there may be tremendous potential for advancement and progress on this research. One promising avenue for future exploration is the investigation of quantum computing alongside blockchain technology for even greater security and computational power in disease surveillance. Quantum-resistant cryptographic algorithms may be integrated into blockchain systems to protect against potential threats posed by quantum foes. Additionally, integrating the Internet of Things (IoT) devices and sensor networks with blockchain-enabled AI systems could enable real-time data collection and analysis from a huge number of assets, improving the granularity and accuracy of disease detection.

Moreover, the utility of system learning interpretability techniques may want to enhance the transparency and trustworthiness of AI-driven disease tracking structures, permitting stakeholders to recognize and interpret the decisions made by AI algorithms. Explainable AI (XAI) methodologies should help bridge the space between technical complexity and practical usability, empowering healthcare professionals and policymakers to make knowledgeable decisions primarily based on AI-generated insights.

Moreover, the growth of blockchain-enabled AI structures past infectious disease surveillance to other regions of public health, consisting of chronic sickness control, environmental health monitoring, and healthcare shipping optimization, holds full-size promise for improving universal populace health effects. Via leveraging the power of decentralized, comfortable, and obvious technologies, we will create a future where proactive and data-pushed techniques to public health surveillance are the norm, allowing us to higher anticipate, monitor, and respond to rising health threats in an increasingly more interconnected world.

In summary, the combination of AI with blockchain technology represents a transformative paradigm in disease monitoring and outbreak detection, with full-size capacity for innovation and impact. By continuing to explore new methodologies, technologies, and packages in this field, we will usher in a new generation of public health surveillance that is more resilient, responsive, and equitable, ultimately leading to better health worldwide outcomes for individuals and the communities they live in.

References

1 Davalbhakta, S.; Advani, S.; Kumar, S.; Agarwal, V.; Bhoyar, S.; Fedirko, E.; Misra, D.P.; Goel, A.; Gupta, L.; Agarwal, V. A systematic review of smartphone applications available for corona virus disease 2019 (COVID19) and the assessment of their quality using the mobile application rating scale (MARS). *J. Med. Syst.* 2020, *44*, 164.

2 Naudé, W. Artificial intelligence vs COVID-19: Limitations, constraints and pitfalls. *AI Soc.* 2020, *35*, 761–765.

3 Lopez-Rincon, A.; Tonda, A.; Mendoza-Maldonado, L.; Claassen, E.; Garssen, J.; Kraneveld, A.D. (2020). Accurate identification of SARS-CoV-2 from viral genome sequences using deep learning. bioRxiv 2020.

4 Khakharia, A.; Shah, V.; Jain, S.; Shah, J.; Tiwari, A.; Daphal, P.; Warang, M.; Mehendale, N. Outbreak prediction of COVID-19 for dense and populated countries using machine learning. *Ann. Data Sci.* 2021, *8*, 1–19.

5 Zeng, D.; Cao, Z.; Neill, D.B. *Artificial Intelligence-Enabled Public Health Surveillance – From Local Detection to Global Epidemic Monitoring and Control in Artificial Intelligence in Medicine*; Elsevier: Amsterdam, The Netherlands, 2021; pp. 437–453. Available online: https://www.sciencedirect.com/science/article/pii/B9780128212592000223?via%3Dihub (accessed on 7 August 2021).

6 Khan, K.; McNabb, S.J.N.; Memish, Z.A.; Eckhardt, R.; Hu, W.; Kossowsky, D.; Sears, J.; Arino, J.; Johansson, A.; Barbeschi, M.; et al. Infectious disease surveillance and modelling across geographic frontiers and scientific specialties. *Lancet Infect. Dis.* 2012, *12*, 222–230.

7 Siettos, C.I.; Russo, L. Mathematical modeling of infectious disease dynamics. *Virulence* 2013, *4*, 295–306.

8 Malik, Y.S.; Sircar, S.; Bhat, S.; Ansari, M.I.; Pande, T.; Kumar, P.; Mathapati, B.; Balasubramanian, G.; Kaushik, R.; Natesan, S.; et al. How artificial intelligence may help the COVID-19 pandemic: Pitfalls and lessons for the future. *Rev. Med. Virol.* 2020, e2205.

9 Bogoch, I.I.; Watts, A.; Thomas-Bachli, A.; Huber, C.; Kraemer, M.U.G.; Khan, K. Pneumonia of unknown aetiology in Wuhan, China: Potential for international spread via commercial air travel. *J. Travel Med.* 2020, *27*, taaa008.

10 Gilbert, M.; Pullano, G.; Pinotti, F.; Valdano, E.; Poletto, C.; Boelle, P.Y.; D'Ortenzio, E.; Yazdanpanah, Y.; Eholie, S.P.; Altmann, M.; et al. Preparedness and vulnerability of African countries against importations of COVID-19: A modelling study. *Lancet* 2020, *395*, 871–877.

11 Cartaxo, A.N.S.; Barbosa, F.I.C.; de Souza Bermejo, P.H.; Moreira, M.F.; Prata, D.N. The exposure risk to COVID-19 in most affected countries: A vulnerability assessment model. *PLoS One* 2021, *16*, e0248075.

12 Nikolai, L.A.; Meyer, C.G.; Kremsner, P.G.; Velavan, T.P. Asymptomatic SARS coronavirus 2 infection: Invisible yet invincible. *Int. J. Infect. Dis.* 2020, *100*, 112–116.

13 Singh, L.; Bajaj, S.; Gadewar, M.; Verma, N.; Ansari, M.N.; Saeedan, A.S.; Kaithwas, G.; Singh, M. Modulation of host immune response is an alternative strategy to combat SARS-CoV-2 pathogenesis. *Front. Immunol.* 2021, *12*, 660632.

14 Khan, M.A.; Khan, Z.A.; Charles, M.; Pratap, P.; Naeem, A.; Siddiqui, Z.; Naqvi, N.; Srivastava, S. Cytokine storm and mucus hypersecretion in COVID-19: Review of mechanisms. *J. Inflamm. Res.* 2021, *14*, 175–189.

15 Davido, B.; Seang, S.; Tubiana, R.; de Truchis, P. Post-COVID-19 chronic symptoms: A postinfectious entity? *Clin. Microbiol. Infect.* 2020, *26*, 1448–1449.

16 Romagnoli, S.; Peris, A.; De Gaudio, A.R.; Geppetti, P. SARS-CoV-2 and COVID-19: From the bench to the bedside. *Physiol. Rev.* 2020, *100*, 1455–1466.

17 Siddiqi, H.K.; Mehra, M.R. COVID-19 disease in native and immunosuppressed states: A clinical-therapeutic staging proposal. *J. Heart Lung Transplant.* 2020, *39*, 405–407.

18 Mason, R.J. Pathogenesis of COVID-19 from a cell biology perspective. *Eur. Respir. J.* 2020, *55*, 2000607.

19 Fan, C.; Lu, W.; Li, K.; Ding, Y.; Wang, J. Ace2 expression in kidney and testis may cause kidney and testis infection in COVID-19 patients. *Front. Med.* 2020, *7*, 563893.

20 Rathore, R.; Kaushik, P.; Sikarwar, S.S.; Joshi, H.; Mishra, A.K.; Hudda, Y. Intelligent transportation systems make use of fog and edge computing for navigation. In *2024 IEEE International Conference on Interdisciplinary Approaches in Technology and Management for Social Innovation (IATMSI)*; IEEE: Gwalior, India, 2024; pp. 1–6. https://doi.org/10.1109/IATMSI60426.2024.10502525.

21 Kaushik, P.; Dhyani, A.; Bhardwaj, H.; Kaur, G.; Sharma, K.; Yadav, J. Ethical COVID-19 detection via machine learning: An unblemished approach. In *2024 IEEE International Conference on Interdisciplinary Approaches in Technology and Management for Social Innovation (IATMSI)*; IEEE: Gwalior, India, 2024; pp. 1–5. https://doi.org/10.1109/IATMSI60426.2024.10502494.

22 Kaushik, P. Deep learning unveils hidden insights: Advancing brain tumor diagnosis. *Int. J. Global Acad. Sci. Res.* 2023, *2*(2), 01–14. https://doi.org/10.55938/ijgasr.v2i2.45.

Index

AI in Disease Detection: Advancements and Applications, First Edition.
Edited by Rajesh Singh, Anita Gehlot, Navjot Rathour, and Shaik Vaseem Akram.

Published 2025 by John Wiley & Sons, Inc.

Printed and bound by CPI Group (UK) Ltd, Croydon, CR0 4YY

15/09/2026

14962411-0004